MEDICAL INSTRUMENTS AND DEVICES
Principles and Practices

MEDICAL INSTRUMENTS AND **DEVICES**
Principles and Practices

Edited by
Steven Schreiner
Joseph D. Bronzino
Donald R. Peterson

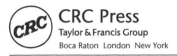

CRC Press
Taylor & Francis Group
Boca Raton London New York

CRC Press is an imprint of the
Taylor & Francis Group, an **informa** business

CRC Press
Taylor & Francis Group
6000 Broken Sound Parkway NW, Suite 300
Boca Raton, FL 33487-2742

First issued in paperback 2017

© 2016 by Taylor & Francis Group, LLC
CRC Press is an imprint of Taylor & Francis Group, an Informa business

No claim to original U.S. Government works

ISBN-13: 978-1-4398-7145-4 (hbk)
ISBN-13: 978-1-138-74852-1 (pbk)

Library of Congress Cataloging-in-Publication Data

Medical instruments and devices : principles and practices / edited by Steven Schreiner, Joseph D. Bronzino, and Donald R. Peterson.
    p. ; cm.
    Abridgement of: The biomedical engineering handbook / edited by Joseph D. Bronzino, Donald R. Peterson. 4th ed. 2014.
    Includes bibliographical references and index.
    ISBN 978-1-4398-7145-4 (hardcover : alk. paper)
    I. Schreiner, Steven, editor. II. Bronzino, Joseph D., 1937- , editor. III. Peterson, Donald R., editor. IV. Biomedical engineering handbook. Abridgement of (work):
    [DNLM: 1. Equipment and Supplies. 2. Biomedical Engineering--instrumentation. W 26]

R857.M3
610.28'4--dc23   2015017088

Visit the Taylor & Francis Web site at
http://www.taylorandfrancis.com

and the CRC Press Web site at
http://www.crcpress.com

Contents

Introduction

Medical Instruments and Devices: Principles and Practices encompasses the broad topic of medical instruments and devices. Given the breadth of this topic, it is an impossible task to include all aspects within the confines of this medium. This book provides information on a range of instruments and devices that span not only a range of physiological systems but also span the physiological scale: from molecule to cell to organ to organ system. Each chapter provides the reader a solid foundation on the topic and offers resources for deeper investigation. I would like to acknowledge the work of the previous editor, Dr. Wolf W. von Maltzahn of Rensselaer Polytechnic Institute, whose editorial prowess is still clearly visible in the design of this section.

Sadly, during the writing of this edition, Dr. Leslie A. Geddes passed away at the age of 88. With BS and MS degrees in electrical engineering from McGill University and a PhD in physiology from Baylor University College of Medicine, Dr. Geddes was a pioneer in biomedical engineering and spent his life teaching and conducting biomedical engineering research. At the time of his death, he was the Showalter Distinguished Professor Emeritus of Bioengineering and the former director of the Hillenbrand Biomedical Engineering Center at Purdue University. Internationally renowned, he was the recipient of numerous awards and prizes, as well as the inventor for many patents. I send my condolences to Dr. Geddes' family; he will be missed by the entire biomedical engineering community. I am pleased to offer you his two foundational chapters on cardiac output and respiration.

MATLAB® and Simulink® are registered trademarks of The MathWorks, Inc. For product information, please contact:

The MathWorks, Inc.
3 Apple Hill Drive
Natick, MA 01760-2098 USA
Tel: 508 647 7000
Fax: 508-647-7001
E-mail: info@mathworks.com
Web: www.mathworks.com

Editors

Steven Schreiner joined the faculty of Western New England College in 1998, where he currently serves as associate professor and chair of biomedical engineering, and chair of the engineering undergraduate admissions committee. He earned a BS in electrical engineering at Western New England College and earned both an MS and PhD in biomedical engineering at Vanderbilt University.

At Western New England College, Dr. Schreiner led the design of the biomedical engineering curriculum and the effort to establish a department of biomedical engineering. He developed and taught a variety of courses, including biomedical systems, engineering physiology, bioinstrumentation, ergonomics, introduction to engineering, advanced bioinstrumentation, and bioengineering. He served on institutional planning and college-wide committees, including college facilities planning, a diversity task force, and the academic standards committee.

A successful leader in his department and in his field, Dr. Schreiner also serves as a medical device consultant, expert witness, and an ABET Accreditation consultant. Also a seasoned grant writer, he has assisted in securing more than $980,000 in grant funding for education programs, engineering research, and laboratory upgrades and renovations.

Dr. Steven Schreiner is currently the dean of the School of Engineering.

Joseph D. Bronzino is currently the president of the Biomedical Engineering Alliance and Consortium (BEACON; www.beaconalliance.org), which is a nonprofit organization dedicated to the promotion of collaborative research, translation, and partnership among academic, medical, and industry people in the field of biomedical engineering to develop new medical technologies and devices. To accomplish this goal, Dr. Bronzino and BEACON facilitate collaborative research, industrial partnering, and the development of emerging companies. Dr. Bronzino earned a BSEE from Worcester Polytechnic Institute, Worcester, Massachusetts, in 1959, an MSEE from the Naval Postgraduate School, Monterey, California, in 1961, and a PhD in electrical engineering from Worcester Polytechnic Institute in 1968. He was recently the Vernon Roosa Professor of Applied Science and endowed chair at Trinity College, Hartford, Connecticut.

Dr. Bronzino is the author of over 200 journal articles and 15 books, including *Technology for Patient Care* (C.V. Mosby, 1977), *Computer Applications for Patient Care* (Addison-Wesley, 1982), *Biomedical Engineering: Basic Concepts and Instrumentation* (PWS Publishing Co., 1986), *Expert Systems: Basic Concepts* (Research Foundation of State University of New York, 1989), *Medical Technology and Society: An Interdisciplinary Perspective* (MIT Press and McGraw-Hill, 1990), *Management of Medical Technology* (Butterworth/Heinemann, 1992), *The Biomedical Engineering Handbook* (CRC Press, 1st Edition, 1995; 2nd Edition, 2000; 3rd Edition, 2006), *Introduction to Biomedical Engineering* (Academic Press, 1st Edition, 1999; 2nd Edition, 2005; 3rd Edition, 2011), *Biomechanics: Principles and Applications* (CRC Press, 2002), *Biomaterials: Principles and Applications* (CRC Press, 2002), *Tissue Engineering* (CRC Press, 2002), and *Biomedical Imaging* (CRC Press, 2002).

Dr. Bronzino is a fellow of IEEE and the American Institute of Medical and Biological Engineering (AIMBE), an honorary member of the Italian Society of Experimental Biology, past chairman of the Biomedical Engineering Division of the American Society for Engineering Education (ASEE), a charter member of the Connecticut Academy of Science and Engineering (CASE), a charter member of the American College of Clinical Engineering (ACCE), a member of the Association for the Advancement of Medical Instrumentation (AAMI), past president of the IEEE-Engineering in Medicine and Biology Society (EMBS), past chairman of the IEEE Health Care Engineering Policy Committee (HCEPC), and past chairman of the IEEE Technical Policy Council in Washington, DC. He is a member of Eta Kappa Nu, Sigma Xi, and Tau Beta Pi. He is also a recipient of the IEEE Millennium Medal for "his contributions to biomedical engineering research and education" and the Goddard Award from WPI for Outstanding Professional Achievement in 2005. He is presently editor-in-chief of the Academic Press/ Elsevier BME Book Series.

Donald R. Peterson is a professor of engineering and the dean of the College of Science, Technology, Engineering, Mathematics, and Nursing at Texas A&M University in Texarkana, Texas, and holds a joint appointment in the Department of Biomedical Engineering (BME) at Texas A&M University in College Station, Texas. He was recently an associate professor of medicine and the director of the Biodynamics Laboratory in the School of Medicine at the University of Connecticut (UConn) and served as chair of the BME Program in the School of Engineering at UConn as well as the director of the BME Graduate and Undergraduate Programs. Dr. Peterson earned a BS in aerospace engineering and a BS in biomechanical engineering from Worcester Polytechnic Institute, in Worcester, Massachusetts, in 1992, an MS in mechanical engineering from the UConn, in Storrs, Connecticut, in 1995, and a PhD in biomedical engineering from UConn in 1999. He has 17 years of experience in BME education and has offered graduate-level and undergraduate-level courses in the areas of biomechanics, biodynamics, biofluid mechanics, BME communication, BME senior design, and ergonomics, and has taught subjects such as gross anatomy, occupational biomechanics, and occupational exposure and response in the School of Medicine. Dr. Peterson was also recently the co-executive director of the Biomedical Engineering Alliance and Consortium (BEACON), which is a nonprofit organization dedicated to the promotion of collaborative research, translation, and partnership among academic, medical, and industry people in the field of biomedical engineering to develop new medical technologies and devices.

Dr. Peterson has over 21 years of experience in devices and systems and in engineering and medical research, and his work on human–device interaction has led to applications on the design and development of several medical devices and tools. Other recent translations of his research include the development of devices such as robotic assist devices and prosthetics, long-duration biosensor monitoring systems, surgical and dental instruments, patient care medical devices, spacesuits and space tools for NASA, powered and non-powered hand tools, musical instruments, sports equipment, computer input devices, and so on. Other overlapping research initiatives focus on the development of computational models and simulations of biofluid dynamics and biomechanical performance, cell mechanics and cellular responses to fluid shear stress, human exposure and response to vibration, and the acoustics of hearing protection and communication. He has also been involved clinically with the Occupational and Environmental Medicine group at the UConn Health Center, where his work has been directed toward the objective engineering analysis of the anatomic and physiological processes involved in the onset of musculoskeletal and neuromuscular diseases, including strategies of disease mitigation.

Dr. Peterson's scholarly activities include over 50 published journal articles, 2 textbook chapters, 2 textbook sections, and 12 textbooks, including his new appointment as co-editor-in-chief for *The Biomedical Engineering Handbook* by CRC Press.

Contributors

Khosrow Behbehani
Department of Biomedical Engineering
University of Texas
Arlington, Texas

and

Southwestern Medical Center
University of Texas
Dallas, Texas

Paul A. Belk
St. Jude Medical
St. Paul, Minnesota

Robert D. Butterfield
IVAC Corporation
San Diego, California

Christopher S. Chen
Department of Bioengineering
University of Pennsylvania
Philadelphia, Pennsylvania

David D. Cunningham
Eastern Kentucky University
Richmond, Kentucky

Gary Drzewiecki
Department of Biomedical Engineering
Rutgers University
Piscataway, New Jersey

Jeffrey L. Eggleston
Covidien Energy-Based Devices
Valleylab Inc.
Boulder, Colorado

Ross Flewelling
Nellcor Inc.
Pleasant, California

Leslie A. Geddes (deceased)
Purdue University
West Lafayette, Indiana

Sverre Grimnes
Department of Physics
University of Oslo
and
Department of Clinical and Biomedical
    Engineering
Oslo University Hospital
Oslo, Norway

Millard M. Judy
Baylor Research Institute
Dallas, Texas

Ørjan G. Martinsen
Department of Physics
University of Oslo
and
Department of Clinical and Biomedical
    Engineering
Oslo University Hospital
Oslo, Norway

Gary C.H. Mo
Departments of Chemical Engineering and
    Applied Chemistry and Biochemistry
and
Institute of Biomaterials and Biomedical
    Engineering
University of Toronto
Toronto, Ontario, Canada

Thomas J. Mullen
Medtronic
Minneapolis, Minnesota

Joachim H. Nagel
Institute of Biomedical Engineering
University of Stuttgart
Stuttgart, Germany

A. William Paulsen
Quinnipiac University
Hamden, Connecticut

P. Hunter Peckham
Case Western Reserve University
Cleveland, Ohio

Pat Ridgely
Medtronic, Inc.
Minneapolis, Minnesota

Richard L. Roa
Baylor University Medical Center
Dallas, Texas

Nathan J. Sniadecki
Department of Mechanical Engineering and
    Department of Bioengineering
University of Washington
Seattle, Washington

Primoz Strojnik
Case Western Reserve University
Cleveland, Ohio

Willis A. Tacker Jr.
Purdue University
West Lafayette, Indiana

Wolf W. von Maltzahn
Rensselaer Polytechnic Institute
Troy, New York

Gregory I. Voss
IVAC Corporation
San Diego, California

Christopher M. Yip
Departments of Chemical Engineering and
    Applied Chemistry and Biochemistry
University of Toronto
Toronto, Ontario, Canada

1

Biopotential Amplifiers

Joachim H. Nagel
University of Stuttgart

1.1 Introduction

Biosignals are recorded as potentials, voltages, and electrical field strengths generated by nerves and muscles. The measurements involve voltages at very low levels, typically ranging between 1 μV and 100 mV, with high source impedances and superimposed high-level interference signals and noise. The signals need to be amplified to make them compatible with devices such as displays, recorders, or analog/digital (A/D) converters for computerized equipments. Amplifiers suitable to measure these signals have to satisfy very specific requirements. They have to provide amplification selective to the physiological signal, reject superimposed noise and interference signals, and guarantee protection from damages through voltage and current surges for both patient and electronic equipment. Amplifiers featuring these specifications are known as biopotential amplifiers. The basic requirements and features as well as some specialized systems will be presented.

1.2 Basic Amplifier Requirements

The basic requirements that a biopotential amplifier has to satisfy are

- The physiological process to be monitored should not be influenced in any way by the amplifier
- The measured signal should not be distorted
- The amplifier should provide the best possible separation of signal and interferences
- The amplifier has to offer protection of the patient from any hazard of electrical shock
- The amplifier itself has to be protected against damages that might result from high input voltages as they occur during the application of defibrillators or electrosurgical instrumentation

A typical configuration for the measurement of biopotentials is shown in Figure 1.1. Three electrodes, two of them detecting the biological signal and the third providing the reference potential, connect the

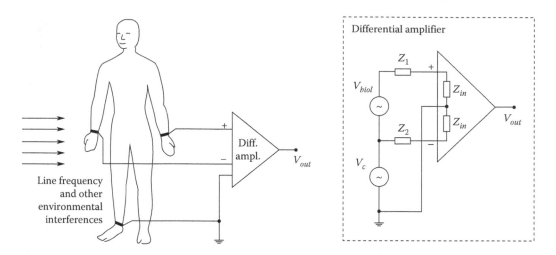

FIGURE 1.1 Typical configuration for the measurement of biopotentials. The biological signal V_{biol} appears between the two measuring electrodes at the right and left arm of the patient, and is fed to the inverting and the noninverting inputs of the differential amplifier. The right leg electrode provides the reference potential for the amplifier with a common mode voltage V_c as indicated.

subject to the amplifier. The input signal to the amplifier consists of five components: the desired biopotential, undesired biopotentials, a power line interference signal of 60 Hz (50 Hz in some countries) and its harmonics, interference signals generated by the tissue/electrode interface, and noise. Accurate design of the amplifier provides rejection of a large portion of the signal interferences. The main task of the differential amplifier as shown in Figure 1.1 is to reject the line frequency interference that is electrostatically or magnetically coupled to the subject. The desired biopotential appears as a voltage between the two input terminals of the differential amplifier and is referred to as the *differential signal*. The line frequency interference signal shows only very small differences in amplitude and phase between the two measuring electrodes, causing approximately the same potential at both inputs, and thus appears only between the inputs and ground and is called the *common mode signal*. Strong rejection of the common mode signal is one of the most important characteristics of a good biopotential amplifier.

The *common mode rejection ratio* or CMRR of an amplifier is defined as the ratio of the differential mode gain over the common mode gain. As seen in Figure 1.1, the rejection of the common mode signal in a biopotential amplifier is both a function of the amplifier CMRR and the source impedances Z_1 and Z_2. For the ideal biopotential amplifier with $Z_1 = Z_2$ and infinite CMRR of the differential amplifier, the output voltage is the pure biological signal amplified by G_D, the differential mode gain: $V_{out} = G_D \cdot V_{biol}$. With finite CMRR, the common mode signal is not completely rejected, adding the interference term $G_D \cdot V_c/CMRR$ to the output signal. Even in the case of an ideal differential amplifier with infinite CMRR, the common mode signal will not completely disappear unless the source impedances are equal. The common mode signal V_c causes currents to flow through Z_1 and Z_2. The related voltage drops show a difference if the source impedances are unequal, thus generating a differential signal at the amplifier input, which, of course, is not rejected by the differential amplifier. With amplifier gain G_D and input impedance Z_{in}, the output voltage of the amplifier is

$$V_{out} = G_D V_{biol} + \frac{G_D V_c}{CMRR} + G_D V_c \left(1 - \frac{Z_{in}}{Z_{in} + Z_1 - Z_2}\right) \tag{1.1}$$

The output of a real biopotential amplifier will always consist of the desired output component owing to a differential biosignal, an undesired component because of incomplete rejection of common mode interference signals as a function of CMRR and an undesired component because of source impedance unbalance allowing a small proportion of a common mode signal to appear as a differential signal to the amplifier. Because source impedance unbalances of 5000–10,000 Ω, mainly caused by electrodes, are not uncommon and sufficient rejection of line frequency interferences requires a minimum CMRR of 100 dB, the input impedance of the amplifier should be at least $10^9\ \Omega$ at 60 Hz to prevent source impedance unbalances from deteriorating the overall CMRR of the amplifier. State-of-the-art biopotential amplifiers provide a CMRR of 120–140 dB.

To provide optimum signal quality and adequate voltage level for further signal processing, the amplifier has to provide a gain of 100–50,000 and needs to maintain the best possible signal-to-noise ratio. The presence of high-level interference signals not only deteriorates the quality of the physiological signals, but also restricts the design of the biopotential amplifier. Electrode half-cell potentials, for example, limit the gain factor of the first amplifier stage because their amplitude can be several orders of magnitude larger than the amplitude of the physiological signal. To prevent the amplifier to go into saturation, this component has to be eliminated before the required gain can be provided for the physiological signal.

A typical design of the various stages of a biopotential amplifier is shown in Figure 1.2. The electrodes that provide the transition between the ionic flow of currents in biological tissue and the electronic flow of current in the amplifier represent a complex electrochemical system that is described elsewhere in this handbook. The electrodes determine to a large extent the composition of the measured signal. The preamplifier represents the most critical part of the amplifier itself as it sets the stage for the quality of the biosignal. With appropriate design, the preamplifier can eliminate, or at least minimize most of the signals interfering with the measurement of biopotentials.

In addition to electrode potentials and electromagnetic interferences, noise—generated by the amplifier and the connection between biological source and amplifier—has to be taken into account when designing the preamplifier. The total source resistance R_s, including the resistance of the biological source and all transition resistances between signal source and amplifier input, causes thermal voltage noise with a root mean square (rms) value of

$$E_{rms} = \sqrt{4kTR_s B} \cdot (V)$$

(1.2)

where k = Boltzmann constant, T = absolute temperature, R_s = resistance in ohms, and B = bandwidth in Hertz.

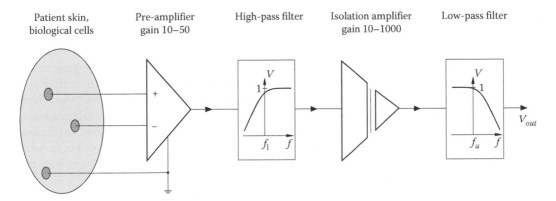

FIGURE 1.2 Schematic design of the main stages of a biopotential amplifier. Three electrodes connect the patient to a preamplifier stage. After removing DC and low-frequency interferences, the signal is connected to an output low-pass filter through an isolation stage that provides electrical safety to the patient, prevents ground loops, and reduces the influence of interference signals.

Additionally, there is the inherent amplifier noise. It consists of two frequency-dependent components, the internal voltage noise source e_n and the voltage drop across the source resistance R_s caused by an internal current noise generator i_n. The total input noise for the amplifier with a bandwidth of $B = f_2 - f_1$ is calculated as the sum of its three independent components:

$$E_{rms}^2 = \int_{f_1}^{f_2} e_n^2 df + R_s^2 \int_{f_1}^{f_2} i_n^2 df + 4kTR_s B \tag{1.3}$$

High signal-to-noise ratios thus require the use of very low noise amplifiers and the limitation of bandwidth. The current technology offers differential amplifiers with voltage noise of less than 10 nV/√Hz and current noise less than 1 pA/√Hz. Both parameters are frequency dependent and decrease approximately with the square root of frequency. The exact relationship depends on the technology of the amplifier input stage. Field effect transistor (FET) preamplifiers exhibit about 5 times the voltage noise density compared to bipolar transistors but a current noise density that is about 100 times smaller.

The purpose of the high- and low-pass filters, shown in Figure 1.2, is to eliminate interference signals such as electrode half-cell potentials and preamplifier offset potentials and to reduce the noise amplitude by the limitation of the amplifier bandwidth. Because the biosignal should not be distorted or attenuated, higher order sharp-cutting linear-phase filters have to be used. Active Bessel filters are preferred filter types because of their smooth transfer function. Separation of biosignal and interference is in most cases incomplete because of the overlap of their spectra.

The isolation stage serves the galvanic decoupling of the patient from the measuring equipment and provides safety from electrical hazards. This stage also prevents galvanic currents from deteriorating the signal to noise ratio, especially by preventing ground loops. Various principles can be used to realize the isolation stage. Analog isolation amplifiers use either transformer, optical, or capacitive couplers to transmit the signal through the isolation barrier. Digital isolation amplifiers use a voltage/frequency converter to digitize the signal before it is transmitted easily by optical or inductive couplers to the output frequency/voltage converter. The most important characteristics of an isolation amplifier are low leakage current, isolation impedance, isolation voltage (or mode) rejection (IMR), and maximum safe isolation voltage.

1.2.1 Interferences

The most critical point in the measurement of biopotentials is the contact between electrodes and biological tissue. Both the electrode offset potential and the electrode/tissue impedance are subject to changes because of relative movements of electrode and tissue. Thus, two interference signals are generated as motion artifacts: the changes of the electrode potential and motion-induced changes of the voltage drop caused by the input current of the preamplifier. These motion artifacts can be minimized by providing high input impedances for the preamplifier, usage of nonpolarized electrodes with low half-cell potentials such as Ag/AgCl electrodes, and by reducing the source impedance by use of electrode gel. Motion artifacts, interferences from external electromagnetic fields, and noise can also be generated in the wires connecting electrodes and amplifier. Reduction of these interferences is achieved by using twisted pair cables, shielded wires, and input guarding.

Recording of biopotentials is often done in an environment that is equipped with many electrical systems that produce strong electrical and magnetic fields. In addition to 60 Hz (or 50 Hz) power line frequency and some strong harmonics, high-frequency electromagnetic fields are encountered. At power line frequency, the electric and magnetic components of the interfering fields can be considered separately. Electrical fields are caused by all conductors that are connected to power, even with no flow

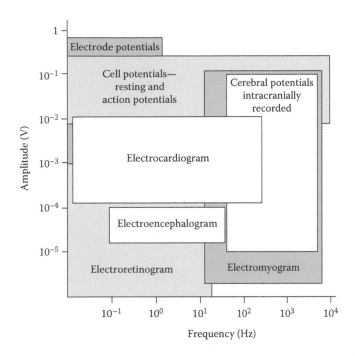

FIGURE 1.3 Amplitudes and spectral ranges of some important biosignals. The various biopotentials completely cover the area from 10^{-6} to almost 1 V and from DC to 10 kHz.

of current. A current is capacitively coupled into the body where it flows to the ground electrode. If an isolation amplifier is used without patient ground, the current is capacitively coupled to the ground. In this case, the body potential floats with a voltage of up to 100 V toward the ground. Minimizing interferences requires increasing the distance between power lines and the body, use of isolation amplifiers, separate grounding of the body at a location as far away from the measuring electrodes as possible, and use of shielded electrode cables.

The magnetic field components produce eddy currents in the body. Amplifier, electrode cable, and the body form an induction loop that is subject to the generation of an interference signal. Minimizing this interference signal requires increasing the distance between interference source and patient, twisting the connecting cables, shielding of the magnetic fields, and relocating the patient to a place and orientation that offers minimum interference signals. In many cases, an additional narrow-band-rejection filter (notch filter) is implemented as an additional stage in the biopotential amplifier to provide sufficient suppression of line frequency interferences.

To achieve optimum signal quality, the biopotential amplifier has to be adapted to the specific application. On the basis of signal parameters, both appropriate bandwidth and gain factor are chosen. Figure 1.3 shows an overview of the most commonly measured biopotentials and specifies the normal ranges for amplitude and bandwidth.

A final requirement for biopotential amplifiers is the need for calibration. Because the amplitude of the biopotential often has to be determined very accurately, there must be provisions to easily determine the gain or the amplitude range referenced to the input of the amplifier. For this purpose, the gain of the amplifier must be well calibrated. To prevent difficulties with calibrations, some amplifiers that need to have adjustable gain use various fixed gain settings rather than providing a continuous gain control. Some amplifiers have a standard signal source of known amplitude built in that can be momentarily connected to the input by the push of a button to check the calibration at the output of the biopotential amplifier. Table 1.1 gives an example for the specifications of a typical electrocardiogram (ECG) amplifier.

TABLE 1.1   Typical Specifications for an ECG Amplifier

Gain	500, 1000, 2000, and 5000
Frequency response	Maximum bandwidth (0.05 Hz–10 kHz)
Low-pass filter	20 Hz, 35 Hz, 50 Hz, 150 Hz, 1 kHz, and 10 kHz
High-pass filter	0.05 Hz, 0.1 Hz, 0.5 Hz, 1.0 Hz, and 10 Hz
Filter type	Slope Butterworth, flattest response, and −12 dB/octave
Notch interference filter	50 dB rejection at 50 or 60 Hz
Noise voltage (0.05–35 Hz)	0.1 μV (rms)
Z_{in}	2 MΩ (differential), 1000 MΩ (common mode)
CMRR	110 dB min (50/60 Hz)
Common mode input voltage range	±10 V
Output range	±10 V (analog)
Input voltage range	
Gain	V_{in} (mV)
500:	±20
1000:	±10
2000:	±5
5000:	±2
AC calibrator	1 mV *P–P* square wave, 10 Hz
Subject isolation	>4 kV

1.2.2 Special Circuits

1.2.2.1 Instrumentation Amplifier

An important stage of all biopotential amplifiers is the input preamplifier that substantially contributes to the overall quality of the system. The main tasks of the preamplifier are to sense the voltage between two measuring electrodes while rejecting the common mode signal and minimizing the effect of electrode polarization overpotentials. Crucial to the performance of the preamplifier is the input impedance that should be as high as possible. Such a differential amplifier cannot be realized using a standard single *operational amplifier* (op-amp) design because this does not provide the necessary high input impedance. The general solution to the problem involves voltage followers or noninverting amplifiers, to attain high input impedances. A possible realization is shown in Figure 1.4a. The main disadvantage

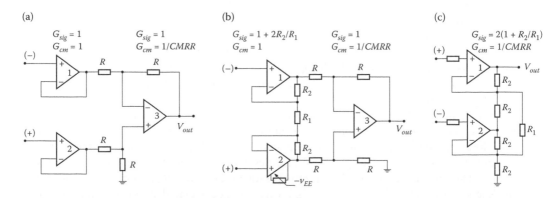

FIGURE 1.4   Circuit drawings for three different realizations of instrumentation amplifiers for biomedical applications. (a) Voltage follower input stage, (b) improved, amplifying input stage, and (c) 2-op-amp version.

of this circuit is that it requires high CMRR both in the followers and in the final op-amp. With the input buffers working at unity gain, all the common mode rejection must be accomplished in the output amplifier, requiring very precise resistor matching. Additionally, the noise of the final op-amp is added at a low signal level, decreasing the signal-to-noise ratio unnecessarily. The circuit in Figure 1.4b eliminates this disadvantage. It represents the standard instrumentation amplifier configuration. The two input op-amps provide high differential gain and unity common mode gain without the requirement of close resistor matching. The differential output from the first stage represents a signal with substantial relative reduction of the common mode signal and is used to drive a standard differential amplifier that further reduces the common mode signal. CMRR of the output op-amp as well as resistor matching in its circuit are less critical than in the follower-type instrumentation amplifier. Offset trimming for the whole circuit can be done at one of the input op-amps. Complete instrumentation amplifier integrated circuits based on this standard instrumentation amplifier configuration are available from several manufacturers. All components except R_1, which determines the gain of the amplifier, and the potentiometer for offset trimming are contained on the integrated circuit chip. Figure 1.4c shows another configuration that offers high input impedance with only two op-amps. For good CMRR, however, it requires precise resistor matching.

In applications where direct current (DC) and very-low-frequency biopotentials are not to be measured, it would be desirable to block those signal components at the preamplifier inputs by simply adding a capacitor working as a passive high-pass filter. This would eliminate the electrode offset potentials and permit a higher gain factor for the preamplifier *and thus a higher CMRR*. A capacitor between electrodes and amplifier input would, however, result in charging effects from the input bias current. Owing to the difficulty of precisely matching capacitors for the two input leads, they would also contribute to an increased source impedance unbalance and thus reduce CMRR. Avoiding the problem of charging effects by adding a resistor between the preamplifier inputs and ground, as shown in Figure 1.5a, also results in a decrease of CMRR because of the diminished and mismatched input impedance. A 1% mismatch for two 1 MΩ resistors can already create a –60 dB loss in CMRR. The loss in CMRR is much greater if the capacitors are mismatched, which cannot be prevented in real systems. Nevertheless, such realizations are used where the specific situation permits. In some applications, a further reduction of the amplifier to a two-electrode amplifier configuration would be convenient, even at the expense of some loss in the CMRR. Figure 1.6 shows a preamplifier design working with two electrodes and providing alternating current (AC) coupling as proposed by Pallás-Areny and Webster (1990).

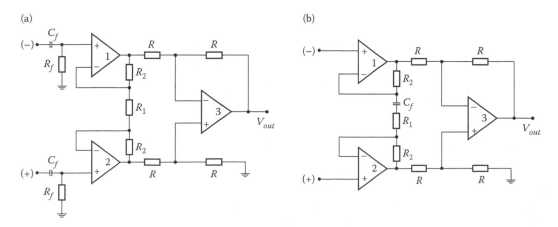

FIGURE 1.5 AC-coupled instrumentation amplifier designs. The classical design using an RC high-pass filter at the inputs (a) and a high CMRR "quasi-high-pass" amplifier as proposed by C.C. Lu (b).

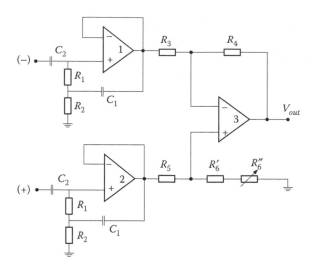

FIGURE 1.6   Composite instrumentation amplifier based on an AC-coupled first stage. The second stage is based on a one op-amp differential amplifier that can be replaced by an instrumentation amplifier.

A third alternative of eliminating DC and low frequencies in the first amplifier stage, a directly coupled quasi-high-pass amplifier design can be used that maintains the high CMRR of DC-coupled high input impedance instrumentation amplifiers (Song et al. 1998). In this design, the gain determining resistor R_1 (Figure 1.5a) is replaced by a first-order high-pass filter consisting of R_1 and a series capacitor C_f. The signal gain of the amplifier is

$$G = 1 + \frac{2R_2}{R_1 + (1/j\omega C)} \tag{1.4}$$

Thus, DC gain is 1, whereas the high-frequency gain remains at $G = 1 + 2R_2/R_1$. A realization using an off-the-shelf instrumentation amplifier (Burr-Brown INA 118) operates at low power (0.35 mA) with low offset voltage (11 μV typical) and low input bias current (1 nA typical), and offers a high CMRR of 118 dB at a gain of $G = 50$. The very high input impedance (10 GΩ) of the instrumentation amplifier renders it insensitive to fluctuations of the electrode impedance. Therefore, it is suitable for bioelectric measurements using pasteless electrodes applied to unprepared, that is, high impedance skin.

The preamplifier, often implemented as a separate device that is placed adjacent to the electrodes or even directly attached to the electrodes, also acts as an impedance converter that allows the transmission of even weak signals to the remote monitoring unit. Owing to the low output impedance of the preamplifier, the input impedance of the following amplifier stage can be low, and still the influence of interference signals coupled into the transmission lines is reduced.

1.3 Isolation Amplifier and Patient Safety

Isolation amplifiers can be used to break ground loops, eliminate source ground connections, and provide isolation protection to the patient and electronic equipment. In a biopotential amplifier, the main purpose of the isolation amplifier is the protection of the patient by eliminating the hazard of electric shock resulting from the interaction among patient, amplifier, and other electric devices in the patient's environment, specifically defibrillators and electrosurgical equipment. It also adds to the prevention of line frequency interferences.

Isolation amplifiers are realized in three different technologies: transformer isolation, capacitor isolation, and optoisolation. An isolation barrier provides a complete galvanic separation of the input side, that is, patient and preamplifier, from all equipment on the output side. Ideally, there will be no flow of electric current across the barrier. The isolation mode voltage is the voltage that appears across the isolation barrier, that is, between the input common and the output common (Figure 1.7). The amplifier has to withstand the largest expected isolation voltages without damage. Two isolation voltages are specified for commercial isolation amplifiers: the continuous rating and the test voltage. To eliminate the need for longtime testing, the device is tested at about 2 times the rated continuous voltage. Thus, for a continuous rating of 2000 V, the device has to be tested at 4000–5000 V for a reasonable period of time.

Because there is always some leakage across the isolation barrier, the isolation mode rejection ratio (IMRR) is not infinite. For a circuit as shown in Figure 1.7, the output voltage is

$$V_{out} = \frac{G}{R_{G1} + R_{G2} + R_{IN}}\left[V_D + \frac{V_{CM}}{CMRR}\right] + \frac{V_{ISO}}{IMRR} \tag{1.5}$$

where G is the amplifier gain, V_D, V_{CM}, and V_{ISO} are differential, common mode, and isolation voltages, respectively, and CMRR is the common mode rejection ratio for the amplifier (Burr-Brown, 1994).

Typical values of IMRR for a gain of 10 are 140 dB at DC, and 120 dB at 60 Hz with a source unbalance of 5000 Ω. The isolation impedance is approximately 1.8 pF || 10^{12} Ω.

Transformer-coupled isolation amplifiers perform on the basis of inductive transmission of a carrier signal that is amplitude modulated by the biosignal. A synchronous demodulator on the output port reconstructs the signal before it is fed through a Bessel response low-pass filter to an output buffer. A power transformer, generally driven by a 400–900 kHz square wave, supplies isolated power to the amplifier.

Optically coupled isolation amplifiers can principally be realized using only a single light-emitting diode (LED) and photodiode combination. Although useful for a wide range of digital applications, this design has fundamental limitations as to its linearity and stability as a function of time and temperature. A matched photodiode design, as used in the Burr-Brown 3650/3652 isolation amplifier, overcomes these difficulties (Burr-Brown, 1994). Operation of the amplifier requires an isolated power supply to drive the input stages. Transformer-coupled low-leakage current-isolated DC/DC converters

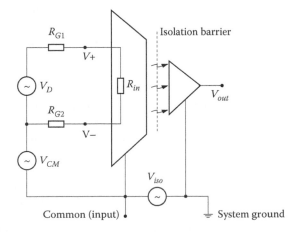

FIGURE 1.7 Equivalent circuit of an isolation amplifier. The differential amplifier on the left transmits the signal through the isolation barrier by a transformer, capacitor, or an optocoupler.

are commonly used for this purpose. In some particular applications, especially in cases where the signal is transmitted over a longer distance by fiber optics, for example, ECG amplifiers used for gated magnetic resonance imaging, batteries are used to power the amplifier. Fiber optic coupling in isolation amplifiers is another option that offers the advantage of higher flexibility in the placement of parts on the amplifier board.

Biopotential amplifiers have to provide sufficient protection from electrical shock to both user and patient. Electrical-safety codes and standards specify the minimum safety requirements for the equipment, especially the maximum leakage currents for chassis and patient leads, and the power distribution system (Webster, 1992; AAMI, 1993).

Special attention to patient safety is required in situations where biopotential amplifiers are connected to personal computers (PCs) that are increasingly used to process and store physiological signals and data. Owing to the design of the power supplies used in standard PCs permitting high leakage currents—an inadequate situation for a medical environment—there is a potential risk involved even when the patient is isolated from the PC through an isolation amplifier stage or optical signal transmission from the amplifier to the computer. This holds especially in those cases where because of the proximity of the PC to the patient, an operator might touch the patient and computer at the same time, or the patient might touch the computer. It is required that a special power supply with sufficient limitation of leakage currents is used in the computer, or that an additional, medical grade isolation transformer is used to provide the necessary isolation between power outlet and PC.

1.4 Surge Protection

The isolation amplifiers described in the preceding section are primarily used for the protection of the patient from electric shock. Voltage surges between electrodes as they occur during the application of a defibrillator or electrosurgical instrumentation also present a risk to the biopotential amplifier. Biopotential amplifiers should be protected against serious damage to the electronic circuits. This is also part of the patient safety because defective input stages could otherwise apply dangerous current levels to the patient. To achieve this protection, voltage-limiting devices are connected between each measuring electrode and electric ground. Ideally, these devices do not represent a shunt impedance and thus do not lower the input impedance of the preamplifier as long as the input voltage remains in a range considered safe for the equipment. They appear as an open circuit. As soon as the voltage drop across the device reaches a critical value V_b, the impedance of the device changes sharply and current passes through it to such an extent that the voltage cannot exceed V_b because of the voltage drop across the series resistor R as indicated in Figure 1.8.

The devices used for amplifier protection are diodes, Zener diodes, and gas-discharge tubes. Parallel silicon diodes limit the voltage to approximately 600 mV. The transition from nonconducting to conducting state is not very sharp and signal distortion begins at about 300 mV that can be within the range of input voltages depending on the electrodes used. The breakdown voltage can be increased by connecting several diodes in series. Higher breakdown voltages are achieved by Zener diodes connected back to back. One of the diodes will be biased in the forward direction and the other in the reverse direction. The breakdown voltage in the forward direction is approximately 600 mV but the breakdown voltage in the reverse direction is higher, generally in the range of 3–20 V, with a sharper voltage–current characteristic than the diode circuit.

A preferred voltage-limiting device for biopotential amplifiers is the gas-discharge tube. Owing to its extremely high impedance in the nonconducting state, this device appears as an open circuit until it reaches its breakdown voltage. At the breakdown voltage that is in the range of 50–90 V, the tube switches to the conducting state and maintains a voltage that is usually several volts less than the breakdown voltage. Although the voltage maintained by the gas-discharge tube is still too high for some amplifiers, it is sufficiently low to allow the input current to be easily limited to a safe value by simple

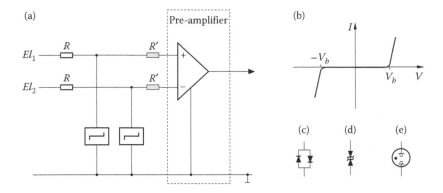

FIGURE 1.8 Protection of the amplifier input against high-voltage transients. The connection diagram for voltage-limiting elements is shown in panel (a) with two optional resistors R′ at the input. A typical current–voltage characteristic is shown in panel (b). Voltage-limiting elements shown are the antiparallel connection of diodes (c), antiparallel connection of Zener diodes (d), and gas-discharge tubes (e).

circuit elements such as resistors like the resistor $R′$ indicated in Figure 1.8a. Preferred gas-discharge tubes for biomedical applications are miniature neon lamps that are very inexpensive and have a symmetric characteristic.

1.5 Input Guarding

The common mode input impedance and thus the CMRR of an amplifier can be greatly increased by guarding the input circuit (Strong 1970). The common mode signal can be obtained by two averaging resistors connected between the outputs of the two input op-amps of an instrumentation amplifier as shown in Figure 1.9. The buffered common mode signal at the output of op-amp 4 can be used as guard voltage to reduce the effects of cable capacitance and leakage.

In many modern biopotential amplifiers, the reference electrode is not grounded. Instead, it is connected to the output of an amplifier for the common mode voltage, op-amp 3 in Figure 1.10, which works as an inverting amplifier. The inverted common mode voltage is fed back to the reference electrode. This

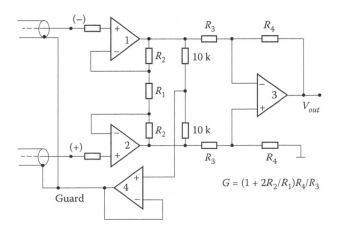

$$G = (1 + 2R_2/R_1)R_4/R_3$$

FIGURE 1.9 Instrumentation amplifier providing input guarding.

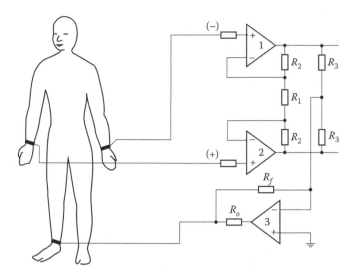

FIGURE 1.10   Driven-right-leg circuit reducing common mode interference.

negative feedback reduces the common mode voltage to a low value (Webster, 1992). Electrocardiographs based on this principle are called driven-right-leg systems replacing the right-leg ground electrode of ordinary electrocardiographs by an actively driven electrode.

1.6 Dynamic Range and Recovery

With an increase of either the common mode or differential input voltage, there will be a point where the amplifier will overload and the output voltage will no longer be representative for the input voltage. Similarly, with a decrease of the input voltage, there will be a point where the noise components of the output voltage cover the output signal to a degree that a measurement of the desired biopotential is no longer possible. The dynamic range of the amplifier, that is, the range between the smallest and largest possible input signal to be measured, has to cover the whole amplitude range of the physiological signal of interest. The required dynamic range of biopotential amplifiers can be quite large. In an application such as fetal monitoring, for example, two signals are recorded simultaneously from the electrodes that are quite different in their amplitudes: the fetal and the maternal ECG. Although the maternal ECG shows an amplitude of up to 10 mV, the fetal ECG often does not reach more than 1 μV. Assuming that the fetal ECG is separated from the composite signal and fed to an A/D converter for digital signal processing with a resolution of 10 bit (signed integer), the smallest voltage to be safely measured with the biopotential amplifier is 1/512 μV or about 2 nV versus 10 mV for the largest signal, or even up to 300 mV in the presence of an electrode offset potential. This translates to a dynamic range of 134 dB for the signals alone and 164 dB if the electrode potential is included into the consideration. Although most applications are less demanding, even such extreme requirements can be realized through careful design of the biopotential amplifier and the use of adequate components. The penalty for using less-expensive amplifiers with diminished performance would be a potentially severe loss of information.

Transients appearing at the input of the biopotential amplifier, such as voltage peaks from a cardiac pacemaker or a defibrillator, can drive the amplifier into saturation. An important characteristic of the amplifier is the time it takes to recover from such overloads. The recovery time depends on the characteristics of the transient, such as amplitude and duration, the specific design of the amplifier, such as bandwidth, and the components used. Typical biopotential amplifiers may take several seconds to recover from severe overload. The recovery time can be reduced by disconnecting the amplifier inputs at the discovery of a transient using an electronic switch.

1.6.1 Passive Isolation Amplifiers

Increasingly, biopotentials have to be measured within implanted devices and need to be transmitted to an external monitor or controller. Such applications include cardiac pacemakers transmitting the intracardiac ECG and functional electrical stimulation where, for example, action potentials measured at one eyelid serve to stimulate the other lid to restore the physiological function of a damaged lid at least to some degree. In these applications, the power consumption of the implanted biopotential amplifier limits the life span of the implanted device. The usual solution to this problem is an inductive transmission of power into the implanted device that serves to recharge an implanted battery. In applications where the size of the implant is of concern, it is desirable to eliminate the need for the battery and the related circuitry by using a quasi-passive biopotential amplifier, that is, an amplifier that does not need a power supply.

The function of passive telemetric amplifiers for biopotentials is based on the ability of the biological source to drive a low-power device such as an FET and the sensing of the biopotentials through inductive or acoustic coupling of the implanted and external devices (Nagel et al. 1982). In an inductive system, an FET serves as a load to an implanted secondary resonator, that is, an LC circuit containing a secondary coil with the inductance L and a capacitor with the capacitance C that is stimulated inductively by an extracorporeal oscillator (Figure 1.11). Depending on the special realization of the system, the biopotential is available in the external circuit from either an amplitude or frequency-modulated carrier signal. The input impedance of the inductive transmitter as a function of the secondary load impedance Z_2 is given by

$$Z_1 = j\omega L_1 + \frac{(\omega M)^2}{Z_2 + j\omega L_2} \tag{1.6}$$

In an amplitude-modulated system, the resistive part of the input impedance Z_1 must change as a linear function of the biopotential. The signal is obtained as the envelope of the carrier signal is measured across a resistor R_m. A frequency-modulated system is realized when the frequency of the signal generator is determined at least in part by the impedance Z_1 of the inductive transmitter. In both cases, the signal-dependent changes of the secondary impedance Z_2 can be achieved by a junction–FET. Using the FET as a variable load resistance changing its resistance in proportion to the source–gate voltage that is determined by the electrodes of this two-electrode amplifier, the power supplied by the biological source is sufficient to drive the amplifier. The input impedance can be in the range of 10^{10} Ω.

Optimal transmission characteristics are achieved with amplitude modulation (AM) systems. Different combinations of external and implanted resonance circuits are possible to realize an AM system, but primary parallel with secondary serial resonance yields the best characteristics. In this case, the input impedance is given by

$$Z_1 = \frac{1}{j\omega C_1} + \left(\frac{L_1}{M}\right)^2 \cdot R_2 \tag{1.7}$$

The transmission factor $(L_1/M)^2$ is optimal because the secondary inductivity, that is, the implanted inductivity L_2 can be small, only the external inductivity determines the transmission factor, and the mutual inductivity M should be small, a fact that favors the loose coupling that is inherent to two coils

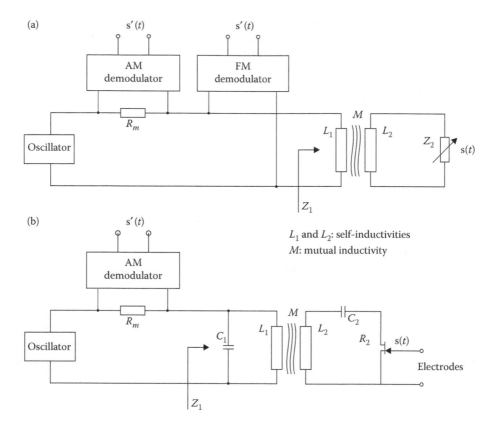

FIGURE 1.11 *Passive* isolation amplifier can be operated without the need for an isolated power supply (a). The biological source provides the power to modulate the load impedance of an inductive transformer. As an easy realization shown in (b), an FET can be directly connected to two electrodes. The source–drain resistance changes as a linear function of the biopotential that is then reflected by the input impedance of the transformer.

separated by skin and tissue. There are, of course, limits to M that cannot be seen from Equation 1.7. In a similar fashion, two piezoelectric crystals can be employed to provide the coupling between input and output.

This two-lead isolation amplifier design is not limited to telemetric applications, it can also be used in all other applications where its main advantage lies in its simplicity and the resulting substantial cost savings as compared to other isolation amplifiers that require additional amplifier stages and an additional isolated power supply.

1.7 Digital Electronics

The ever-increasing density of integrated digital circuits together with their extremely low-power consumption permits digitizing and preprocessing of signals already on the isolated patient side of the amplifiers, thus improving signal quality and eliminating the problems normally related to the isolation barrier, especially those concerning isolation voltage interferences and long-term stability of the isolation amplifiers. Digital signal transmission to a remote monitoring unit, a computer system, or computer network can be achieved without any risk of detecting transmission line interferences, especially when implemented with fiber optical cables.

Digital techniques also offer easy means of controlling the front end of the amplifier. Gain factors can be easily adapted, and changes of the electrode potential resulting from electrode polarization or from interferences that might drive the differential amplifier into saturation can be easily detected and compensated.

1.8 Summary

Biopotential amplifiers are a crucial component in many medical and biological measurements, and largely determine the quality and information content of the measured signals. The extremely wide range of necessary specifications with regard to bandwidth, sensitivity, dynamic range, gain, CMRR, and patient safety leaves only little room for the application of general-purpose biopotential amplifiers and mostly requires the use of special-purpose amplifiers.

Defining Terms

Common mode rejection ratio (CMRR): CMRR of a differential amplifier is defined as the ratio between the amplitude of a common mode signal and the amplitude of a differential signal that would produce the same output amplitude or as the ratio of the differential gain over the common mode gain: CMRR = GD/GCM. Expressed in decibels, the common mode rejection is 20 log 10 CMRR. The common mode rejection is a function of frequency and source impedance unbalance.

Isolation mode rejection ratio (IMRR): IMRR of an isolation amplifier is defined as the ratio between the isolation voltage, V_{ISO}, and the amplitude of the isolation signal appearing at the output of the isolation amplifier or as isolation voltage divided by output voltage V_{OUT} in the absence of differential and common mode signal: IMRR = V_{ISO}/V_{OUT}.

Operational amplifier (op-amp): Op-amp is a very high-gain DC-coupled differential amplifier with single-ended output, high-voltage gain, high input impedance, and low output impedance. Owing to its high open-loop gain, the characteristics of an op-amp circuit only depend on its feedback network. Therefore, the integrated circuit op-amp is an extremely convenient tool for the realization of linear amplifier circuits (Horowitz and Hill, 1980).

References

AAMI. 1993. *AAMI Standards and Recommended Practices, Biomedical Equipment*, Vol. 2, 4th ed. AAMI, Arlington, VA.

Burr-Brown. 1994. *Burr-Brown Integrated Circuits Data Book, Linear Products*, Burr-Brown Corp., Tucson, AZ.

Horowitz, P. and W. Hill. 1980. *The Art of Electronics*, Cambridge University Press, Cambridge, UK.

Nagel, J.H., M. Ostgen, and M. Schaldach. 1982. Telemetriesystem. *German Patent Application*, P3233240. 8–15.

Pallás-Areny, R. and J.G. Webster. 1990. Composite instrumentation amplifier for biopotentials. *Annals of Biomedical Engineering.* 18, 251–262.

Song, Y., O. Ozdamar, and C.C. Lu. 1998. Pasteless electrode/amplifier system for auditory brainstem response (ABR) recording. *Annals of Biomedical Engineering.* 26, S-103.

Strong, P. 1970. *Biophysical Measurements*, Tektronix, Inc., Beaverton, OR.

Webster, J.G. (ed.), 1992. *Medical Instrumentation, Application and Design*, 2nd ed. Houghton Mifflin Company, Boston, MA.

Further Information

Detailed information on the realization of amplifiers for biomedical instrumentation and the availability of commercial products can be found in the references and in the data books and application notes of various manufacturers of integrated circuit amplifiers, such as Burr-Brown, Analog Devices, and Linear Technology Corporation, as well as manufacturers of laboratory equipment, such as Biopac Systemy Inc., Gould, and Grass.

2

Bioimpedance Measurements

Sverre Grimnes
University of Oslo
Oslo University Hospital

Ørjan G. Martinsen
University of Oslo
Oslo University Hospital

2.1 What Is Bioimpedance?

Bioimpedance is an electrical property of a biomaterial: the ability to oppose alternating current (AC) flow. Impedance is a physical variable, which may be of interest as such, but often, it is converted into another variable or parameter of special, for example, clinical interest. Active electrodes are always used in bioimpedance sensors; the method is exogenous with two current-carrying (CC) electrodes sending the measuring current through the tissue volume of interest. This is in contrast to measuring, for example, a biopotential difference caused by living tissue activity (bioelectricity) with passive pickup (PU) electrodes, an endogenous method.

The biomaterial may be living tissue measured *in situ* and *in vivo*, or it may be dead, for example, hair or meat. The biomaterial may also be excised tissue or cell suspensions kept alive outside the body (*ex vivo*) or passively dying or dead tissue in a glass container (*in vitro*). In this chapter, we will focus on living person and patient tissue.

The books that include our field are, for instance: Malmivuo and Plonsey (1995), which also covers magnetic aspects; Schwan (2001), which is a collection of many of the classical papers by Herman P.

Schwan; Plonsey and Barr (2000), which focuses on bioelectricity; and Grimnes and Martinsen (2008) on bioimpedance and bioelectricity.

2.2 Conductors and Dielectrics

A tissue as a biomaterial may be considered as a conductor or a dielectric. Figure 2.1 shows a model of the biomaterial between two metal electrode plates. In principle, a dielectric is dry without direct current (DC) conductance and living tissue is wet with appreciable DC conductance and polarization impedance caused by the double layer at the surface of the wetted metal plates. Charge carriers are electrons in metal, but ions in tissue.

Let us consider the AC case in Figure 2.1. The AC is a sinusoidal signal with voltage u and current i. Admittance **Y** and impedance **Z** are found by measuring i and u.

However, as illustrated in Figure 2.2, living tissue has capacitive properties because of, for example, cell membranes. Therefore, the u and i signals are not in-phase, and impedance and admittance are complex quantities. They are written in **bold** characters and can be decomposed in their in-phase and quadrature components

$$\mathbf{Y} = \mathbf{i}/u = G + jB = G + j\omega C_p \qquad \text{[siemens]} \quad (2.1)$$

$$\mathbf{Z} = \mathbf{u}/i = R + jX = R - j/\omega C_s \qquad \text{[ohm]} \quad (2.2)$$

where j is the imaginary unit, G is the conductance, B is the susceptance, ω is the angular frequency, and C_p is the parallel capacitance. R is the resistance, X is the reactance, and C_s is the series capacitance.

Material constants such as conductivity can be used instead of conductance if geometrical dimensions such as A and d are known

$$\mathbf{Y} = (\sigma' + j\sigma'') \, A/d \qquad (2.3)$$

where σ is the conductivity [siemens/m], σ' the in-phase part, and σ'' the 90° (capacitive) part.

$$\mathbf{Z} = 1/\mathbf{Y} = (\rho' - j\,\rho'')d/A \qquad (2.4)$$

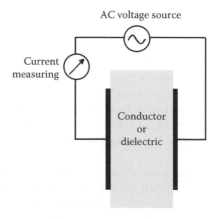

FIGURE 2.1   Basic model of a conductor or a dielectric placed between two metal plates of contact area *A* and distance *d*.

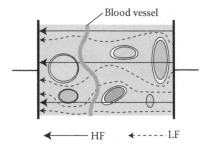

FIGURE 2.2 Tissue, cells, membranes, and a blood vessel. Note the difference between (<1 kHz) and HF (>100 kHz) current flow lines.

where ρ is the resistivity [ohm m], ρ' the in-phase part, and ρ'' the 90° (capacitive) part.

$$\varepsilon = \varepsilon' - j\varepsilon'' = (C' - jC'')d/A \qquad \text{[farad/m]} \quad (2.5)$$

where ε is complex permittivity, ε' capacitive permittivity expressing the capacitor's ability to store electric energy, ε'' dielectric loss permittivity, and **C** complex capacitance.

Equations 2.3 through 2.5 show that if a biomaterial is to be regarded as a conductor, complex resistivity or conductivity parameters are used; if the material is to be regarded as a dielectric, permittivity parameters are used. In linear cases, the information content is the same.

The circuit of Figure 2.1 is an AC circuit. Capacitance and permittivity cannot be measured at frequency 0 Hz; they are instead defined with static values (ε_s) found from capacitor DC voltage U and charge Q ($C = Q/U$).

Without phase data, the modulus of the quantities is simple and useful. If the biomaterial is considered as an ideal, dry capacitor ($C'' = 0$), the capacitance C is

$$C = \varepsilon \, A/d \qquad \text{[farad]} \quad (2.6)$$

If it is considered as an ideal conductor, the conductance is

$$G = \sigma \, A/d \qquad \text{[siemens]} \quad (2.7)$$

Material constants may be derived from measured values if the biomaterial is measured *in vitro* in simple geometries, such as circular or rectangular tubes. Tissue is a very heterogeneous material and *in vivo* measurements are not sharply limited to a defined volume. It may be very difficult or virtually impossible to go from, for example, measured conductance, resistance, and capacitance to conductivity, resistivity, and permittivity.

Living tissue is neither an ideal capacitor nor an ideal conductor. Many types of membranes with special electrical properties are found—from the dead, horny layer at the human skin surface to cell membranes and the large peritoneum membrane in the abdominal cavity. At a frequency of, for example, 1000 Hz, an imposed current may partly pass the extracellular electrolytes and partly the intracellular electrolytes through the capacitive cell membranes. This is illustrated in Figure 2.2, showing how a high-frequency (HF) current passes right through the intracellular volume, whereas the low-frequency (LF) current must go around the membrane obstacles. The current division leads to a frequency-dependent phase shift between measured voltage and current, and by measuring a frequency spectrum, additional data can be obtained.

2.3 Living Tissue Electrical Models

Electrical circuits with lumped components are often used as models mimicking the electrical properties of tissue. The simplest models are with three components. If all components are ideal (not frequency-dependent values), the model is a Debye model.

2.3.1 Debye Models

The model to the left in Figure 2.3 is often used to model skin impedance. For instance, R may represent the deeper viable parts and the parallel R and C components represent the poorly conducting stratum corneum (SC). The model to the right may be used for tissue as shown in Figure 2.2. Then G models the extracellular electrolyte, C_m the cell membranes, and R the intracellular resistance. Fixed component values in the two models can be found so that they have exactly the same impedance spectrum.

Figure 2.4 shows dielectric models of the same tissue as shown in Figure 2.2. They have no DC conductance and basically have quite different spectra than the models of Figure 2.4. Fixed component values in the two dielectric models can be found so that they have exactly the same impedance spectrum. The same impedance spectrum with 2R-1C and 1R-2C models is not possible.

2.3.2 Dispersions

Take a look again at Figure 2.2. At LF, the membrane impedances are high and AC current through the membranes is very small; the tissue behaves as a frequency-independent AC conductor without contribution from the cell membranes and intracellular electrolytes. At HF, the membranes have low impedance and the current contribution of the intracellular electrolytes is high. The tissue also then behaves as an AC conductor but with a higher conductance than at LF.

Both the models of Figure 2.3 have the same general impedance spectrum as the one shown in Figure 2.5. Such a spectrum represents a *dispersion,* characterized by the following behavior: At LF and

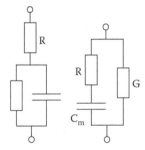

FIGURE 2.3 Two popular *impedance* models (2R-1C).

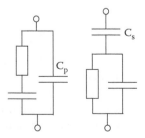

FIGURE 2.4 Two popular *dielectric* models (1R-2C).

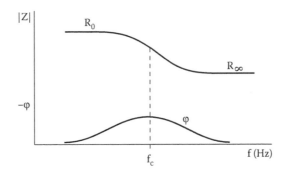

FIGURE 2.5 Frequency spectrum of the tissue electrical model shown in Figure 2.3.

HF, the impedance is resistive with zero phase shift. The resistance R_∞ at HF is lower than the LF value R_0. At a characteristic frequency, the phase shift is maximum (and negative) and the impedance is complex. Because the capacitor is ideal in a Debye model, all energy dissipation occurs in the two resistors.

2.3.3 Memristive Systems and Constant Phase Elements

Traditionally, special components have been used for making bioimpedance electrical models. A new component that appeared recently is the memristor (memory resistor). It was first described by Chua (1971). It is a passive two-terminal circuit element, which complements the resistor, coil, and capacitor. There is a relationship between charge and magnetic flux in the memristor in such a way that the resistance is dependent on the net amount of charge having passed the device in a given direction. The theory was extended to memristive systems (Chua and Kang 1976), comprising memristors, memcapacitors, and meminductors. All these elements typically show pinched hysteretic loops in the two constitutive variables that define them: current–voltage for the memristor, charge–voltage for the memcapacitor, and current–flux for the meminductor (Di Ventra et al. 2009). Memristor theory has, for example, been used within bioimpedance for the modeling of electro-osmosis in the human epidermis (Johnsen et al. 2011).

Constant phase elements (CPEs) have been used in bioimpedance models since the late 1920s. A CPE can be modeled by a resistor and capacitor, both having frequency-dependent values, in such a way that the phase angle is frequency independent. A CPE is mathematically simple, but not so simple as to realize with discrete, passive components in the real world. A particular type of CPE is the Warburg element, known from electrochemistry and solid state physics. It is diffusion controlled with a constant phase angle of 45° (Warburg 1899).

2.3.4 Cole Models

The similarity between the spectra of a model with just three components and a complex material such as tissue is of course limited. The first step of refinement is often to replace an ideal capacitor found in the Debye models of Figures 2.3 and 2.4 with a CPE. They are then called Cole impedance models (Cole 1940) and Cole–Cole permittivity models (Cole and Cole 1941).

2.3.5 Schwan Multiple α, β, and γ Dispersion Model

Schwan published his dispersion models many times, sometimes only with permittivity ε', sometimes also with ε'', or σ' as shown on Figure 2.6. Schwan (1957) named the LF part α dispersion. It is caused by cell-surface processes. The medium-frequency (MF) part is called β dispersion and is caused by

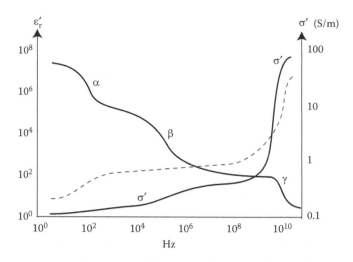

FIGURE 2.6 Schwan general model of α, β, and γ dispersions. Dashed curve is an example of measured muscle longitudinal conductivity.

capacitive membranes dividing intracellular and extracellular electrolytes. The HF part is called γ dispersion and is caused by water and protein processes. A clear separation between the dispersions is of course only possible if their characteristic frequencies are sufficiently apart. If this is not the case, dispersions may merge into a more or less straight line. The difference between tissue electrical parameters may be very large, from SC (low conductivity) to blood tissue (high conductivity). In addition to the generic curves shown in Figure 2.6, an example of measured conductivity from longitudinal muscle tissue (Gabriel et al. 1996) is shown.

In the literature, there is abundant data on conductivity/resistivity dispersions of biomaterials (Gabriel et al. 1996), biopolymers and membranes (Takashima 1989), dielectric and electronic properties (Pethig 1979), and physical properties (Duck 1990). Table 2.1 shows a few examples of LF (<1 kHz) data, followed by some comments on different tissues to illustrate the complexity of giving the exact data. As the tissue is so heterogeneous both on the micro- and macro- (organ) scale, the given values must be regarded as some sort of mean values of a given volume. Also, the question of difference between normal and pathological tissue is of great interest.

Tissue anisotropy may be strong, as shown in Table 2.1 for a muscle with 10 times higher longitude than perpendicular conductivity (Epstein and Foster 1983). They found that the anisotropy almost disappeared at 1 MHz; it is an LF phenomenon. The conductivity of muscle tissue is dependent on other factors such as mechanical contraction (Shiffman et al. 2003).

Tissue values change rapidly if the tissue becomes ischemic or dies (Gersing 1998; Schäfer et al. 1998; Casas et al. 1999; Martinsen et al. 2000).

2.3.5.1 Skin

SC resistivity in Table 2.1 is quoted from Yamamoto and Yamamoto (1976). The resistivity is higher the lower the water content of the SC. This is also the case with many (dead) protein powders (Takashima and Schwan 1965; Smith and Foster 1985). The water content of SC is dependent on the relative humidity of the air in contact with the SC surface. Methods for diagnosis of, for example, cancer tissue by information extraction from impedance dispersions in skin and oral mucosa have been found (Ollmar 1998), or correlation of impedance response patterns to histological findings in irritant skin reactions induced by various surfactants (Nicander et al. 1996).

TABLE 2.1 Conductivity and Resistivity Data

Material	Conductivity σ (S/m)	Resistivity ρ (Ω m)
Metals (implants)	5×10^6	2×10^{-7}
Saline (0.9% NaCl 37°C)	2	0.5
Muscle (longit/perpend)	0.6/0.06	1.6/16
Skin (SC)	10^{-5}	10^5
Diamond	10^{-14}	10^{14}

2.3.5.2 Cell Suspensions

Electrical properties of tissue and cell suspensions were reviewed by Schwan (1957). Membrane capacitance and conductance for pancreatic β-cells were measured by an electrokinetic method (Pethig et al. 2005; Grimnes and Martinsen 2008). The conductivity of blood is dependent on blood velocity; this is the Sigman effect (Sigman et al. 1937).

Also, deoxyribonucleic acid (DNA) molecules and their electrical conduction have been examined: the electrical conduction through DNA molecules (Fink and Schönenberger 1999) and resonances in the dielectric absorption of DNA (Foster et al. 1987). Recently, the Pethig group (Chung et al. 2011) has shown that measurement results in a cell suspension up to 10 MHz that is dependent on the cytoplasma membrane capacitance and resistance, the cell diameter, and the suspension conductivity. By using special interdigitated electrodes, the cell membrane capacitive reactance sort out the resistance above 100 MHz so that the electric field penetrates into the cell interior and intracellular dielectric properties can be measured.

2.4 Electrodes and Electrode Polarization

Electrodes are the most important part of an impedance-measuring system (Geddes 1972). They determine the sensitivity field (Section 2.5), which determines the contribution of each small voxel to the overall result. Three- and four-electrode systems are more complicated because, as we shall see, they introduce volumes of negative sensitivity because they measure *transfer* impedance.

2.4.1 Electrode Types

2.4.1.1 Skin Surface Electrodes

Skin electrodes have the largest commercial product volume, most of them are pregelled ready-to-use nonsterile products. Some of them have a snap-action wire contact; others are prewired, for instance, adapted for babies. There is a contact electrolyte between the skin and the electrode metal. Dry SC is a poor conductor and this easily results in poor (high impedance) contact and noise. The contact area with the skin should be as large as practically possible, and reducing the SCs thickness by sandpaper abrasion is useful. Hydrating the skin with contact electrolyte or by the covering effect of the electrode will usually reduce the contact impedance with time (minutes to hours).

Figure 2.7 shows to the left a classical wet gel type with an adhesive foam ring holding a sponge with gel in position and pressed against the skin. The AgCl metal part is recessed to reduce movement artifacts. If the electrolyte has higher salt concentration than, for example, seawater, it may irritate the skin and should be used as a short-time (hours) electrode. Long-term use (days) must have weaker electrolytes to be nonirritating on the skin. Often, the adhesive part of the foam is more irritating to the skin than the electrolyte. The wet electrolyte penetrates the SC and may fill the sweat ducts steadily increasing the electrical contact with the body.

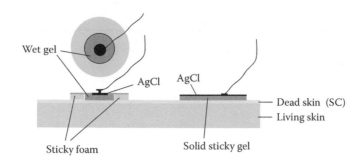

FIGURE 2.7   Two common types of skin surface electrodes.

Figure 2.7 to the right shows a solid gel electrode where the gel is also the sticky part. The gel (solid- or hydrogel) does not penetrate the skin but may to a small extent participate in receiving and storing water from the skin or delivering water to the skin (Tronstad et al. 2010).

2.4.1.1.1 Needle and Catheter Sterile Electrodes

With an invasive needle, it is possible to obtain rapid low impedance contact with the body. In neurology, the needles may be in the form of a tube with thin noble metal wires coming out through perpendicular holes on the shaft or coaxially at the tube end. The catheter version is often with metal rings and a metal tip at the end. They are used as CC or PU electrodes. If the needle shaft is insulated, the contact area can be small and the space resolution high in CC or PU applications. The needle tip position can be guided by measuring impedance spectra with the tip (Kalvøy et al. 2009). The needle may be of massive metal or hollow allowing liquid infusion together with impedance measurements.

2.4.1.1.2 Micro- and Nanotechnology Electrodes

By using interdigitated microelectrodes, it is possible to sort different cells in a suspension (Becker et al. 1994); it is a parallel to the Coulter counter technique described in Section 2.8 Micromachined electrodes for biopotential measurements are described in Griss et al. (2001). Pethig's group (Chung et al. 2011) describes interdigitated nanoelectrodes in a cellular suspension being able to measure intracellular dielectric properties.

2.4.2 Electrode Polarization

Electrode polarization is an important source of error in tissue impedance measurements (Schwan 1968). Current carriers in the electrode metal are electrons and those in living tissue are ions. The electric contact between metal and electrolyte (tissue liquids or applied electrolyte) has special electric nonlinear properties because of the formation of a double layer in the electrolyte. The double layer is very thin (nanometer) and depleted of current carriers. It generates a DC voltage and generates special polarization impedance. Figure 2.8 shows the polarization spectrum of an electrode with wet gel and AgCl metal surface. They have been obtained with two pregelled electrodes face to face and are taking half the impedance value. The Bode plot (Section 2.7) in Figure 2.8 shows a maximum phase shift of about 25° at 20 kHz. The impedance modulus is from about 300 Ω (1 Hz) down to 25 Ω (1 MHz). Above about 500 kHz, the phase goes through zero and the impedance becomes inductive. This is because of the self-inductance of the lead wires. Figure 2.9 shows a Wessel plot (Section 2.7) of the impedance. It reveals that the polarization impedance has two dispersions. The HF dispersion has a characteristic frequency of 46 kHz, determined by a circular arc drawn by regression analysis. Electrode polarization impedance dispersions are dependent on the metal, surface geometrical properties, and contact electrolyte (Mirtaheri et al. 2005) (Figure 2.9).

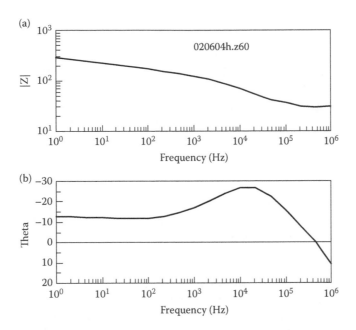

FIGURE 2.8 Polarization impedance by Bode plot. Two electrodes face to face, contribution of one electrode. Commercial ECG skin electrode with wet gel and AgCl metal surface of 0.7 cm².

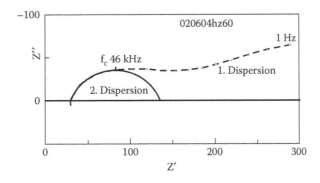

FIGURE 2.9 Polarization impedance Wessel plot showing a part of a first dispersion, and a second dispersion with a complete circular arc regression line. Same data as Figure 2.8a.

2.5 Electrode Systems and Their Sensitivity Fields

Bipolar (Figure 2.10) means that two electrodes contribute equally to the measurement result. Used as DC CC electrodes, they are polarized and become anode and cathode with different electrolytic processes. Measured AC impedance will include the polarization impedance of each electrode and the contribution of the tissue in between each electrode. As signal PU electrodes, they are used with negligible current flow and are then not polarized. They measure the potential difference between the electrodes. The potential difference may be generated as a result of remote organ activity setting up a volume current flow spreading out from the organ (endogenous currents generating, e.g., ECG or EMG). The potential difference may also be neurogenic, for example, originating from a sweat gland being excited by a nerve signal from a remote source.

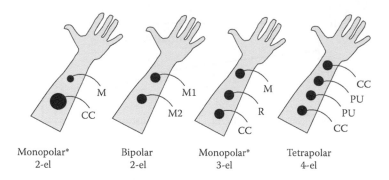

FIGURE 2.10 Skin surface electrode systems. Monopolar* systems are usually not ideally monopolar, see text below. The three- and four- electrode systems measure transfer immittance. Electrode functions: M, measuring; CC, current carrying; R, reference; PU, pick up.

A bipolar PU electrode system is also a local electric field strength sensor because $\mathbf{E} \cdot \mathbf{d} = U$ where $\mathbf{E}$ is he local electric field strength (V/m) in magnitude and direction (space vector), $\mathbf{d}$ the distance and direction between the electrodes (space vector), and U the potential difference. By using two bipolar electrode systems perpendicular to each other, the direction of the E-field can be determined. And if tissue conductivity σ is known, the local current density $\mathbf{J}$ can be estimated according to $\mathbf{J} = \sigma\,\mathbf{E}$.

Monopolar means that one of the electrodes contributes more to the measurement result than the other.

An *ideal* monopolar two-electrode system means that the large electrode has negligible influence on the result. The monopolar system shown in Figure 2.10 (left) has two very different electrode areas. With DC current flow, they are polarized and will become anode and cathode with different electrolytic processes. However, the large electrode will have much smaller current density and is, therefore, often regarded as an indifferent or neutral electrode. AC impedance will be dominated by the impedance of the small electrode (electrode polarization impedance included). As PU electrodes with negligible current flow, the size of the electrodes is not important but the metal of each electrode is very important. A potential difference will be measured if the large electrode is positioned at an indifferent skin site and the small electrode at a nerve-activated skin site. If both electrodes are placed on an active site, the recorded voltage difference may be very low.

Monopolar three-electrode system (Figure 2.10, number 3 to the right) means that it functions as a monopolar system when used on high-resistivity SC, cf. Figure 2.16. Then the *M* electrode contributes much more to the measurement result than the two other electrodes. However, in direct contact with low resistivity, the living tissue in Figure 2.13 shows that the *R* electrode is surrounded by high-sensitivity zones (and also small negative sensitivity zones) even if the *R* electrode is not CC.

The four-electrode tetrapolar system of Figure 2.10 is very different from the two-electrode mono- and bipolar systems (Grimnes and Martinsen 2007). It measures *transfer* impedance because the potential is recorded at a separate PU port and not at the CC port. If the two ports are far apart, no signal will be transferred from the CC to the PU port and the transfer impedance will be virtually 0 Ω.

2.5.1 Sensitivity Field

When measuring the impedance of a material with, for example, surface electrodes, it is obvious that not all small subvolumes in the material contribute equally to the measured impedance. Volumes between and close to the electrodes contribute more than volumes far away from the electrodes. Hence, a careful choice of electrode size and placement will enable the user to focus the measurements on the desired part of the material.

It is sometimes assumed that if the electrodes are placed in a linear fashion, with the voltage PU electrodes between the CC electrodes, only the volume between the PU electrodes is measured. Not only is this wrong, but there will also be zones of negative sensitivity between the PU electrodes and the CC electrodes (Grimnes and Martinsen 2007). Negative sensitivity means that if the complex resistivity is increased in that specific volume, lower total impedance will be measured.

The sensitivity of a small volume *dv* (voxel) within a material is a measure of how much this volume contributes to the total measured impedance (Geselowitz 1971), provided that the electrical properties (e.g., resistivity) are uniform throughout the material. If, in this case, the resistivity varies within the material, the local resistivity must be multiplied with the sensitivity to give a measure of the volume's contribution to the total measured resistance.

If we look at a simple example of a DC resistance measurement with a four-electrode system, the sensitivity will be computed in the following manner:

1. Imagine that you inject a current *I* between the two CC electrodes. Compute the current density J_1 in each small volume element in the material as a result of this current.
2. Imagine that you instead inject the same current between the PU electrodes and again compute the resulting current density J_2 in each small volume element.
3. The vector dot product between J_1 and J_2 in each volume element, divided by the current squared, is now the sensitivity of the volume element and if we multiply with the resistivity ρ in each volume, we will directly obtain this volume's contribution to the total measured resistance *R*.

Hence, the local (voxel) sensitivity *S* and the total measured volume resistance *R* will be

$$S = J_1 \cdot J_2 / I^2 \qquad R = \int_V \rho S \, dv \qquad (2.8)$$

Note that sensitivity is not dependent on voxel resistivity. These equations demonstrate the reciprocal nature of tetrapolar systems (or any other electrode system where this theory applies); under linear conditions, the CC electrodes and PU electrodes can be interchanged without any change in measured values.

A positive value for the sensitivity means that if the resistivity of this volume element is increased, a higher total resistance will be measured. The higher the value of sensitivity, the greater the influence on measured resistance. A negative value for the sensitivity, however, means that increased resistivity in that volume gives a lower total resistance. Two-electrode systems will not have volumes with negative sensitivity, but both the three- and four-electrode systems will typically have volumes with negative sensitivity. The commercial software package Comsol Multiphysics has been used for making Figures 2.11 through 2.14. All the finite-element calculations were made with half-cylinders immersed into the surface of the tissue and with the tissue volume extending far outside the figure in side and bottom directions.

Figure 2.11 is with a vertical slice with a resistivity 5 times that of the surrounding medium. It has little influence on the sensitivity field. Multiplying the sensitivity field with the local resistivity yields the volume resistance density field, as shown in Figure 2.12. The result is quite different and illustrates that with respect to the overall transfer resistance of the system, the increased resistivity of the slice is very important. The transfer resistance is not determined by the sensitivity value alone, the sensitivity is to be multiplied by the resistivity to obtain resistance values.

Sensitivity calculations can be utilized equally well for two-, three-, and four-electrode systems. In each case, you must identify the two CC electrodes used for driving an electrical current through the

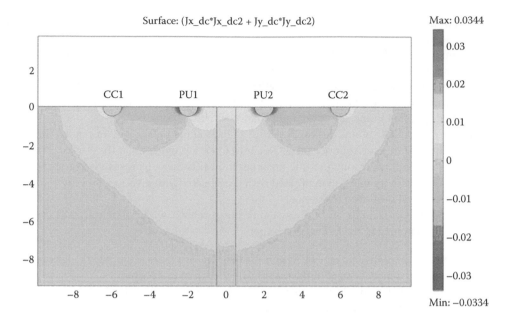

FIGURE 2.11 Volume sensitivity field of a biomaterial with a tetrapolar electrode system with two CC electrodes and two PU electrodes. Two homogeneous biomaterial regions, the vertical slice has 5 times the resistivity of the surrounding medium.

material and the two PU electrodes used for measuring the potential drop in the material. Figure 2.13 shows the sensitivity field for a three-electrode system (Grimnes 1983a).

In the case of a two-electrode system, the driving and PU electrode pairs are the same, and the sensitivity in a given volume will hence be the square of the current density divided by the square of the total injected current. The sensitivity can only have positive values (Figure 2.14).

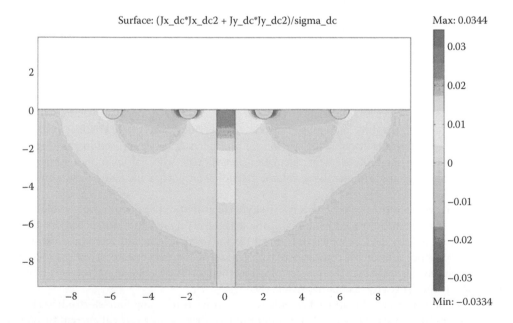

FIGURE 2.12 Volume *resistance density* plot of the model shown in Figure 2.11.

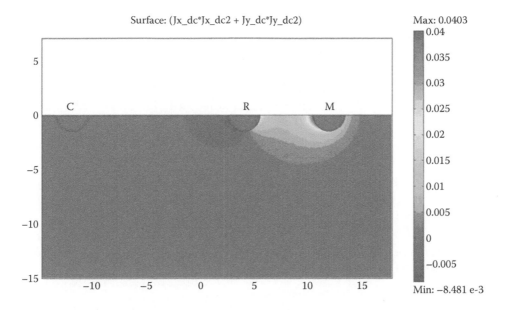

FIGURE 2.13 Volume *sensitivity* field of a quasi-monopolar three-electrode system. Notice zones of negative sensitivity at the left side of the *R* electrode.

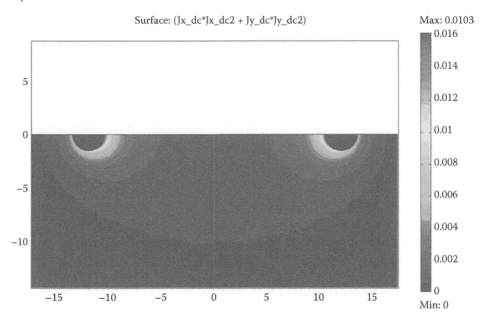

FIGURE 2.14 Volume *sensitivity* field of a bipolar two-electrode system. Notice the lack of negative sensitivity volumes.

2.6 Instrumentation and Quality Controls

With two electrodes, impedance or admittance can be calculated by measuring the voltage u and current i in the electrode wires. The two electrodes function as both CC and PU pairs. It is often practical to monitor *admittance* directly by applying a constant (amplitude) voltage and measuring current because the admittance is then proportional to current according to Y = i/u. *Impedance* is measured

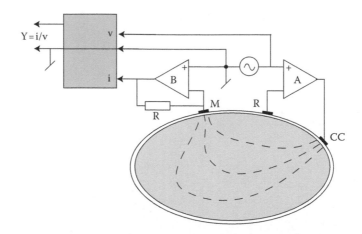

FIGURE 2.15 Monopolar admittance measuring circuit with three skin surface electrodes. SC thickness is exaggerated. Current flow lines are shown as dashed lines.

directly by applying a constant current i and measuring voltage because it is proportional to the voltage, $Z = u/i$.

Figure 2.15 shows an example of a skin surface admittance measuring circuit. It is a quasi-monopolar system with three electrodes: M is the measuring electrode, R a potential recording reference electrode, and CC is a current-carrying control electrode.

Two operational amplifiers are used: amplifier A for setting up a current through the body so that the voltage recorded by R becomes equal to the excitation voltage (30 mV). Amplifier B is an ideal (zero-voltage drop) current-reading amplifier. If the skin has sufficiently high resistivity, the R and CC electrodes are merely control electrodes with negligible influence on the admittance result (this is in contrast to Figure 2.13 because there the skin was not modeled). The well-conducting living body is considered isopotential. There is no current flow through the R electrode so that amplifier A brings the internal body potential to be equal to the excitation voltage. As the M electrode is on reference potential, $Y = i/u$ where i is the measured current and u is the constant AC potential difference across the SC.

Because of the capacitive properties of the skin, the measured current will be phase shifted with respect to the excitation voltage. By using a synchronous rectifier circuit with the excitation voltage as reference, the admittance can be decomposed so that only the in-phase conductance component G is measured. Susceptance B can be measured simultaneously according to $Y = G + jB$ by using a second synchronous rectifier with the reference signal 90° phase shifted.

More detailed descriptions of measuring methods can be found in Schwan (1963), Grimnes (1983a), Yelamos et al. (1999), and Grimnes and Martinsen (2008).

2.6.1 Synchronous Rectifiers

To measure impedance, an external current must be applied; it is an exogenous method. Thus, impedance measurements are ideally suited for synchronous rectification (SR) because the external excitation signal is available. The SR acts as a sort of sharp tracking filter with a bandwidth dependent on the time constant of the output of the low-pass filter. The result is a very noisy robust system.

SR is obtained by multiplying the input signal with the reference signal. Two types of circuit are in common use: the simplest method (Figure 2.16a) is with a reference signal in the form of a square wave. The multiplier circle may contain only on–off switches. The most elaborate method (Figure 2.16b) is with the reference signal as a sinusoidal waveform and the multiplication may be done digitally after

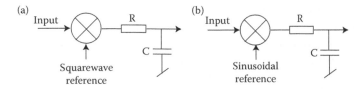

FIGURE 2.16 Synchronous rectifier circuits (a) with square wave and (b) with sinusoidal reference signal. Each circle mathematically multiplies the input signal with the reference signal.

both signals have been sampled and *A–D* converted. Such a circuit can be made insensitive to the DC level of the input signal (Grimnes and Martinsen 2008).

2.6.2 Quality Controls

2.6.2.1 Linearity

Bioimpedance is measured with an electric current applied to the CC electrodes. If the current waveform is sinusoidal, the signal from the PU electrodes should also be a sine. If it is not, the system is nonlinear and the current amplitude should then be reduced until the PU signal is sinusoidal. Signal-to-noise ratio is also reduced; so, a trade-off may be necessary in the choice of the best amplitude.

There are sources of nonlinearity both in electrode polarization and tissue impedance (Schwan 1992). Onaral and Schwan (1982) studied electrode *polarization impedance* and found that the limit voltage of linearity was about 100 mV and frequency independent. The corresponding limit current is of course impedance dependent and therefore frequency dependent, and may be about 5 μA/cm^2 at a frequency of 1 Hz.

Yamamoto and Yamamoto (1981) studied *human skin tissue* and found the limit current of linearity to be about 10 μA/cm^2 at a frequency of 10 Hz. Grimnes (1983b) studied electro-osmosis in human skin *in vivo* and found a strong polarity-dependent nonlinearity. The effect was stronger; the lower the frequency, Figure 2.17 shows the dramatic effect with ±20 V and 0.2 Hz, soon leading to skin breakdown. Nonlinearity of cardiac pacemaker CC electrodes made of noble metals and intended for use with pulses has been extensively studied (Jaron et al. 1969).

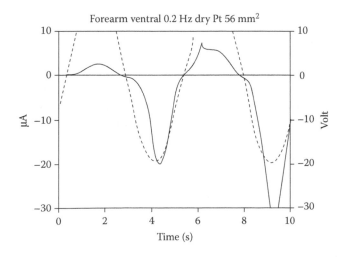

FIGURE 2.17 Electro-osmotic nonlinearity on the skin. Dashed line shows the applied voltage.

2.6.2.2 Kramers–Kronig Control

The Kramers–Kronig theorem in linear systems links, for example, the modulus spectrum of the impedance $|Z|$ to the phase spectrum (Grimnes and Martinsen 2008). Take a look at the Bode plot of Figure 2.8a. The steeper the fall of the Z-modulus with frequency, the more negative the phase. Phase zero means that the impedance level is constant. The change to positive phase corresponds to increasing impedance with higher frequency. The results shown in Figure 2.8a are Kramers–Kronig compatible. Noncompatibility may be because of nonlinearity, change of measured volume, or drift in volume properties (e.g., temperature) during spectrum recording.

2.6.2.3 Reciprocity Control of Transfer Impedance

According to the theorem, PU and CC electrodes can be swapped without change in measured transfer impedance. This may sound contraintuitive, but it is so. Reciprocity is destroyed if the system is nonlinear, for example, if the CC electrodes have larger contact area than the PU electrodes. After swapping, the small CC electrodes may then be driven into nonlinearity because of the increased current density. Reciprocity may also be destroyed if the properties of the biomaterial have changed.

2.6.3 Electrical Safety

For humans, bioimpedance methods use currents, which are not perceptible and of course not harmful. Only AC sinusoidal currents and DC are considered in this section, not pulse excitation. The biological effects of externally applied electromagnetic fields (through the air) are treated elsewhere (Polk and Postow 1996). For practical reasons, perception and hazard levels are usually quoted as current, energy, or charge in the external circuit (Dalziel 1954, 1972). The current density field in the tissue is usually unknown.

2.6.3.1 Threshold of Perception

2.6.3.1.1 Direct Current

The sensation of AC and DC currents is quite different. DC produces electrolytic products in the tissue near the electrode metal. The sensation may come after minutes, and after the DC has been switched off, the sensation may persist for a long time (minutes and more). Such perception is, therefore, not related to direct electric current nerve excitation. If a DC current is suddenly switched on or off, a transient sensation may be felt on the skin; this is direct nerve excitation. Table 2.2 shows that the maximum 10 μA DC is allowable auxiliary current.

2.6.3.1.2 Sine Waves

The lowest level (<1 μA) of 50/60 Hz perception is caused by *electrovibration* (Grimnes 1983c). It is perceived when dry skin slides on a CC conductor; the frictional force is modulated by the electrostatic force and can be felt as a lateral mechanical vibration.

The second level (1 mA) of 50/60 Hz is due to the *direct electric excitation* of nerves. The level increases as frequency is increased above 1 kHz (Figure 2.18). For example, 10 mA at 100 kHz is without perception, but temperature rise caused by the current may then be a limiting factor. Interpersonal variations

TABLE 2.2 Allowable Values of Continuous Leakage and Patient Auxiliary Currents (μA) (IEC-60601 2005)

	Type B		Type BF		Type CF		
Currents	NC	Single fault	NC	Single fault	NC	Single fault	
Patient leakage	100	500	100	500	10	50	
Patient auxiliary	100	500	100	500	10	50	AC
Patient auxiliary	10	50	10	50	10	50	DC

Note: NC = normal conditions.

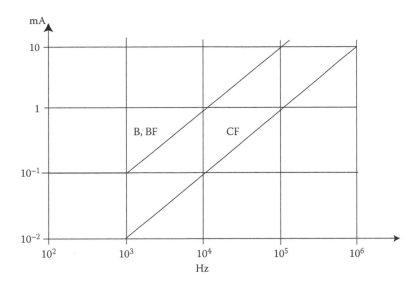

FIGURE 2.18 Allowable excitation (auxiliary) currents, AC (>0.1 Hz) rms values (according to IEC-60601 (2005)).

and the dependence on age and sex are small. The skin condition is not important as long as there are no wounds. The skin site may be important.

2.6.3.2 Electrical Hazards

If the current density is sufficiently high, an electric current triggers nerve and muscle tissue. If the current flow is through the heart or the brain stem, this may be lethal.

2.6.3.2.1 Macroshock

A macroshock situation is when current is applied to tissue far away from the heart or brain stem. The current is spread out more or less uniformly, and rather, large currents are needed in the external circuit (usually quoted >50 mA at 50/60 Hz) to attain dangerous levels in local tissue volumes such as heart and lungs.

2.6.3.2.2 Microshock

Small area contacts occur, for example, with pacemaker electrodes, catheter electrodes, and CC fluid-filled cardiac catheters. Small area contact implies a monopolar system with possible high local current densities but low current levels in the external circuit. This is called a *microshock* situation. The 50/60 Hz safe current limit for a small area contact with the heart is 10 μA in normal modes. The difference between macro- and microshock dangerous current levels is, therefore, more than three orders of magnitude.

2.6.3.3 Electrical Safety of Electromedical Equipment

Special safety precautions are taken for *electromedical equipment* and its use in the patient environment and in physical contact with the patient. Safety is regulated by international standards such as (IEC-60601 2005) used in Table 2.2.

The part of the equipment intended to be in physical contact with the patient is called the *applied part*. The applied part may ground the patient (type B) or keep the patient floating with respect to ground (BF—body floating or CF—cardiac floating) by *galvanic separation* circuitry (magnetic or optical coupling, battery-operated equipment).

Leakage currents are currents at power line frequency (50 or 60 Hz), they may be because of capacitive currents even with perfect insulation, and are thus difficult to avoid completely. *Patient leakage currents* are the leakage currents flowing to the patient via the applied part. Patient *auxiliary currents* are important for bioimpedance measurements. They are functional currents flowing *between* leads of the applied part, for example, as used with impedance plethysmography. They are not leakage currents and therefore usually not at power line frequency. It can be seen that not more than 10 μA DC can be used in an applied part under normal conditions, but 100 μA AC (>0.1 Hz) can be used except in CF (cardiac) applications.

Nerve and muscle tissue is less sensitive at higher frequencies. The allowable currents increase (Figure 2.18), for example, to 10 mA at 100 kHz in B and BF applications.

2.7 Result Presentations

2.7.1 Spectrum Plots

Bode plots are with logarithmic frequency and impedance scales, and with linear phase scale. An example is given in Figure 2.8a. The advantage is that a broad frequency spectrum can be shown combined with frequency-independent resolution.

Wessel (Argand, Nyquist, and Cole) plots are plots in the imaginary plane with real and imaginary axes (Figure 2.8b). The frequency scale is along the curve. The advantage is easily discernible dispersion arcs. The problem is the lack of linear frequency scale and the narrow high-resolution zone around the characteristic frequency.

2.7.2 Time-Series Plots

These plots are with fixed measuring frequency. An important parameter may be the sampling frequency because the recording of an LF spectrum may take a minute or more.

2.7.3 Converting Measured Variables to Clinical Variables or Parameters

Living tissue is a very heterogeneous and complex biomaterial. Impedance as a quantity is valid for a tissue volume and the contribution of the different volume elements (voxels) can be very different according to the electrode system sensitivity field. The results always represent some sort of mean values valid for a body region.

Geddes and Baker (1989) used the expression "Detection of Physiological Events by Impedance." The physiological variable may, for instance, be blood volume or flow and air volume or flow as described in Section 2.8.1. Impedance-based transducers convert the measured variable online into a signal from which the clinical parameter can be continuously calculated. Users are often not aware of which variable is the primary (actually measured) variable.

The measured variable can also be converted into the clinical parameter by a process of combining information from more than one sensor (polygraphy). Such calculation may be based on multivariate analysis. The result may be a numerical value or be placed in a group, for example, "normal" or "pathological." The end result may be variables such as CO_2 level, glucose level, lactic acid level, sweat activity (SA), total body water (TBW), meat quality, fruit freshness, and so on. For an interesting clinical parameter, it is often necessary to define a range of normal values to find a diagnosis or prognosis. To evaluate a proposed measuring method, a protocol is set up describing how measurements on healthy persons or organs are to be performed. The results are compared with a golden standard giving correct answers; for example, the hope is that lactic acid level can be measured with bioimpedance. Healthy persons are selected for impedance measurement, for example, of a large muscle performing mechanical work. Blood samples are taken and examined *in vitro* in a biochemical instrument (golden standard). Correlation coefficients between *in vivo* and *in vitro* results give the answer.

2.8 Application Examples

The application field of bioimpedance is very wide—from single-cell measurements with micro- and nanoelectrodes to whole-body composition analysis; from healthy to ischemic, pathological, and dead tissue. We have selected some typical bioimpedance application examples.

2.8.1 Volume and Flow Measurements

Volume measurements by impedance were proposed early and became one of the first widespread impedance applications in hospital instrumentation. It is a part of the usual bedside patient monitor present in all intensive-care units; impedance adds respiration to the ECG and blood pressure channels. It is embedded in the monitors rather anonymously, uses the ECG electrodes already there, and passes unnoticed as a clinical bioimpedance method by most users.

2.8.1.1 Plethysmographic *One-Compartment Model*

Plethysmography is a volume-measuring method, for example, of blood or air volumes in the lungs. Figure 2.19 illustrates a basic one-compartment model of a blood vessel segment of length L. As a one-compartment model, the electrical contribution of the vessel wall has been neglected. The resistance R of the blood volume is $R = \rho L/A$, where A is the cross-sectional area and ρ is the resistivity of the blood. The volume $v = LA$ and $A = v/L$ is put into the equation so that $v = \rho L^2/R$.

The variable G is preferred to variable R because it is directly proportional to v; so, the equation above is changed to

$$v = G\,\rho L^2 \qquad [\text{m}^3] \text{ or } [\text{L}] \text{ liter}$$
$$\text{Validity: A is constant along the length and } \rho \text{ is uniformly distributed.} \qquad (2.9)$$

2.8.1.2 Volume Sensor

In our simplified model, a choice must now be made: Let us consider that the segment volume is increased by a blood pressure increase. The elastic vessel wall is stretched so that a volume Δv is added to the tube content; does it result in a swelling of length or cross-sectional area? A blood vessel is usually considered to swell in cross-sectional area. Then L is constant and by measuring G, we have a calibrated volume-measuring system if ρ is considered constant with a known value.

Equation 2.9 represents a basic example of an impedance-based sensor in the form of a transducer. The transducer is the vessel segment, which is biological. It converts the volume variable into an electrical signal in a way so that the measured quantity is conductance G [siemens S]. By multiplying the conductance value with the constant ρL^2 [ohm m³], the measured result can be presented as volume [m³]. It is a common misunderstanding that the transducer measures volume. The measured variable, however, is electrical conductance. The elasticity of the wall determines the compliance $C = \Delta v/\Delta p$ of the vessel segment volume, with p as blood pressure. $C = 0$ is a stiff wall with no volume increase with increasing blood pressure and so no plethysmography.

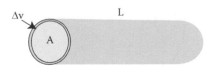

FIGURE 2.19   One-compartment blood vessel plethysmographic model.

2.8.1.3 Flow Sensor

Consider that the vessel segment is closed in one end. From Equation 2.9, $\Delta v = \Delta G\ \rho L^2$ and

$$dv/dt = (dG/dt)\ \rho L^2 \qquad \text{for example, [L/s].} \qquad (2.10)$$

The time derivative of volume is flow, flow into, or out of a closed segment.

2.8.1.4 Plethysmographic Two-Compartment Model

In the two-compartment model, the inner volume is, for example, a blood volume and the outer volume is the surrounding tissue volume.

Figure 2.20 shows the two-compartment model with a volume increase Δv. All tissue is considered incompressible (no air). If the inner volume $vA = A \cdot L$ is supplied with extra volume Δv, it swells to $\Delta v + vA$. The outer tube also swells to an increased outer diameter, but the volume vt remains constant. If all the volumes have the same resistivity, it can be shown that

$$\Delta G/G = \Delta v/(\Delta v + v_A + v_t) \qquad (2.11)$$

where v_A is the volume of the inner cylinder and v_t is the volume of the outer tissue cylinder. It is evident that the surrounding tissue also diminishes the sensitivity of the method because the compliance of the blood vessel is reduced by the support of the tissue surroundings. Further details can be found (Grimnes and Martinsen 2008), also for the case when the resistivities of the compartments are unequal and when the Sigman effect is relevant.

2.8.2 Three Different Variables Measured with Two Electrodes

With only two chest ECG electrodes, it is possible to monitor

- Blood: Mechanical pumping action of the heart
- Electrical activity of the heart
- Air: Mechanical respiration activity

The two electrodes are attached to the skin of the chest. As ECG PU electrodes, they record the signal corresponding to the electrical activity of the heart. It is well known that electrical activity is not necessarily followed by mechanical blood pumping. For the impedance measurement, an AC current of, for example, 50 kHz is applied to the same electrodes. The impedance as a function of time shows two different signals (Figure 2.21). The large-amplitude signal is due to the emptying and filling of the lungs with air. The smaller waves correspond to the mechanical emptying of the heart with well-conducting blood (ICG—impedance cardiography). Figure 2.21 shows a result also comprising an *apnea* period of about eight heartbeats where only the mechanical pumping activity of the heart is visible. The division

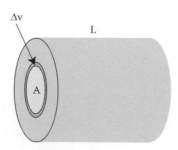

FIGURE 2.20   Two-compartment plethysmographic model.

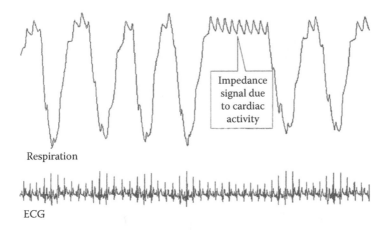

FIGURE 2.21 Simultaneous registration of (1) heart mechanical pumping activity, (2) heart electrical activity, and (3) lung mechanical ventilation, using only two electrodes. (From Patterson R. 1995. *The Biomedical Engineering Handbook*. Boca Raton, FL, CRC Press, 3rd edition, pp. 1223–1230.)

between the air and blood plethysmographies is only possible because the two variables have rather different repetition frequencies.

2.8.3 Bioimpedance in Electrosurgery

Electrosurgery (ES) units are used in all operating rooms throughout the world. HF currents are used for tissue cutting, coagulation, desiccation, and sealing. Several bioimpedance systems are used to increase performance and safety.

2.8.3.1 Monitoring Return Electrode Safety

In monopolar ES, the safe functioning of the return electrode is most important. If the HF current (often around 500 kHz) does not have a safe return path back to the unit, the current spreads uncontrolled into the air (antenna effect) and jump to metal objects of all kinds because of capacitive coupling. Patients being in touch with such objects will also couple current from the patient body to the metal, resulting in tissue burns. One method to reduce the risk of accidents is to split the return electrode plate in two halves and monitor by impedance that both halves have good contact with the skin. The halves are coupled with a HF capacitor and both function as the return electrode for the ES HF current. A small sensing current is sent out to the halves to check the continuity of leads and skin contact. The current is supposed to go through one half-electrode and the skin to the other half. If the contact area is too small or a lead is broken, the impedance becomes too high and a trigger alarm is activated. During alarm, the surgeon cannot activate the ES unit any longer.

Figure 2.22 shows how the impedance is measured at 50 kHz and the impedance value is sampled at the start of the procedure. The sampled value is used as reference for the remaining procedure, and the impedance is continuously monitored and compared with the reference. If the deviation is too large, an alarm is triggered and further activation of the ES unit is inhibited. There are two alarm levels. The low level gives warning of a short-circuit condition, the high level gives warning of poor skin contact or wire break.

2.8.3.2 Bipolar Forceps Activation

Forceps are used for bipolar microsurgery and the unit is activated by a pedal or a microswitch on the forceps. However, some surgeons prefer impedance-based activation so that when both tips have sufficient tissue contact, a low impedance level is reached, which triggers activation.

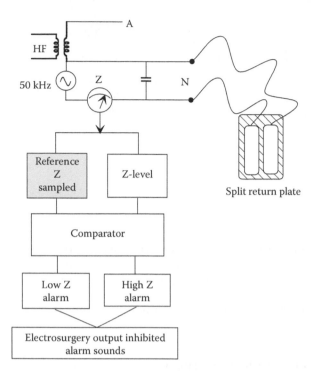

FIGURE 2.22 Impedance-based ES safety monitoring of the return plate system.

2.8.3.3 Vessel Sealing

Safe sealing of blood vessels is very important to prevent postoperative bleeding and reoperations. A special technique for sealing is based on the discovery that under tight control, it is possible to prevent too much tissue destruction and obtain a melting process between connective protein tissue parts of the blood vessel walls. The method is based on a special bipolar jaw with large contact surfaces and a high mechanical pressure to the tissue between the surface blades (Figure 2.23). The electrical contact to the tissue between the upper and lower jaw is very efficient, and it is possible to use much lower voltage and higher current than in ordinary cut and coagulation procedures. The impedance of the tissue is monitored during the clamping and current flow, and within a few seconds, the sealing process starts and this is registered by the impedance system. The impedance system registers when melting is optimum and activation is automatically stopped by the system, not the surgeon. The cutting device is used immediately after activation stops so that both vessel ends can be effectively sealed.

2.8.4 Body Composition

The parameters of interest in body composition analysis (bioelectric impedance analysis, BIA) are (a) TBW, (b) extracellular/intracellular fluid balance, (c) muscle mass, and (d) fat mass. Application areas are as diversified as sports, medicine, nutrition, and fluid balance in renal dialysis and transplantations.

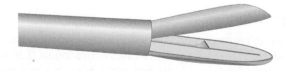

FIGURE 2.23 Vessel-sealing bipolar electrode system with cutting device. (Courtesy: Tormod Martinsen.)

2.8.4.1 Method

The most validated method is prediction of TBW from four-electrode whole-body transfer impedance measurements at 50 kHz. It is not really a whole-body measurement because the results are dominated by the wrist and ankle segments with very little influence from the chest because of the large cross-sectional area. By using more than four electrodes, it is possible to measure more than one body segment. With two electrodes at each hand and foot, the body impedance can, for instance, be modeled in five segments: arms, legs, and chest.

Either the series impedance electrical model (often with the reactance component X neglected) or the parallel equivalent has been used. Several indexes have been introduced to increase the accuracy. Gender, age, and anthropometric results, such as total body weight and height, are parameters used. An often-used index is H^2/R_{segm}, where H is the body height and R_{segm} the resistance of a given segment. Because of the $1/R_{segm}$ term, this is therefore actually a *conductance* index. Calibration, for example, can be done by determining the k-constants in the equation

$$TBW = k_1 \frac{H^2}{R_{segm}} + k_2 \qquad (2.12)$$

Such an equation is not directly derived from biophysical laws, but has been empirically selected because it gives the best correlation.

2.8.4.2 Results

The correlation according to Equation 2.12 can be better than 0.95. Hundreds of validation studies with isotope dilution have established a solid relation between whole-body impedance at 50 kHz and body fluid volume (Kyle et al. 2004). Improved prediction of extracellular and TBW has been obtained using impedance loci generated by multiple-frequency BIA (Cornish et al. 1993). Predicting body cell mass with bioimpedance by using more theoretical methods has also been proposed (De Lorenzo et al. 1997). Assessment of hydration change in women during pregnancy and postpartum with bioelectrical impedance vectors has been used (Lukaski et al. 2007).

Complex impedance data can also be given as modulus and phase. Phase has been used as an index of *nutrition*. This is true only in comparison between vectors with the same modulus. For instance, short vectors with a small phase angle are associated with edema, whereas long vectors with an increased phase angle indicate dehydration. The prediction error of fat mass is too high for clinical use (standard error of the estimate in the order of 3–4 L for TBW and 3–4 kg for the fat-free mass) (Sun et al. 2003).

2.8.4.3 Calibration

Calibration can be done with alternative but cumbersome methods using, for example, deuterium, underwater weighing, or dual-energy x-ray absorption. Standardization of the type of electrodes used and their placement is a major concern (Cornish et al. 1999; Kyle et al. 2004).

2.8.5 Electrical Impedance Tomography

There are many examples in medicine where the spatial distribution of a variable is more important than a single value valid for the whole body or just one small volume. For example, in cancer, the spread (metastases) must be mapped; in lungs, it is not just the vital capacity, but how different parts of the lung respond to treatment differently and where in the airway or blood perfusion obstructions occur; with impedance, it is possible to map a tissue layer (EIT, electrical impedance tomography) defined by a skin surface multiple-electrode system; clinical application areas are imaging and imaging of small regions, which can be parameterized and compared (e.g., left and right lung); with thorax imaging,

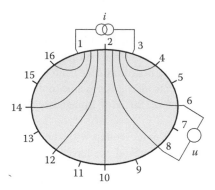

FIGURE 2.24 EIT 16-electrode skin surface system. Current is applied to one bipolar electrode pair; the corresponding equipotential lines are shown. Signals are picked up with all six corresponding bipolar pairs. A homogeneous material model is shown.

determining stroke volume (cardiac output [CO]), pulmonary blood perfusion, and regional lung function; and furthermore, imaging for brain function, breast cancer screening, gastrointestinal function, and hyperthermia (Holder 2005).

Electric current is typically injected in one CC electrode pair and the voltages of all the other PU electrode pairs are recorded. Current injection can then be successively shifted until all electrode pairs have been used as a CC pair. The quantity measured is a group of transfer impedances.

Typical EIT systems involve 16–32 electrodes in any one plane and operate at frequencies between 10 kHz and 1 MHz. The Sheffield Mark III system (Brown et al. 1994a,b) uses 16 electrodes and injects current and measures potential drop between interleaved neighboring electrodes to reduce cross talk (Figure 2.24). Figure 2.24 shows equipotential lines because of a single CC electrode pair. A total of 64 measurements are made at each frequency when driving odd-numbered electrodes and measuring at even-numbered electrodes. Because of reciprocity (see Section 2.5), this gives 32 independent measurements. Voltage differences can be sampled from all PU electrode pairs (not just neighboring) with any combination of single or multiple CC electrode pair combinations.

As explained in Section 2.5, the sensitivity to a given local change in resistivity is given by the dot product of the current vectors resulting from injecting current through the two CC pairs and two PU pairs, respectively. The sensitivity may hence be highest close to the CC or PU electrodes and lowest toward the center of the medium. Figure 2.24 shows the equipotential lines, not the sensitivity field of the CC–PU four-electrode system.

2.8.5.1 Multifrequency EIT

One of the fundamental problems of anatomical imaging based on single-frequency impedance measurements was that the absolute impedance is difficult to determine sufficiently accurately because of the errors in the positioning of the electrodes, boundary shape, and contact impedance density. Impedance imaging was, therefore, concerned with impedance changes because of physiological or pathological processes. With the introduction of multifrequency EIT, the possibility of tissue characterization based on impedance spectroscopy was introduced. If the frequency response varies significantly between different organs and tissues, it will be easier to achieve anatomical images because the images will be based on characteristic impedance changes rather than the absolute value of impedance. Indexes, that is, the relation between measured data at two frequencies may be used, but because of the different characteristic frequencies for different tissues, it has been proved difficult to choose only two frequencies to match all types of tissue. Hence, typically 8–16 frequencies are used (Brown et al. 1994a) computed from the measured data several parameters from a three-component electrical model. They also adapted the measured data to the Cole impedance equation (Cole 1940). Furthermore, indexes were made by using the lowest frequency of 9.6 kHz data as a reference and Brown et al. concluded that it may be possible to identify tissues on the basis of their impedance spectrum and the spectrum of the changes in impedance.

2.8.5.2 Contactless Data-Acquisition Techniques

Contactless data-acquisition techniques can also be used in EIT. Such systems may involve coils for inducing currents but with usual PU electrodes. Totally, contactless circuitry is also possible with magnetic coils or capacitive coupling both for the current excitation and for measuring the tissue current response. Contactless systems have been presented at frequencies up to 20 MHz.

2.8.5.3 Invasive EIT

Classical EIT in medicine is with surface electrodes. However, an array with insulated needles but exposed tips can perform a two-dimensional (2D) recording when measuring during rapid withdrawal of the array. Intended use is in resuscitation outside hospitals (Martinsen et al. 2010).

2.8.5.4 Image Reconstruction

The algorithms for image reconstruction started with the Sheffield group using back-projection methods. On the basis of the equipotential lines shown in Figure 2.24, a conformal transformation could be performed so that the equipotential lines became straight lines. Through many refinement steps, the end result was that uniform resolution across the image was not possible, the spatial accuracy was about 15% of the body diameter; best at the edge (12%) and gradually worse toward the center where the spatial accuracy may be 20% (Holder 2005). The back projection is based on some conditions that are not fulfilled: that the problem can be treated as a 2D problem and that the initial resistivity is uniform. Even if back projection had little theoretical support, it gave the best *in vivo* results. An alternative to back projection was the use of a sensitivity matrix. The sensitivity matrix is the matrix of values by which the conductivity values can be multiplied to give the electrode voltages. The matrix describes how different parts of the measured object influence on the recorded voltages because of the geometrical shape of the object. Iterative methods can be used for static imaging; an intelligent guess of the distribution of, for example, conductivities in the tissue is made initially. The forward problem is then solved to calculate the theoretical boundary potentials that are compared to the actual measured potentials. The initial guess is then modified to reduce the difference between calculated and measured potentials and this process is repeated until the difference is acceptably small. The sensitivity matrix has to be inverted to enable image reconstruction. This operation is not uncomplicated and many techniques have been suggested.

2.8.5.5 Advantages and Problems

EIT is basically not tomographic in the way, for instance, computer tomography (CT) is. Photons reaching a CT detector have followed straight lines after scattered photons have been absorbed in collimators. Electric current lines out from a CC electrode spread out in all directions and do not clearly define a tomographic plane and its thickness. Some important achievements in the pursuit of three-dimensional (3D) EIT were presented in *Nature* (Metherall et al. 1996). This leads to a 3D multilayer aspect as a parallel to the magnetic resonance imaging (MRI) volume-imaging technique. However, the complexity of both the EIT hardware and software increases considerably by introducing this third dimension.

A sufficiently precise positioning of the electrodes is difficult and it is easier to work with dynamic images, which do not depend so much on absolute impedance values. If the tissue shows sufficient dispersion, a multifrequency approach has been found useful. Also, time series from changes in the tissue during recording, for instance, respiration, has proven useful.

EIT is a fast technique because an image uptake can take less than 1/10 s. The sensors are small and low priced, and the instrumentation can also be low priced, small, and light weighted.

A new and very interesting application is the monitoring of the distribution of ventilation in the lungs. Dräger has developed a special EIT application using 15 or 16 electrodes around the chest. It is used in intensive-care and neonatal units. To operate ventilators in a manner that is correct for each patient, doctors need reliable data not only on classical respiration parameters valid for the lung volume, but also on the distribution of the ventilation to assess treatment. The EIT instrumentation is small and well suited for bedside use delivering information directly in real time. This is in contrast to x-ray, CT, and MRI instrumentation where the patient usually must be brought to a special examination room.

New application examples are coming up all the time, such as imaging of gastric function, pulmonary ventilation, perfusion, brain hemorrhage, hyperthermia, swallowing disorders, and breast cancer. A fundamental difficulty is the considerable anisotropy found in the electrical properties of, for example, muscle tissue.

2.8.6 Some Additional Applications

2.8.6.1 Impedance Cardiography and Cardiac Output

ICG has been around for a long time (Kubicek et al. 1970) and appreciable activity has been going on toward clarifying the best method (Hettrick and Zielinski 2006). The electrode systems consist of either four band electrodes, two in the region of the neck and two around the thorax, or the use of spot electrodes (Kauppinen et al. 1998). The origin of the impedance changes during the cardiac cycle is known. Physiologically, it is the filling and emptying of the heart, the opening and closing of the valves, the rapid filling and slow emptying of the aorta, the filling and emptying of the lung vessels, lung tissue, and surrounding tissue. Clinically, the need for a bedside CO monitor has resulted in intensive research and many interventional trials (Bernstein 1986). New ways, for example, with the use of the Sigman effect are still under development (Bernstein 2010).

2.8.6.2 Intrathoracic Impedance and Fluid Status

Active implants, such as pacemakers, cardioverters (ICDs), and neurostimulators, are increasingly using impedance measurements (Yu et al. 2005; Vollmann et al. 2007). The implants are already equipped with advanced electronic circuitry and advanced multielectrode catheter systems together with data storage and communication facilities. Parameters of interest are, for instance, CO, myocardial contractility, ischemia, and thoracic fluid accumulation.

2.8.6.3 Implant Rejection Monitoring

Transplanted organs, such as heart or kidney, can be followed with impedance measurements using skin electrodes or implanted leads or catheters (Ollmar 1997).

2.8.6.4 Cancer Detection

For many years, there has been hope that the impedance difference between normal and cancerous tissue is sufficiently large to clinically obtain useful diagnoses. An impedance method is rapid and practical, but cancer is a serious diagnosis and both sensitivity and specificity must be high. Interesting results have been obtained with the cervix in nonpregnant and pregnant women. Skin cancer in the breast has been examined (Jossinet 1996). Perhaps, the most promising results have been presented by Stig Ollmar's group (Ollmar et al. 1995) on skin cancer, using a special electrode surface with many very small and very short needles as a microinvasive technique (Emtestam et al. 1998; Åberg et al. 2004).

2.8.6.5 Sweat Activity

Human skin conductance is very dependent on SA. The SA instrumentation uses skin surface electrodes for unipolar admittance measurements (Tronstad et al. 2008). Small, portable, and multichannel loggers are now available enabling recording of SA under circumstances such as daily errands, exercise, and sleep. Results show that SA is related to physical exercise, dermatomes, distribution of sweat glands, and sympathetic activity. With the normal sweating patterns of the healthy population better known, measurements on hyperhidrosis patients can yield a distinguishing parameter, which can be used for diagnosis and treatment evaluation.

2.8.6.6 Skin Hydration

SC complex resistivity is very dependent on SC hydration. The hydration is dependent on the SA and also the relative humidity of the surrounding air in contact with the SC surface. They both influence the measured admittance but in different ways. The capacitive part of the skin admittance (susceptance) gives information on SC hydration (Martinsen and Grimnes 2001).

Gravimetric and other methods have been used for *in vitro* calibration of skin hydration measurements (Martinsen et al. 2008).

2.8.6.7 Needle Positioning

The method is based on precise determinations of local impedance values in tissue surrounding the tip of a needle (Kalvøy et al. 2009). Such impedance spectra allow determination of the tissue type and thereby an anatomical positioning of the needle. In some clinical applications, the separation of fat and muscle is, for instance, crucial. For clinical use, sufficient spatial resolution is obtained cause of the small sensitivity zone. A needle may be a solid needle or a cannula for simultaneous infusion or biopsy taking. The method requires a needle with an insulated shaft and a conducting tip in galvanic contact with the tissue. The method may also be applied in further characterization of tissue state, for example, oxygenation, content of substances such as lactic acid, and so on.

2.8.6.8 Electrodermal Response

Palmar skin changes both skin potential level and skin conductance as a response to psychophysiological stimuli (answering questions, doing mathematical calculations, taking a deep breath, being in a stressed situation, etc.). A committee report (Fowles et al. 1981) recommended the use of DC conductance and this has been the most popular method since. 0.5 V DC is applied to two electrodes, the current is measured and the DC conductance calculated. However, a new committee report also recommends using AC conductance for electrodermal response measurements (Boucsein et al. 2012). By using AC conductance, it is possible to measure skin potential simultaneously with the same electrode (Grimnes et al. 2011). The waves are very dependent on the electrode contact and electrolyte used (Tronstad et al. 2010). Potential response waves may be different from AC response waves and the generation mechanism is unknown.

2.8.6.9 Cell- and Bacteria Suspensions, Coulter Counter

Schwan (1957) wrote an introduction to impedance measurement on cell and bacteria suspensions. A Coulter counter is a streaming blood cell counter. Two different electrolyte reservoirs equipped with impedance CC electrodes are connected via a short capillary. The reservoir with the cell suspension is on higher pressure so that the electrolyte with cells stream through the capillary. Measured impedance is dominated by the capillary because of its very small diameter. At passage, the impedance goes through a peak because of the cell membrane. The frequency of the peaks is the number of cells passed per second; the impedance waveforms are characteristic for different cell types. The cell suspension must have a concentration so that the probability of two cells in the capillary at the same time is low. The electrolyte concentration must be adapted to the impedance increase caused by each cell.

2.8.6.10 Rheoencephalography

Although not evident from the title, rheoencephalography is a plethysmographic technique based on bioimpedance and with focus on cerebral blood flow (Bodo et al. 2004; Grimnes and Martinsen 2008; Bodo 2010).

2.8.6.11 Cell Nanometer Motion

Some cells must be in contact with a surface to thrive. When a cell is in contact with a small electrode surface, the cell's covering effect results in an impedance increase. The electrode can be of gold and can have a surface area not very larger than the spread of a single cell. The suspension can contain protein molecules, which first cover the golden surface so that the cell is attracted to the protein surface. The basic polarization impedance is, therefore, modified by the protein layer. The impedance is measured, for example, at 4 kHz. Living cells that are attached to a surface will move around on the electrode surface giving varying impedance. This cell motion corresponds to nanometer movements giving information about cell status and behavior (Giaever and Keese 1993).

2.8.6.12 EMG and Neurology Impedance

The action potential is the endogenous bioelectric signal from an excited nerve cell. The process can be followed by impedance changes as well (Sauter et al. 2009) and in electrical impedance myography (EIM) (Nie et al. 2006).

2.8.6.13 Electroporation

Electroporation is generation of pores in the cell membranes by short voltage pulses (Weaver and Chizmadzhev 1996; Pliquett et al. 2007). The cells may die (a sort of nonthermal ablation) or survive. The generation of pores implies an impedance decrease, which can be detected by an impedance reduction. Bioimpedance can, therefore, monitor the pore-generating process. In the Coulter counter the cells pass rapidly through a capillary connecting two electrolytic chambers and are counted and analyzed. Here, a single cell is mechanically trapped in a hole between two chambers and by pulsing the two chambers the cell can be electroporated even with low voltages pulses, and the process can be followed in the stationary cell.

References

Åberg P, Nicander I, Hansson J, Geladi P, Holmgren U, Ollmar S. 2004. Skin cancer identification using multi-frequency electrical impedance—A potential screening tool. *IEEE Trans Biomed Eng* 51, 2097–2102.

Becker FF, Wang X-B, Huang Y, Pethig R, Vykoukal J, Gascoyne PRC. 1994. The removal of human leukaemia cells from blood using interdigitated microelectrodes. *J Phys D: Appl Phys* 27, 2659–2662.

Bernstein DP. 1986. A new stroke volume equation for thoracic electrical bioimpedance: Theory and rationale. *Crit Care Med* 14 (10), 904–909.

Bernstein, DP. 2010. Impedance cardiography: Pulsatile blood flow and the biophysical and electrodynamic basis for the stroke volume equations. *J Electr Bioimp* 1, 2–17.

Bodo M. 2010. Studies in rheoencephalography (REG). *J Electr Bioimp* 1, 18–40.

Bodo M, Pearce FJ, Armonda RA. 2004. Cerebrovascular reactivity: Rat studies in rheoencephalography. *Physiol Meas* 25, 1371–1384.

Boucsein W, Fowles DC, Grimnes S, Ben-Shakhar G, Roth WT, Dawson ME, Filion DL. 2012. Publication recommendations for electrodermal response. *Psychophysiology*, 49, 1017–1034.

Brown BH, Barber DC, Leathard AD, Lu L, Wang W, Smallwood RH, Wilson AJ. 1994b. High frequency EIT data collection and parametric imaging. *Innov Tech Biol Med* 15(1), 1–8.

Brown BH, Barber DC, Wang W, Lu L, Leathard AD, Smallwood RH, Hampshire AR, Mackay R, Hatzigalanis K. 1994a. Multi-frequency imaging and modeling of respiratory related electrical impedance changes. *Physiol Meas.* 15(suppl.), 1–12.

Casas O, Bragos R, Riu P, Rosell J, Tresanchez M, Warren M, Rodriguez-Sinovas A, Carreño A, Cinca J. 1999. *In-vivo* and *in-situ* ischemic tissue characterisation using electrical impedance spectroscopy. *Ann N Y Acad Sci* 873, 51–59.

Chua LO. 1971. Memristor—The missing circuit element. *IEEE Trans Circuit Theory* CT-18(5), 507–519.

Chua LO, Kang SM. 1976. Memristive devices and systems. *Proc IEEE*, 64, 209–223.

Chung C, Waterfall M, Pells S, Menachery A, Smith S, Pethig R. 2011. Dielectrophoretic characterisation of mammalian cells above 100 MHz. *J Electr Bioimp* 2, 64–71.

Cole KS. 1940. Permeability and impermeability of cell membranes for ions. *Cold Spring Harbor Sympos Quant Biol* 8, 110–122.

Cole KS, Cole RH. 1941. Dispersion and absorption in dielectrics. I. Alternating current characteristics. *J Chem Phys* 9, 341–351.

Cornish BH, Jacobs A, Thomas BJ, Ward LC. 1999. Optimising electrode sites for segmental bioimpedance measurements. *Physiol Meas* 20, 241–250.

Cornish BH, Thomas BJ, Ward LC. 1993. Improved prediction of extracellular and total body water using impedance loci generated by multiple frequency bioelectrical impedance analysis. *Phys Med Biol* 38, 337.

Dalziel CF. 1954. The threshold of perception currents. *AIEE Trans Power App Syst* 73, 990–996.

Dalziel, CF. 1972. Electric shock hazard. *IEEE Spectr*, 9, 41.

De Lorenzo A, Andreoli A, Matthie J, Withers P. 1997. Predicting body cell mass with bioimpedance by using theoretical methods: A technology review. *J Appl Physiol* 82, 1542–1558.

Di Ventra M, Pershin YV, Chua LO. 2009. Circuit elements with memory: Memristors, memcapacitors, and meminductors. *Proc IEEE* 97, 1717–1724.

Duck FA.1990. *Physical Properties of Tissue. A Comprehensive Reference Book*. London, Academic Press.

Emtestam L, Nicander I, Stenström M, Ollmar S. 1998. Electrical impedance of nodular basal cell carcinoma: A pilot study. *Dermatology* 197, 313–316.

Epstein BR, Foster KR. 1983. Anisotropy in the dielectric properties of skeletal muscles. *Med Biol Eng Comp* 21, 51.

Fink H-W, Schönenberger C. 1999. Electrical conduction through DNA molecules. *Nature* 398, 407–410.

Foster KR, Epstein BR, Gealt MA. 1987. "Resonances" in the dielectric absorption of DNA? *Biophys J* 52, 421–425.

Fowles DC, Christie MJ, Edelberg R, Grings WW, Lykken DT, Venables PH. 1981. Publication recommendations for electrodermal measurements. *Psychophysiology* 18, 232–239.

Gabriel S, Lau RW, Gabriel C. 1996. The dielectric properties of biological tissue: II. Measurements in the frequency range 10 Hz to 20 GHz. *Phys Med Biol* 41, 2251–2269.

Geddes LA. 1972. *Electrodes and the Measurement of Bioelectric Events*. New York, Wiley-Interscience.

Geddes LA, Baker LE. 1989. *Applied Biomedical Instrumentation*. New York, Wiley Interscience.

Gersing E. 1998. Impedance spectroscopy on living tissue for determination of the state of organs. *Bioelectrochem Bioenerg* 45(2), 145–149.

Geselowitz DB. 1971. An application of electrocardiographic lead theory to impedance plethysmography. *IEEE Trans Biomed Eng* 18, 38–41.

Giaever I, Keese CR. 1993. A morphological biosensor for mammalian cells. *Nature 366*, 591–592.

Grimnes S. 1983a. Impedance measurement of individual skin surface electrodes. *Med Biol Eng Comput* 21, 750–755.

Grimnes S. 1983b. Skin impedance and electro-osmosis in the human epidermis. *Med Biol Eng Comput* 21, 739–749.

Grimnes S. 1983c. Electrovibration, cutaneous sensation of microampere current. *Acta Physiol Scand* 118, 19–25.

Grimnes S, Jabbari A, Martinsen ØG, Tronstad C. 2011. Electrodermal activity by DC potential and AC conductance measured simultaneously at the same skin site. *Skin Res Technol* 17, 26–34.

Grimnes S, Martinsen ØG. 2007. Sources of error in tetrapolar impedance measurements on biomaterials and other ionic conductors. *J Phys D: Appl Phys* 40, 9–14.

Grimnes S, Martinsen ØG. 2008. *Bioimpedance and Bioelectricity Basics*. Amsterdam, Elsevier-Academic Press.

Griss P, Enoksson P, Tolvanen-Laakso HK, Meriläinen P, Ollmar S, Stemme G. 2001. Micromachined electrodes for biopotential measurements. *IEEE J Microelectro-mechanical Systems* 10, 10–16.

Hettrick DA, Zielinski TM. 2006. *Bioimpedance in Cardiovascular Medicine. Encyclopedia of Medical Devices and Instrumentation*, 2nd edition. New York, John Wiley & Sons, Inc. pp. 197–216.

Holder DS (ed). 2005. *Electrical Impedance Tomography. Method, History and Applications.* Bristol, Institute of Physics Publishing (IoP).

IEC-60601. 2005. Medical electrical equipment. General requirements for basic safety and essential performance. International standard.

Jaron D, Briller A, Schwan HP, Geselowitz DB. 1969. Nonlinearity of cardiac pacemaker electrodes. *IEEE Trans Biomed Eng* 16, 132–138.

Johnsen GK, Lütken CA, Martinsen ØG, Grimnes S. 2011. Memristive model of electro-osmosis in skin. *Phys Rev E* 83, 031916.

Jossinet J. 1996. Variability of impedivity in normal and pathological breast tissue. *Med Biol Eng Comput* 34(5), 346–350.

Kalvøy H, Frich L, Grimnes S, Martinsen ØG, Hol PK, Stubhaug A. 2009. Impedance-based tissue discrimination for needle guidance. *Physiol Meas* 30, 129–140.

Kauppinen PK, Hyttinen JA, Malmivuo JA. 1998. Sensitivity distributions of impedance cardiography using band and spot electrodes analyzed by a three-dimensional computer model. *Ann Biomed Eng* 26(4), 694–702.

Kubicek WG, Patterson RP, Witsoe DA, Mattson RH. 1970. Impedance cardiography as a non-invasive method for monitoring cardiac function and other parameters of the cardiovascular system. *Ann NY Acad Sci* 170, 724–732.

Kyle UG, Bosaeus I, De Lorenzo AD, Deurenberg P, Elia M, Gomez JM, Heitmann BL et al. 2004. Bioelectrical impedance analysis—Part I: Review of principles and methods. *Clin Nutr* 23, 1226–1243.

Lukaski HC, Hall CB, Siders WA. 2007. Assessment of change in hydration in women during pregnancy and postpartum with bioelectrical impedance vectors. *Nutrition* 8, 543–550.

Malmivuo J, Plonsey R. 1995. *Bioelectromagnetism.* New York, Oxford University Press.

Martinsen ØG, Grimnes S. 2001. Facts and myths about electrical measurement of stratum corneum hydration state. *Dermatology*, 202, 87–89.

Martinsen ØG, Grimnes S, Mirtaheri P. 2000. Non-invasive measurements of post mortem changes in dielectric properties of haddock muscle—A pilot study. *J Food Eng* 43, 189–192.

Martinsen ØG, Grimnes S, Nilsen JK, Tronstad C, Jang W, Kim H, Shin K. 2008. Gravimetric method for *in vitro* calibration of skin hydration measurements. *IEEE Trans Biomed Eng* 55(2), 728–732.

Martinsen ØG, Kalvøy H, Grimnes S, Nordbotten B, Hol PK, Fosse E, Myklebust H, Becker LB. 2010. Invasive electrical impedance tomography for blood vessel detection. *Open Biomed Eng J* 4, 135–137.

Metherall P, Barber DC, Smallwood RH, Brown BH. 1996. Three dimensional electrical impedance tomography. *Nature* 380(6574), 509–512.

Mirtaheri P, Grimnes S, Martinsen ØG. 2005. Electrode polarization impedance in weak NaCl aqueous solutions. *IEEE Trans Biomed Eng.* 52(12), 2093–2099.

Nicander I, Ollmar S, Eek A, Lundh Rozell B, Emtestam L. 1996. Correlation of impedance response patterns to histological findings in irritant skin reactions induced by various surfactants. *Br J Dermatol* 134, 221–228.

Nie R, Chin AB, Lee KS, Sunmonu NA, Rutkove SB. 2006. Electrical impedance myography: Transitioning from human to animal studies. *Clin Neurophys* 117, 1844–1849.

Ollmar S. 1997. Noninvasive monitoring of transplanted kidneys by impedance spectroscopy—A pilot study. *Med Biol Eng Comput* 35 (suppl.), Part 1, 336.

Ollmar S. 1998. Methods for information extraction from impedance spectra of biological tissue, in particular skin and oral mucosa—A critical review and suggestions for the future. *Bioelectrochem Bioenerg* 45, 157–160.

Ollmar S, Eek A, Sundstrøm F, Emtestam L. 1995. Electrical impedance for estimation of irritation in oral mucosa and skin. *Med Prog Technol* 21, 29–37.

Onaral B, Schwan HP. 1982. Linear and nonlinear properties of platinum electrode polarisation. Part I: Frequency dependence at very low frequencies. *Med & Biol Eng & Comp* 20, 299–306.

Patterson R. 1995. Bioelectric impedance measurement. In: Bronzino JD (ed.) *The Biomedical Engineering Handbook*. Boca Raton, FL, CRC Press, 3rd edition, pp. 1223–1230.

Pethig R. 1979. *Dielectric and Electronic Properties of Biological Materials*. Chichester, John Wiley.

Pethig R, Jakubek LM, Sanger RH, Heart E, Corson ED, Smith PJS. 2005. Electrokinetic measurements of membrane capacitance and conductance for pancreatic β-cells. *IEE Proc Nanobiotechnol* 152(6), 189–193.

Pliquett U, Joshi RP, Sridhara V, Schoenbach KH. 2007. High electric field effects on cell membranes. *Bioelectrochemistry* 27, 275–282.

Plonsey, R, Barr C. 2007. *Bioelectricity, a Quantitative Approach*. 3rd edition, New York, Springer.

Polk C, Postow E. 1996. *Biological Effects of Electromagnetic Fields*. Boca Raton, FL, CRC Handbook.

Sauter AR, Dodgson MS, Kalvøy H, Grimnes S, Stubhaug A, Klaastad Ø. 2009. Current threshold for nerve stimulation depends on electrical impedance of the tissue: A study of ultrasound-guided electrical nerve stimulation of the median nerve. *Anesth Analog* 108(4), 1338–1343.

Schäfer M, Schlegel C, Kirlum H-J, Gersing E, Gebhard MM. 1998. Monitoring of damage to skeletal muscle tissue caused by ischemia. *Bioelectrochem Bioenerg* 45, 151–155.

Schwan HP. 1957. Electrical properties of tissue and cell suspensions. In: *Advances in Biological and Medical Physics*. Lawrence JH, Tobias CA, eds. Vol. V, pp. 147–209, Academic Press.

Schwan HP. 1963. Determination of biological impedances. In: *Physical Techniques in Biological Research*. Nastuk WL, ed. Vol. 6, pp. 323–406, Academic Press.

Schwan HP. 1968. Electrode polarization impedance and measurements in biological materials. *Ann NY Acad Sci* 148, 191–208.

Schwan HP. 1992. Linear and non-linear electrode polarisation and biological materials. *Ann Biomed Eng* 20, 269–288.

Schwan HP. 2001. In: *Selected Papers by Herman P. Schwan*. Grimnes S, Martinsen ØG, eds. Medisinkteknisk avdelings forlag (Oslo). ogm//www.med-tek.no/t-Bokhandel.aspx

Shiffman CA, Aaron R, Rutkove SB. 2003. Electrical impedance of muscle during isometric contraction. *Physiol Meas* 24, 213–234.

Sigman E, Kolin A, Katz LN, Jochim K. 1937. Effect of motion on the electrical conductivity of the blood. *Am J Physiol* 118, 708–719.

Smith SR, Foster KR. 1985. Dielectric properties of low-water content tissues. *Phys Med Biol* 30, 965.

Sun SS, Chumlea WC, Heimsfield SB et al. 2003. Development of bioelectrical impedance analysis prediction equations for body composition with the use of a multicomponent model for use in epidemiological surveys. *Am J Clin Nutr* 77, 331–340.

Takashima S. 1989. *Electrical Properties of Biopolymers and Membranes*. Bristol, Adam Hilger.

Takashima S, Schwan HP. 1965. Dielectric dispersion of crystalline powders of amino acids, peptides and proteins. *J Phys Chem* 69, 4176–4182.

Tronstad C, Gjein GE, Grimnes S, Martinsen ØG, Krogstad A-L, Fosse E. 2008. Electrical measurement of sweat activity. *Physiol Meas* 29(6), S407–S415.

Tronstad C, Johnsen GK, Grimnes S, Martinsen ØJ. 2010. A study on electrode gels for skin conductance measurements. *Physiol Meas* 31, 1395–1410.

Vollmann D, Nagele H, Schauerte P et al. 2007. Clinical utility of intrathoracic impedance monitoring to alert patients with an implanted device of deteriorating chronic heart failure. *Eur Heart J* 19, 1835–1840.

Warburg E. 1899. Über das Verhalten sogenannte unpolarisierbare Elektroden gegen Wechselstrom. *Ann Phys Chem* 67, 493–499.

Weaver JC, Chizmadzhev YA. 1996. Theory of electroporation: A review. *Bioelectrochem. Bioenerg.* 41, 135–160.

Yamamoto T, Yamamoto Y. 1976. Electrical properties of the epidermal stratum corneum. *Med Biol Eng* 14, 592–594.

Yamamoto T, Yamamoto Y. 1981. Non-linear electrical properties of the skin in the low frequency range. *Med Biol Eng Comp* 19, 302–310.

Yelamos D, Casas O, Bragos R, Rosell J. 1999. Improvement of a front end for bioimpedance spectroscopy. *Ann N Y Acad Sci* 873, 306–312.

Yu C, Wang L, Chau E et al. 2005. Intrathoracic impedance monitoring in patients with heart failure. Correlation with fluid status and feasibility of early warning preceding hospitalization. *Circulation* 112, 841–848.

3

Implantable Cardiac Pacemakers

Pat Ridgely
Medtronic, Inc.

3.1 Introduction

The practical use of an implantable device for delivering a controlled, rhythmic electric stimulus to maintain the heartbeat is now approximately 50 years old and has become a standard cardiac therapy. During this period, circuit density has increased by a factor of more than a million, and devices have become steadily smaller (from 250 g in 1960 to less than a tenth of that today). Early devices provided only single-chamber, asynchronous, nonprogrammable pacing coupled with questionable reliability and short device longevity. Today, advances in a variety of technologies provide dual-chamber multiprogrammability, rate response, data collection, diagnostic functions, and exceptional reliability. Moreover, lithium-iodide power sources have extended device longevity to beyond a decade.

The modern pacing system still comprises three distinct components: pulse generator, lead, and programmer (Figure 3.1). The pulse generator houses the battery; the circuitry, which senses electrical (and in some cases, physical) activity, configures an appropriate response, and generates the stimulus; and a transceiver. The lead is an insulated wire that carries the stimulus from the generator to the heart and relays intrinsic cardiac signals back to the generator. The programmer is a telemetry device used to provide two-way communications between the generator and the clinician. It can alter the therapy delivered by the pacemaker and retrieve diagnostic data that are essential for optimally titrating that therapy over time. Ultimately, the therapeutic success of the pacing prescription rests on the clinician's choice of an appropriate system, the use of sound implant technique, and programming focused on patient outcomes.

This chapter discusses in further detail the components of the modern pacing system and the significant evolution that has occurred since its inception. The emphasis here is on system operation; an in-depth discussion of the fundamental electrophysiology of tissue stimulation can be found in Ellenbogen et al. (2007).

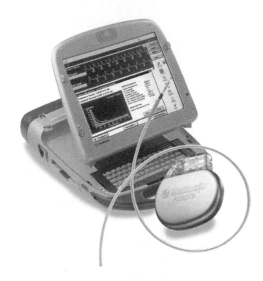

FIGURE 3.1   A pacing system comprises a programmer, pulse generator, and lead.

3.2 Indications

The decision to implant a permanent pacemaker usually is based on the major goals of symptom relief (at rest and with physical activity), restoration of functional capacity and quality of life, and reduced mortality. As with other healthcare technologies, the appropriate use of pacing is the intent of indications guidelines published by professional societies in cardiology. (The most recent version of guidelines for the United States can be found on the website of the Heart Rhythm Society.)

Historically, pacing has been indicated when there is a dramatic slowing of the heart rate or a failure in the connection between the atria and ventricles, resulting in decreased cardiac output manifested by symptoms such as syncope, light-headedness, fatigue, and exercise intolerance. Though this failure of impulse formation and/or conduction resulting in bradycardia has been the overriding theme of pacemaker indications, two additional uses have become important:

- Antitachycardia pacing to terminate inappropriately fast rhythms, typically in the ventricle
- Cardiac resynchronization therapy (CRT) to restore the normal activation sequence of contraction in the hearts of some patients with heart failure

3.3 Pulse Generators

The pulse generator contains a power source, output circuit, sensing circuit, and a timing circuit.

A telemetry coil is used to send and receive information between the generator and the programmer. Rate-adaptive pulse generators include the sensor components, along with the circuit, to process the information measured by the sensor (Figures 3.2 and 3.3).

Modern pacemakers use both read-only memory (ROM) and random-access memory (RAM). Although RAM provides the ability to store diagnostic data and change feature sets after implantation, the need to minimize device size and current drain keeps RAM typically on the order of tens of kilobytes in older devices. (Newer devices may have a megabyte or more.) ROM is less susceptible to data errors; therefore, it is typically used to store essential execution codes. Pacemakers usually have less ROM than RAM.

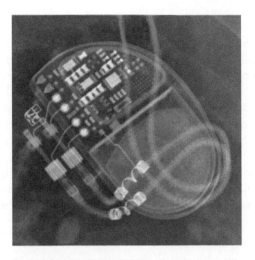

FIGURE 3.2 X-ray view of a pulse generator and two leads.

All components of the pulse generator are housed in a hermetically sealed titanium case with an epoxy header block that accepts the lead(s). Because pacing leads are available with a variety of connector sites and configurations, the pulse generator is available with an equal variety of connectors. The outer casing is laser etched with the manufacturer, model name, type (e.g., single- versus dual-chamber), model number, serial number, and the lead-connection diagram for each identification. Once implanted, it may be necessary to use an x-ray to reveal the identity of the generator. Some manufacturers use radiopaque symbols and ID codes for this purpose, whereas others give their generators characteristic shapes.

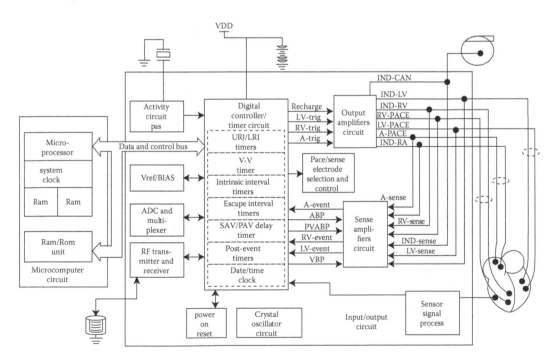

FIGURE 3.3 Sample block diagram of a pacemaker.

3.3.1 Sensing Circuit

Pulse generators have two basic functions, sensing and pacing. Sensing refers to the recognition of intrinsic cardiac depolarization from the chamber or chambers in which the leads are placed. It is imperative for the sensing circuit to discriminate between these intracardiac signals and unwanted electrical interference such as far-field cardiac events, diastolic potentials, skeletal muscle contraction, and pacing stimuli. Because the desired signals are low-amplitude, extensive amplification and filtering are typically required. An intracardiac electrogram shows the waveform as seen by the pacemaker; it is typically quite different from the corresponding event as shown on the surface ECG (Figure 3.4).

Sensing (and pacing) is accomplished with one of two configurations, bipolar and unipolar (Figure 3.5). In bipolar configuration, the anode and cathode are close together, with the anode at the tip of the lead and the cathode a ring electrode about 2 cm proximal to the tip. In unipolar configuration, the

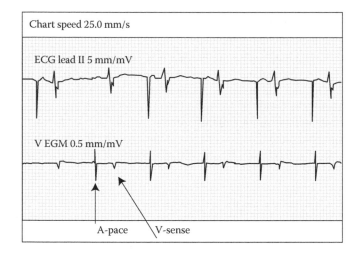

FIGURE 3.4 The surface ECG (ECG LEAD II) represents the sum total of the electrical potentials of all depolarizing tissue. The intracardiac electrogram (V EGM) shows only the potentials measured between the lead electrodes. This allows the evaluation of signals that may be hidden within the surface ECG.

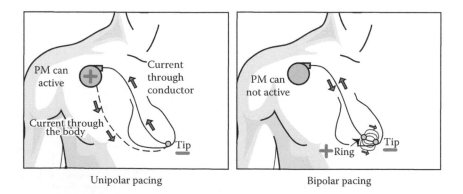

FIGURE 3.5 Unipolar versus bipolar pacing.

anode and cathode may be 5–10 cm apart. The anode is at the lead tip and the cathode is the pulse generator itself (usually located in the pectoral region).

In general, bipolar and unipolar sensing configurations have equal performance. A drawback of the unipolar approach is the increased possibility of sensing noncardiac signals. The large electrode separation may, for example, sense myopotentials from skeletal muscle movement, leading to inappropriate inhibition of pacing. Many newer pacemakers can be programmed to sense or pace in either configuration.

Once the electrogram enters the sensing circuit, it is scrutinized by a bandpass filter. The frequency of an R-wave is 10–30 Hz. The center frequency of most sensing amplifiers is 30 Hz. T-waves are slower, broad signals that are composed of lower frequencies (approximately 5 Hz or less). Far-field signals are also lower frequency signals, whereas skeletal muscle falls in the range of 10–200 Hz (Figure 3.6).

At implant, the voltage amplitude of the R-wave (and the P-wave, in the case of dual-chamber pacing) is measured to ensure the availability of an adequate signal. R-wave amplitudes are typically 5–25 mV, and P-wave amplitudes are 2–6 mV. The signals passing through the sense amplifier are compared to an adjustable reference voltage called the sensitivity; some pacemakers allow sensitivity settings as low as a tenth of a millivolt. Any signal below the reference voltage is not sensed, and those above it are sensed. Higher sensitivity settings (high reference voltage) may lead to substandard sensing, and a lower reference voltage may result in oversensing. A minimum 2:1 safety margin should be maintained between the sensitivity setting and the amplitude of the intracardiac signal. The circuit is protected from extremely high voltages by a Zener diode.

The slope of the signal is also surveyed by the sensing circuit and is determined by the slew rate (the time rate of change in voltage). A slew rate that is too flat or too steep may be eliminated by the bandpass filter. On average, the slew rate measured at implant should be between 0.75 and 2.50 V/s.

The most drastic way to deal with undesirable signals is to "blind" the circuit at specific times during the cardiac cycle. This is accomplished with blanking and refractory periods. Some of these periods

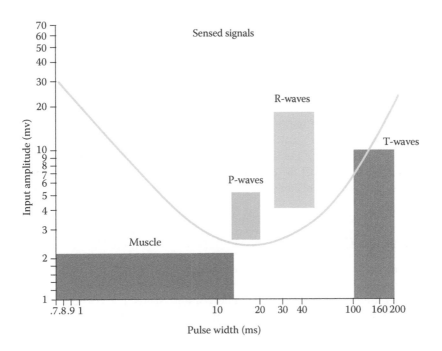

FIGURE 3.6 A conceptual depiction of the bandpass filter, demonstrating the typical filtering of unwanted signals by discriminating between those with slew rates that are too low and/or too high.

are programmable. During the blanking period, the sensing circuit is turned off; during the refractory period, the circuit can see the signal but does not initiate any of the basic timing intervals. Virtually all paced and sensed events begin concurrent blanking and refractory periods, typically ranging from 10 to 400 ms. These are especially helpful in dual-chamber pacemakers in which there exists the potential for the pacing output of the atrial side to inhibit the ventricular pacing output, with dangerous consequences for patients in complete heart block.

Probably, the most common question asked by the general public about pacing systems is the effect of electromagnetic interference (EMI) on their operation. EMI outside of the hospital is an infrequent problem, although patients are advised to avoid sources of strong electromagnetic fields such as arc welders, high-voltage generators, and radar antennae. Some clinicians suggest that patients avoid standing near antitheft devices used in retail stores. Airport screening devices are generally safe. Microwave ovens, ham radio equipment, video games, computers, and office equipment rarely interfere with the operation of modern pacemakers. A common recommendation regarding cell phones is to keep them 15 cm from the pacemaker.

Several medical devices and procedures can affect pacemakers, however: electrocautery, cardioversion and defibrillation, lithotripsy, diathermy, neurostimulation units, RF ablation, radiation therapy, and MRI, among others. MRI can have effects through multiple mechanisms other than EMI: force and torque, current induction, and heating (Al-Ahmad et al. 2010).

Pacemakers affected by interference typically respond with temporary loss of output or temporary reversion to asynchronous pacing (pacing at a fixed rate, with no inhibition from intrinsic cardiac events). The usual consequence for the patient is a return of symptoms that originally led to the pacemaker implant, and pacemaker-dependent patients are placed at clinical risk. Pacemaker manufacturers provide extensive information on interference issues via their websites and technical service phone centers.

3.3.2 Output Circuit

Pacing stimuli are of low energy and short duration: on the order of 10 μJ, delivered in pulses lasting on the order of a millisecond. Modern permanent pulse generators use a constant-voltage approach: the voltage remains at the programmed value while the current varies. Pulse amplitudes are typically on the order of a volt, but in some generators can be as high as 10 V (used for troubleshooting or for pediatric patients).

The output pulse is generated from the discharge of a capacitor charged by the battery. Most modern pulse generators contain a 2.8 V battery. The higher voltages are achieved using voltage multipliers (smaller capacitors used to charge the large capacitor). The voltage can be doubled by charging two smaller capacitors in parallel, with the discharge delivered to the output capacitor in series. Output pulses are emitted at a rate controlled by the timing circuit; output is commonly inhibited by sensed cardiac signals.

3.3.3 Timing Circuit

The timing circuit regulates parameters such as the pacing cycle length, refractory and blanking periods, pulse duration, and specific timing intervals between atrial and ventricular events. A crystal oscillator generating frequencies in the kilohertz range sends a signal to a digital timing and logic control circuit, which in turn operates internally generated clocks at divisions of the oscillatory frequency.

A rate-limiting circuit is incorporated into the timing circuit to prevent the pacing rate from exceeding an upper limit, should a random component failure occur (an extremely rare event). This is also referred to as "runaway" protection and is typically 180–200 pulses per minute.

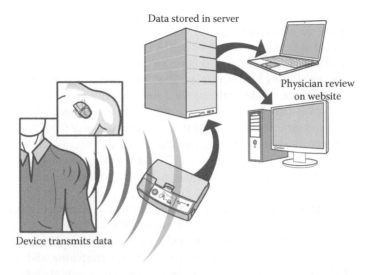

Data stored in server

Physician review
on website

Device transmits data

FIGURE 3.7 Remote monitoring systems connect cardiac device patients from home or other location to their clinics via a secure Internet website.

3.3.4 Telemetry Circuit

Pulse generators have long been capable of two-way communication using near-field inductive coupling between the pulse generator and the programmer. This has enabled real-time telemetry in which the pulse generator during clinic visits provides information such as pulse amplitude, pulse duration, lead impedance, battery impedance, lead current, charge, and energy. The programmer, in turn, delivers coded messages to the pulse generator to alter any of the programmable features and to retrieve diagnostic data. Signal fidelity is accomplished by using pulse-strings, typically 16 digital pulses in length; each manufacturer's devices communicate only with programmers from that manufacturer.

Historically, device monitoring away from the clinic was accomplished transtelephonically. In these sessions, the patient dons wristband electrodes attached to a device that transmits a rhythm strip over a landline. More recently, advances in telecommunication technology have enabled the use of cell-phone-based transmission of essential data directly to a clinic, where it can be viewed via the Internet. This remote monitoring can provide valuable alerts when certain clinical criteria are met (Figure 3.7).

Most manufacturers in the United States use the medical implant communications service (MICS) band, established since 1999. This band sets aside the 402–405 MHz frequency range, a range that has reasonable signal-propagation characteristics in the human body. The increase in wireless and network connectivity has led to concerns over data privacy and security, and calls to the FDA to establish a policy in this area (Maisel and Kohno 2010).

3.3.5 Power Source

The longevity of very early pulse generators was measured in hours, but current devices can function for more than a decade before they need to be replaced due to battery depletion. The clinical desire to have a generator that is small and full featured, yet also long-lasting, poses a formidable challenge to battery designers.

Over the years, several different battery technologies have been tried, including mercury-zinc, rechargeable silver-modified-mercuric-oxide-zinc, rechargeable nickel-cadmium, radioactive plutonium or promethium, and lithium with a variety of different cathodes. Lithium-cupric-sulfide and mercury-zinc batteries were associated with corrosion and early failure. Mercury-zinc produced hydrogen gas as a by-product of the battery reaction; the venting required made it impossible to hermetically seal the generator. This led to fluid infiltration followed by the risk of sudden failure.

Lithium-iodide technology has been the workhorse for pacemaker battery applications, with more than 10 million such devices having been implanted. Their high energy density (on the order of 1 W-h/cc) and low rate of self-discharge enable small size and good longevity, and their simplicity contributes to excellent reliability. Typical capacity is in the range of 1–3 A-h. The semisolid layer of lithium-iodide that separates the anode and the cathode gradually thickens over the life of the cell, increasing the internal resistance of the battery. The voltage produced by lithium-iodide batteries is inversely related to this resistance and is linear from 2.8 V to approximately 2.4 V, representing about 90% of the usable battery life. It then declines exponentially to 1.8 V as the internal battery resistance increases dramatically to 10,000 Ω or more.

When the battery reaches between 2.0 and 2.4 V (depending on the manufacturer), certain functions of the pulse generator are altered so as to alert the clinician. These alterations are called the elective replacement indicators (ERI). They vary from one pulse generator to another and include signature decreases in rate, a change to a specific pacing mode, pulse duration stretching, and the telemetered battery voltage. When the battery voltage reaches 1.8 V, the pulse generator may operate erratically or cease to function and is said to have reached "end of life." The time period between appearance of the ERI and end-of-life status averages about 3–4 months (Figure 3.8).

More recently, demands for higher power (e.g., for faster, longer range telemetry) have led to the emergence of newer battery technologies. One example is the lithium/hybrid-cathode battery, which has an energy density similar to that of lithium-iodide batteries but power output that is roughly two orders of magnitude greater. An excellent discussion of battery technology is given in Ellenbogen et al. (2007).

Many factors besides battery capacity affect longevity, for example, pulse amplitude and duration, pacing amount and rate, single- versus dual-chamber pacing, use of specialized algorithms, lead design, and so-called housekeeping functions (those functions other than actual delivery of pacing stimuli). The total current drain is typically on the order of 10 μA, with most of this in the form of housekeeping current rather than stimulus current. The programming choices made by clinicians can have a dramatic effect on longevity: a pacemaker with a projected longevity of 8 years under nominal settings could have an actual longevity several years more or less than that value.

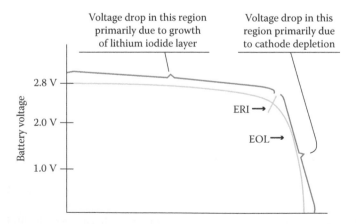

FIGURE 3.8 The initial decline in battery voltage is slow and then more rapid after the battery reaches the ERI voltage. An important aspect of battery design is the predictability of this decline so that timely generator replacement can be anticipated.

3.4 Leads

Standard pacing has traditionally involved the stimulation of one or both chambers (dual-chamber) on the right side of the heart. Cardiac resynchronization therapy (CRT) typically involves pacing at least three chambers (currently the right atrium, right ventricle, and left ventricle), and is thus sometimes called biventricular pacing (Figures 3.9 and 3.10).

Regardless of the specific configuration, implantable pacing leads must be designed not only for consistent performance within the hostile environment of the body but also for easy handling by the implanting physician. Every lead has four major components: electrode, conductor, insulation, and connector pin(s) (Figure 3.11). The electrode is located at the tip of the lead and is in direct contact with the myocardium. Bipolar leads have a tip electrode and a ring electrode (located about 2 cm proximal to the tip); unipolar leads have tip electrodes only. A small-radius electrode provides increased current density, resulting in lower stimulation thresholds; it also increases impedance at the electrode–myocardium interface, thus lowering the current drain further and improving battery longevity. A "high-impedance" lead may have a tip surface area as low as 1.5 mm², whereas standard leads have areas four times as large. A typical value for the impedance "seen" by the pulse generator is 500–1000 Ω; of this, most arises at the electrode–myocardium interface rather than in the lead itself.

Small electrodes, however, historically have been associated with inferior sensing performance. Lead designers were able to achieve both good pacing and good sensing by creating porous-tip electrodes containing thousands of pores in the 20–100 μm range. The pores allow the ingrowth of tissue, resulting in

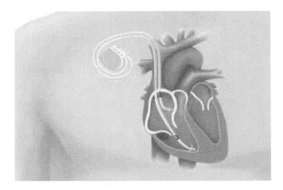

FIGURE 3.9 Illustration of a dual-chamber pacing system.

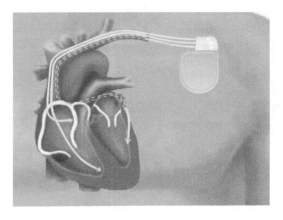

FIGURE 3.10 Illustration of a CRT pacing system.

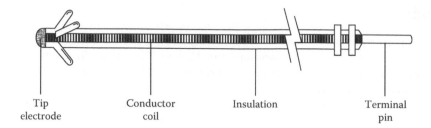

Tip   Conductor   Insulation   Terminal
electrode   coil   pin

FIGURE 3.11   The four major lead components.

necessary increase in the effective sensing area while maintaining a small pacing area. Some commonly used electrode materials include platinum-iridium, Elgiloy (an alloy of cobalt, iron, chromium, molybdenum, nickel, and manganese), platinum coated with platinized titanium, and vitreous or pyrolytic carbon coating a titanium or graphite core.

Another major breakthrough in lead design is the steroid-eluting electrode (Figure 3.12). About 1 mg of a corticosteroid (dexamethasone sodium phosphate) is contained in a silicone core that is surrounded by the electrode material. The "leaking" of the steroid into the myocardium occurs slowly over several years and reduces the inflammation that results from the lead placement. It also retards the growth of the fibrous sack that forms around the electrode, which separates it from viable myocardium. As a result, the dramatic rise in acute thresholds that is seen with nonsteroid leads during the 8–16 weeks postimplant is nearly eliminated.

Once a lead has been implanted, it must remain stable (or fixated). The fixation device is either active or passive. Active-fixation leads incorporate corkscrew mechanisms, barbs, or hooks to attach themselves to the myocardium. Passive-fixation leads are held in place with tines that become entangled in the net-like lining (trabeculae) of the heart. Passive-fixation leads generally have better acute pacing and sensing performance but are difficult to remove chronically. Active-fixation leads are easier to remove chronically and have the advantage of unlimited placement sites. Some implanters prefer to use active-fixation leads in the atrium and passive-fixation leads in the ventricle.

The conductor carries electric signals to the pulse generator and delivers the pacing pulses to the heart. It must be strong and flexible to withstand the repeated flexing stress placed on it by the beating

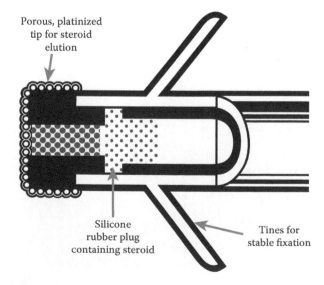

Porous, platinized
tip for steroid
elution

Silicone
rubber plug
containing steroid

Tines for
stable fixation

FIGURE 3.12   The steroid-eluting electrode.

heart. The early conductors were a single, straight wire that was vulnerable to fracturing. They have evolved into conductors that are coiled (for increased flexibility) and multifilar (to prevent complete failure with partial fractures). Common conductor materials are Elgiloy and MP35N (an alloy of cobalt, nickel, chromium, and molybdenum). Because of the need for two conductors, bipolar leads are usually larger in diameter than unipolar leads. Current bipolar leads have a coaxial design that has significantly reduced the overall lead diameter.

Insulation materials (typically silicone and polyurethane) are used to isolate the conductor. Silicone has high biostability and a longer history. Because of low tear strength, however, silicone leads historically tended to be thicker than polyurethane leads. Another relative disadvantage of silicone is its high coefficient of friction in blood, which makes it difficult for two leads to pass through the same vein; a coating applied during manufacturing has diminished this problem. Some forms of polyurethane have shown relatively high failure rates.

A variety of generator-lead connector configurations and adapters are available. Because incompatibility can result in disturbed (or even lost) pacing and sensing, an international standard (IS-1) has been developed in an attempt to minimize incompatibility and allow leads from one manufacturer to be used with generators from another.

Leads can be implanted epicardially and endocardially. Epicardial leads are placed on the outer surface of the heart and require the surgical exposure of a small portion of the heart. They are used when venous occlusion makes it impossible to pass a lead transvenously, when abdominal placement of the pulse generator is needed (as in the case of radiation therapy to the pectoral area), or in children (to allow for growth). Endocardial leads are far more common and perform better in the long term. These leads are passed through the venous system and into the right side of the heart. The subclavian or cephalic veins in the pectoral region are common entry sites. Positioning is facilitated by a thin, firm wire stylet that passes through the central lumen of the lead, stiffening it. Fluoroscopy is used to visualize lead positioning and to confirm the desired location.

Improvements in lead design are often overlooked, as compared to improvements in generator design, but the leads used in 1960 required a pulse generator output of 675 μJ for effective stimulation. The evolution in lead technology since then has reduced that figure by two orders of magnitude.

3.5 Programmers and Ongoing Follow-Up

Noninvasive, reversible alteration of the functional parameters of the pacemaker is critical to ongoing clinical management. For a pacing system to remain effective throughout its lifetime, it must be able to adjust to the patient's changing clinical status. The programmer is the primary clinical tool for changing settings, retrieving diagnostic data, and conducting noninvasive tests.

The pacing rate for programmable pacemakers of the early 1960s was adjusted via a Keith needle manipulated percutaneously into a knob on the side of the pacemaker; rotating the needle changed the pacing rate. Through the late 1960s and early 1970s, magnetically attuned reed switches in the pulse generator made it possible to noninvasively change certain parameters, such as rate, output, sensitivity, and polarity. The application of a magnet could alter the parameters, which were usually limited to only one of two choices. It was not until the late 1970s that RF-technology-enabled programmability began realizing its full potential.

Manufacturers have moved away from dedicated special-use programmers toward a PC-based design. The newer designs are more flexible, intuitive to use, and easily updated when new devices are released. They also enable the use of diagnostic and programming options of increasing complexity (Figure 3.13).

Manufacturers and clinicians alike are becoming more sensitive to the role that time-efficient programming and follow-up can play in the productivity of pacing clinics, which may provide follow-up for thousands of patients a year. The management of the resulting mountains of data is a major challenge, and sophisticated systems are appearing to help with this task.

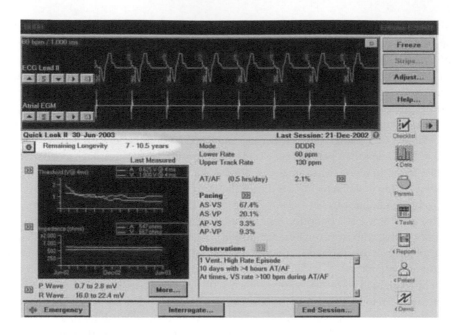

FIGURE 3.13   Typical programmer screen seen during a pacemaker check.

3.6 System Operation

Much of the apparent complexity of the timing rules that determine pacemaker operation is because of a design goal of mimicking normal cardiac function without interfering with it. One example is the dual-chamber feature that provides a sequential stimulation of the atrium before the ventricle. Another example is rate response, designed for patients who lack the normal ability to increase their heart rate in response to a variety of physical conditions (e.g., exercise). Introduced in the mid-1980s, rate-responsive systems use some sort of a sensor to measure the change in a physical variable correlated to heart rate. The sensor output is signal-processed and then used by the output circuit to specify a target pacing rate. The clinician controls the aggressiveness of the rate increase through a variety of parameters (including a choice of transfer function). Pacemaker-resident diagnostics provide data helpful in titrating the rate-response therapy, but most systems operate in "open-loop" fashion: that is, the induced rate changes do not provide negative feedback to the sensor parameter.

The most common sensor is the activity sensor, which uses any of a variety of technologies (e.g., piezo-electric crystals and accelerometers) to detect body movement. Systems using a transthoracic-impedance sensor to estimate pulmonary minute ventilation or cardiac contractility are also commercially available. Numerous other sensors (e.g., stroke volume, blood temperature or pH, oxygen saturation, and right ventricular pressure) have been researched or market-released at various times. Some systems are dual-sensor, combining the best features of each sensor in a single pacing system.

To make it easier to understand the gross-level system operation of modern pacemakers, a five-letter code was developed in 1987 by the North American Society of Pacing and Electrophysiology (NASPE) and the British Pacing and Electrophysiology Group (BPEG), and was subsequently revised (Bernstein et al. 2002). In this "Revised NBG Code," the first letter indicates the chamber (or chambers) that are paced (Table 3.1). The second letter reveals those chambers in which sensing takes place, and the third letter describes how the pacemaker will respond to a sensed event. The pacemaker will "inhibit" the pacing output when intrinsic activity is sensed or will "trigger" a pacing output based on a specific previously sensed event. For example, in the DDD mode:

TABLE 3.1   The NASPE/BPEG Generic (NBG) Pacemaker Code

Position	I	II	III	IV	V
Category	Chamber(s) paced	Chamber(s) sensed	Response to sensing	Rate modulation	Multisite pacing
	O = None	O = None	O = None	O = None	O = None
	A = Atrium	A = Atrium	T = Triggered	R = Rate modulation	A = Atrium
	V = Ventricle	V = Ventricle	I = Inhibited		V = Ventricle
	D = Dual (A+V)	D = Dual (A+V)	D = Dual (T+I)		D = Dual (A+V)
Mfr designation only	S = Single	S = Single			
	(A or V)	(A or V)			

Source: Bernstein, A., Daubert J., Fletcher R. et al. 2002. The revised NASPE/BPEG generic code for antibradycardia, adaptive-rate, and multisite pacing. *PACE* 23:260–64.

D: Pacing takes place in the atrium and the ventricle.

D: Sensing takes place in the atrium and the ventricle.

D: Both inhibition and triggering are the response to a sensed event. An atrial output is inhibited with an atrial-sensed event, whereas a ventricular output is inhibited with a ventricular-sensed event; a ventricular pacing output is triggered by an atrial-sensed event (assuming no ventricular event occurs during the A–V interval).

The fourth letter in the code reflects the ability of the device to provide a rate response. For example, a DDDR device is one that is programmed to pace and sense in both chambers and is capable of sensor-driven rate variability. The fifth letter is used to indicate the device's ability to do multisite pacing.

Pacing in the right ventricle can have deleterious effects in terms of the development of heart failure and atrial fibrillation. This has led to the development of algorithms that minimize ventricular pacing in patients whose bradycardia is because of the dysfunction of their sinus node (which functions as the heart's natural pacemaker), rather than the dysfunction of their heart's intrinsic conduction system. Excellent discussions of this issue and other sophisticated pacemaker algorithms can be found in Al-Ahmad et al. (2010).

3.7 Performance and Reliability

Standard pacing is remarkably effective in treating bradycardia, a condition for which there is no acceptable pharmacological therapy for chronic use. Biventricular pacing is effective in the majority of patients for which it is indicated, but as many as a third of patients who receive the device are the so-called non-responders; major efforts at better defining patient selection criteria are ongoing.

Pacemakers are among the most reliable electronic devices ever built: device survival probabilities of 99.9% (excluding normal battery depletion) at 10 years are not unheard of. But despite intensive quality assurance efforts by manufacturers, the devices do remain subject to occasional failures: the annual pacemaker replacement rate due to generator malfunction has been estimated at roughly one per 1000 devices implanted, a marked improvement in reliability since the early 1980s (Maisel et al. 2006; Maisel 2006). There have been multiple major advisories and recalls issued by the FDA regarding pacing leads, with more of these because of problems with the lead insulation than with the lead conductor.

Manufacturers maintain product performance reports on their websites; reports from the largest manufacturer (Medtronic) date back to the early 1980s. Manufacturers have also established processes by which a product can be returned to them for failure analysis.

3.8 Future of Pacing Technology

Permanent cardiac pacing is the beneficiary of four decades of advances in a variety of key technologies: biomaterials, electrical stimulation, sensing of bioelectrical events, power sources, microelectronics, transducers, signal analysis, telecommunications, and software development. These advances, informed and guided by a wealth of clinical experience acquired during that time, have made pacing a cost-effective cornerstone of cardiac arrhythmia management.

The development of biological pacemakers through the use of, for example, gene therapy, is an active area of cutting-edge pacing research. Other areas of likely evolution include the following:

- Increased automaticity and optimization of arrhythmia monitoring and therapy delivery, with greater provision of feedback to clinicians on their programming choices
- More efficient integration of device-generated data into electronic medical record (EMR) systems
- Increased sophistication of resynchronization therapy, with broader ranges of multisite pacing
- Integration of sensors for monitoring a broader range of patients' clinical status in areas such as cardiac hemodynamics and ischemia status. (At least one manufacturer already provides a feature that uses monitoring of transthoracic impedance as a way to assess pulmonary congestion in heart failure patients with a CRT device)
- Improved battery technology and circuit density, enabling higher power features without increasing device size
- Greater attention to obtaining cost-effectiveness data for new and existing features

References

Al-Ahmad, A., Ellenbogen, K.A., Natale, A., and Wang, P.J. (eds). 2010. *Pacemakers and Implantable Cardioverter Defibrillators: An Expert's Manual.* Minneapolis: Cardiotext.

Bernstein, A., Daubert J., Fletcher R. et al. 2002. The revised NASPE/BPEG generic code for antibradycardia, adaptive-rate, and multisite pacing. *PACE* 23:260–64.

Ellenbogen, K.A., Kay, G.N., Lau, C.P., and Wilkoff B.J. (eds). 2007. *Clinical Cardiac Pacing, Defibrillation, and Resynchronization Therapy.* Philadelphia: Saunders Elsevier.

Heart Rhythm Society website (www.hrsonline.org).

Maisel, W.H. 2006. Pacemaker and ICD generator reliability: Meta-analysis of device registries. *JAMA* 295:1929–34.

Maisel, W.H. and Kohno, T. 2010. Improving the security and privacy of implantable medical devices. *NEJM* 362:1164–66.

Maisel, W.H., Moynahan M., Zuckerman B.D. et al. 2006. Pacemaker and ICD generator malfunctions: Analysis of Food and Drug Administration annual reports. *JAMA* 295:1901–06.

4

Model Investigation of Pseudo-Hypertension in Oscillometry

Gary Drzewiecki
Rutgers University

4.1 Pseudo-Hypertension

Pentz (1999) and Osler (1892) defined pseudo-hypertension as a condition in which the cuff pressure is higher than the intra-arterial pressure resulting from the presence of an atheromatosis. He hypothesized that a higher cuff pressure was needed to compress a calcified and sclerotic artery than a normal vessel. Osler suggested a method for diagnosis of pseudo-hypertension, which was named as Osler's Maneuver by Messerli et al. in 1985. The method is as follows: by palpating the pulse less radial or brachial artery distal to the point of occlusion of the artery with a sphygmomanometer cuff, one can perform the Osler's maneuver. The patient is Osler positive if either of these arteries remains palpable despite being pulse less. However, the patient is Osler negative if the artery collapses and becomes impalpable. In 1985, Messerli et al. assessed "the palpability of the pulse less radial, or brachial artery distal to a point of occlusion of the artery manually or by cuff pressure." They then measured the intra-arterial pressure, arterial compliance, and systemic hemodynamics of the Osler-positive and Osler-negative patients. The degree of pseudo-hypertension in the Osler-positive patients, those with pseudo-hypertension, ranged from 10 to 54 mmHg, which was the difference between cuff and intra-arterial pressure. Osler-positive subjects had lower arterial compliance, which related to the difference between the cuff and intra-arterial pressures. This explained the fact that the stiffer the artery, the higher the degree of pseudo-hypertension. Pseudo-hypertension is thought to occur mostly in the elderly. It advances as arterial compliance decreases and the sclerosis of the arteries increases with age.

Messerli et al. believed that Osler's maneuver was the simplest and best test to discriminate patients with true hypertension from those with a false elevation in blood pressure. However, automatic blood pressure monitors are currently not capable of discriminating the presence of pseudo-hypertension. The frequency of pseudo-hypertension is not certain, but the prevalence of pseudo-hypertension among the adult population has been estimated to be 7% of the adult population (Oparil et al. 1988). Because the total healthcare costs of treating hypertension and its complications range from $15.0 billion to $60.0 billion (Balu and Thomas 2006), the cost of pseudo-hypertension therapy in the United States is estimated to be $4 billion. Other clinical features of pseudo-hypertension are postural hypotension in spite of antihypertensive therapy, drug-resistant hypertension, and the absence of end-organ damage. Pseudo-hypertension may also result in dangerous outcome of unnecessary treatments if it is not recognized (Campbell et al. 1994). The main theory of pseudo-hypertension is the artery disease and stiffening theory.

There has not been any prior analytical investigation of the arterial stiffening theory of pseudo-hypertension. The low arterial compliance theory is tested in this chapter via a mathematical model of oscillometric blood pressure measurement. The computational model will be used to evaluate measurement error introduced by arterial disease or alterations in arterial mechanics in general. Once these errors are established, the model will then be used to investigate the means by which automated blood pressure monitor may detect the occurrence of pseudo-hypertension or provide a correction method by which blood pressure accuracy is improved even in the presence of arterial disease.

4.2 Automatic Oscillometry

Current automatic oscillometric blood pressure monitors use an occlusive arm cuff wrapped around the subject's upper arm. The air tubing of the cuff is connected to a pump, a pressure transducer, and an air-release valve all under computer control. Drzewiecki et al. (1994) proposed a mathematical model of the oscillometric method in addition to the systolic and diastolic ratios. The oscillometric model included the mechanics of the occlusive arm cuff, the arterial pressure pulse waveform, and the mechanics of the brachial artery. The buckling of an artery under a cuff occurred near −2 to 0 mmHg transmural pressure. This effect resulted in a maximum arterial compliance and maximum cuff pressure oscillations when the cuff pressure was nearly equal to mean arterial pressure. The model indicated the basic features of experimental oscillometry: the increasing and decreasing amplitude in oscillations as cuff pressure decreases, the oscillations corresponding to cuff pressure above systolic pressure, maximum oscillation amplitudes in the range of 1–4 mmHg, and an oscillatory maximum at cuff pressure equal to mean arterial pressure, or MAP. This model computed values for the systolic and diastolic detection ratios of 0.593 and 0.717, respectively, that compared well to the experimental values determined by other researchers (Geddes 1983). This model is applied to study pseudo-hypertension in this chapter.

4.3 Modeling Methods

The mathematical model of the oscillometry was implemented in MATLAB® according to the details provided by Drzewiecki et al. (1994). The main elements of the model are brachial artery mechanics, arterial pressure pulse, and automatic blood pressure detection. A brief review of these elements is now provided (Pedley 1980, Shapiro 1977).

4.3.1 Artery Mechanics Model

An empirical relation describing nonlinear geometric collapse and nonlinear elastic distension of an artery is given by

$$A = (d \log ((a^* p) + b))/(1 + \exp (-cp)) \qquad (4.1)$$

where A is the area of the lumen, p transmural pressure, and a, b, c, d are empirical constants calibrated for the normal human brachial artery (Drzewiecki et al. 1994, Brower and Noordergraaf 1978).

4.3.2 Arterial Pulse Pressure Model

The arterial pulse pressure Fourier series of the first two terms of the Fourier series of the human arterial blood pressure pulse is given by

$$Pa(t) = MAP + A0 \sin(2\Pi \, Fhr/60) + A1 \, (\sin(4\Pi \, Fhr)/60 + \emptyset 1) \tag{4.2}$$

where Pa(t) is the Fourier synthesized arterial pressure as a function of time, Fhr the heart rate, $\emptyset 1$ the phase angle, $A0$ and $A1$ are the Fourier constants that approximate the waveform of a human brachial artery pulse.

It is assumed that arterial blood pressure is independent of any other quantity. This results in systolic and diastolic pressures that are constant at this location.

Transmural pressure is given by

$$P = Pa - Pc \tag{4.3}$$

where P is the transmural pressure, Pa arterial pressure, and Pc cuff pressure. Cuff pressure simulates a blood pressure recording such that the cuff is inflated to 150 mmHg and then allowed to decrease at a linear rate according to

$$Pc = -13/3 \, t + 150 \tag{4.4}$$

4.4 Model Parameters

Table 4.1 provides the control values of the model constants that we have applied in the MATLAB model. Parameters a and b are related to the arterial wall stiffness and parameters c and d are related to the arterial closure due to disease and external pressure.

4.5 Computer Modeling

On the basis of the above Drzewiecki et al. mathematical model, a MATLAB program was generated to model oscillometry for normal and diseased arteries. Pressure was input to Equation 4.1 to generate the pulsatile lumen area at each value of cuff pressure. The lumen area pulse is then computed continuously while cuff pressure falls.

The local minimum and maximum of the area pulse were found, and their difference provided the area pulse amplitudes. It was assumed that cuff pressure oscillations are proportionate to the area pulse so that cuff pressure was not computed directly. This is a good approach because it was shown that the

TABLE 4.1 Control Parameters for Oscillometric Model for Typical Normal Human

Quantity	Value	Units	Function
a	0.03	mmHg	Arterial stiffness
b	3.30		Arterial stiffness
c	0.10		Closure stiffness
d	0.08		Closure stiffness
MAP	95.0	mmHg	Mean arterial pressure
A0	10.0		First Fourier pulse magnitude
A1	9.0		Second Fourier pulse magnitude
$\emptyset 1$	1.2	rad	First Fourier pulse phase
Fhr	75.0	beats/min	Heart rate frequency

cuff pressure is simply responding as an arterial volume transducer. The pulse amplitudes were normalized by maximum pulse amplitude to provide the pressure detection ratios. Spline interpolation was used to accurately calculate the detection ratios: 0.55 and 0.85 that correspond to a diastolic pressure of 68.4 mmHg and a systolic pressure of 107.3 mmHg, respectively. These values are equal to those found experimentally by Geddes et al. (1983). The arterial pressure input values were a diastolic reading of 82.5 mmHg and a systolic reading of 114 mmHg that corresponded to 0.88 and 0.67, respectively. Hence, for normal control conditions the oscillometric simulation resulted in 100% accuracy in arterial pressure measurement.

4.5.1 Control Condition Model (Normal Artery)

The control model of the oscillometric blood pressure measurement was represented by the normal parameters of Table 4.1.

4.5.2 Experimental Condition Model (Pseudo-Hypertension)

To develop the experimental model (stiff artery theory), the arterial mechanics was completely modeled by Equation 4.1. The parameters of this equation represent the artery stiffness over varied ranges of pressure. Because it was not fully understood how the arterial mechanics and its pressure area function change with disease, the approach taken here was to perform an evaluation of parametric sensitivity. The mechanical parameters a, b, c, and d were varied to detect their influence on blood pressure accuracy. The results of the model for control and experimental conditions are provided below.

4.6 Results

The arterial pressure pulse as a function of time is illustrated in Figure 4.1. It has fixed waveform that sets systolic pressure at 112 mmHg and diastolic pressure at 73 mmHg.

Hence, this pulse is the input to the model and is only dependent on time. For any model condition, the systolic and diastolic pressure would remain fixed at these values. The modeled computer subject will always have a constant known blood pressure of 112/73 mmHg so that accuracy of blood pressure measurement can be easily assessed.

Cuff pressure and arterial pressure are input to the arterial mechanics model to yield the arterial lumen area pulse which is also related to the cuff pressure oscillations as shown in Figure 4.2. In this example, the cuff pressure was allowed to linearly decrease in pressure according to Equation 4.4.

The control and experimental models each generate lumen area data similar to that of Figure 4.2 because oscillometry is only concerned with the lumen pulse magnitude and lumen area is further analyzed to find blood pressure.

1. *Normal conditions.* The maximum and minimum values of each area pulse was computed and then subtracted from each other to obtain the pulse amplitude at all values of cuff pressure. The amplitude curve is then normalized by the maximum overall amplitude. This analysis yields the oscillation amplitude curve shown in Figure 4.3. The amplitudes of the oscillations may be further analyzed to determine the arterial blood pressure provided the systolic and diastolic detection ratios are known. Hence, the oscillation amplitude curve is all that is required to determine blood pressure by means of oscillometry. If the oscillation amplitude curve is altered by any parameter, it will result in blood pressure determination error.
2. *Experimental conditions.* To identify sources of blood pressure error, the model parameters were varied to discover their effect on the oscillation amplitude curve. The model parameters that are related to arterial mechanics are the parameters a, b, c, d of Equation 4.1. The variation in

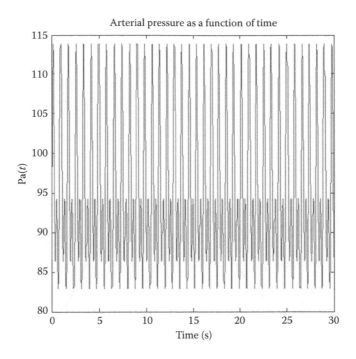

FIGURE 4.1 Arterial pressure pulse versus time. Pressure is in mmHg.

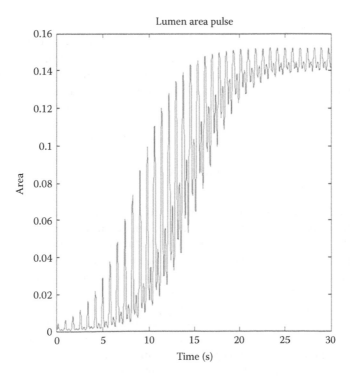

FIGURE 4.2 Lumen area pulse as a function of time and transmural pressure.

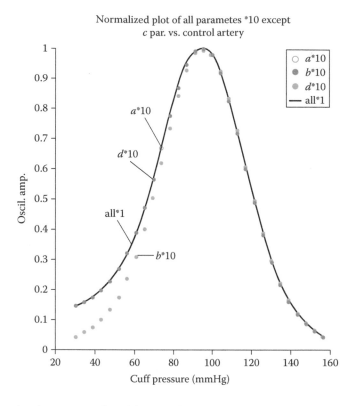

FIGURE 4.3   Control and experimental models: control artery diseased.

parameters *a*, *b*, and *d* by any number did not change their resulting oscillation amplitude curves. They are shown to be superimposed with the control curve and after normalization. This can be seen in Figure 4.3 for the results of both the control model shown and variation parameters *a*, *b*, and *d*. In summary, it is clear that the oscillation amplitude curve is independent of the arterial mechanics following the normalization process. Because actual experimental oscillometry always applies normalization before blood pressure determination, it is clear that this aspect of arterial mechanics does not result in blood pressure errors and is not responsible for pseudo-hypertension. However, the variation of parameter *c* resulted in a very different oscillation amplitude curve as compared to control. Because parameter *c* alters the closure mechanics of an artery it is most closely reflecting arterial disease.

Figure 4.4 shows the control of an experimental oscillation amplitude curve for parameter *c*. The blood pressure determination errors resulting from *c* parameter included pseudo-systolic hypotension and pseudo-diastolic hypertension. These errors are evident from Figure 4.4 as a shift of the parameter curve *c* toward higher cuff pressure in both the systolic and diastolic ranges.

To illustrate the change in arterial mechanics, the cuff pressure area curve was graphed for the model of the control and diseased arteries in Figures 4.5 and 4.6.

In Figures 4.5 and 4.6, positive and negative values of the pressure are because of dilation and constriction of the brachial artery, respectively. In comparison with the normal artery shown in Figure 4.5, the lumen area of the diseased artery is less at all pressures and especially for negative pressures.

The pulse error is the problem of every blood pressure monitor, therefore, by varying the pulse error in the first derivative of the control and experimental models, we observe that for the small and large pulses, the derivative goes below 0.1 only for the diseased artery. Hence, one can conclude that if

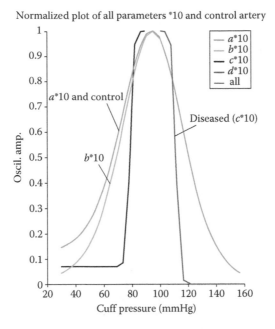

FIGURE 4.4 Control and experimental models: Control and arteries.

oscillations and maximum derivatives are less than 0.1, the artery is diseased, and it collapses easily and we also know that artery collapses in pseudo-hypertension (Figures 4.7 through 4.10).

Because the arterial pressure pulse sets the systolic and diastolic pressure at 112 and 73 mmHg, respectively, the effect of any artery parameter may be easily observed. To discover the effect of each arterial parameter on blood pressure determination accuracy, each artery parameter was varied separately by a

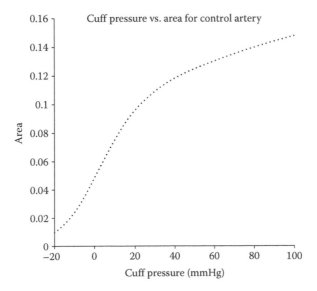

FIGURE 4.5 Cuff pressure versus area for control artery.

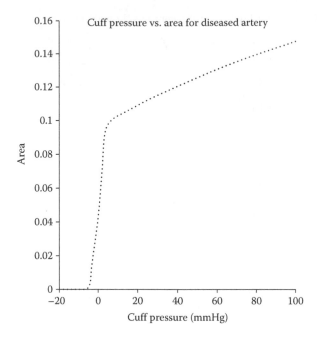

FIGURE 4.6　Cuff pressure versus area for diseased artery.

factor of 10. Therefore, variations in *a*, *b*, *c*, and *d* parameters will not affect the above values for systolic and diastolic pressure. The results are shown in Table 4.2.

Table 4.2 includes the values of systolic and diastolic pressure, % error for the derivative of the oscillometric model for control and the cases when each parameter is multiplied by 10. The negative% errors correspond to a decrease in pressure, whereas the positive ones correlate with an increase in pressure. The *c* parameter causes the largest positive error in blood pressure for diastolic pressure.

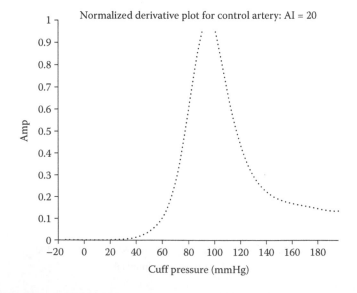

FIGURE 4.7　Normalized arterial oscillations of the control model for control artery: AI = 20.

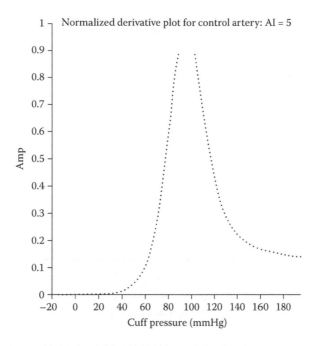

FIGURE 4.8 Normalized oscillations of the control model for control artery: AI = 5.

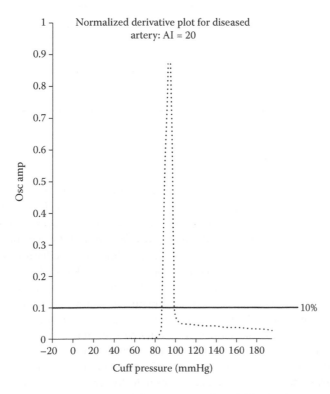

FIGURE 4.9 Normalized arterial oscillations of the experimental model for the diseased artery: AI = 20.

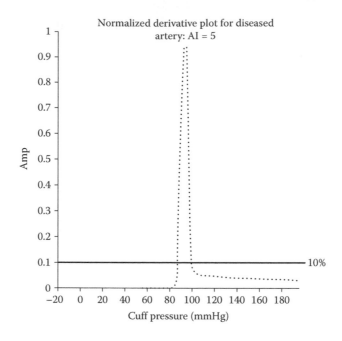

FIGURE 4.10   Normalized arterial oscillations of the model of the DISEASED artery AI = 5.

TABLE 4.2   Derivative of the Oscillometric Model for Control and Diseased Arteries

Multiplier	Parameter	Ps	Pd	% error (Ps)	% error (Pd)
*1 (control)	a, b, c, and d	105.2	74.9	−6.07	2.71
*10	d	107.3	68.3	−4.2	−6.44
*10	c	108.9	78.7	−2.77	7.8
*10	b	107.6	70.8	−3.85	−4.1
*10	a	107.3	68.3	−4.2	−6.8

4.7 Discussion and Analysis

The alteration of parameters a, b, c, or d represent some alteration in the arterial mechanics of the subject under study. The analysis here reveals that the parameters a, b, and d caused very little error in blood pressure measurement and no pseudo-hypertension. This result was also evident from Figure 4.3, in which the oscillometric oscillation curves for a, b, and d superimposed on the control curve and expect no change in error. Conversely, the oscillometric oscillations for the c parameter (Figure 4.4) looked very different from the control oscillations. Parameter c resulted in pseudo-hypertension for diastolic pressure as seen in Table 4.2. Referring to Figure 4.5 and the arterial model, parameters a, b, and d affect the positive pressure region, whereas only parameter c affects the negative pressure portion of the lumen area curve. Negative transmural pressure corresponds with high cuff pressure and the mechanics of arterial closure and collapse. The presence of arterial disease is most likely to affect the arterial closure because it would enable the artery to close at higher transmural pressure. Hence, the c parameter is most closely related to artery disease and the model thereby confirms that artery disease causes pseudo-hypertension in oscillometry as suggested earlier in this section.

In the cuff pressure VS area model, the c parameter was still the source of error, especially for diastolic pressure. It caused pseudo-systolic hypotension and pseudo-diastolic hypertension. By comparing a large pulse to a small one, we noticed that the derivative went low in the high-pressure zone for the diseased artery and this did not happen for the normal artery; therefore, we came up with a new rule that we call the oscillometry of false hypertension. At high blood pressure zone with the derivative less than 0.1, the artery is diseased and stiff, and it collapses easily. As mentioned earlier, the true measurement of the blood pressure should be independent of the arterial mechanics. However, in every modeling experiment, it was found that c was the source of error and its related plot was very different from the rest. Other parameters like a, b, and d did not change the accuracy of blood pressure measurement before and after normalization. Normalization did not even correct the inaccuracy caused by the c parameter. In the case of the diseased artery, the arterial stiffness did increase diastolic pressure by almost 8% (Table 4.2) and this was consistent with the theory of pseudo-hypertension.

Acknowledgment

The author would like to thank the Rutgers' graduate student Farah Rahimy for her work in completing the oscillometric blood pressure model computations related to pseudo-hypertension for this chapter that also resulted in the completion of her MS in biomedical engineering.

References

Balu, S., Thomas, J. Incremental expenditures of treating hypertension in U.S. Al. *Am. J. Hypertens.* 19:810–816, 2006.

Brower, R.W., Noordergraaf, A. Theory of steady flow in collapsible tubes and veins. In: Baan, J., Noordergraaf, A., Raines, J. eds, *Cardiovascular System Dynamics*. Cambridge, MA: Cambridge, pp. 256–265, 1978.

Campbell N.R., Hogan D.B., McKay D.W. Pitfalls to avoid in the measurement of blood pressure in the elderly. *Can. J. Public Health* 85(Suppl 2):S26–28, 1994.

Drzewiecki G., Hood R., Apple H. Theory of the oscillometric maximum and the systolic and diastolic detection ratios. *Ann. Biomed. Eng.* 22(1):88–96, 1994.

Geddes, L.A., Voelz, M., Combs, C., Reiner, D. Characterization of the oscillometric method for measuring indirect blood pressure. *Ann. Biomed. Eng.* 10:271–280, 1983.

High Blood Pressure: Heart & Blood Vessel Disorders. 2007. www.merck.com/mmhe/sec022/ch022a.html

Messerli F.H., Ventura H.O., Amodeo C. Osler's maneuver and Pseudohypertension. *New Eng. J. of Med.* 312:1548–1551, 1985.

Oparil S., Calhoun D.A. Managing the patient with hard-to-control hypertension. *Am. Fam. Physician.* 57(5):1007–1014, 1988.

Osler, W. *The Principles and Practice of Medicine: Designed for the Use of Practitioners and Students of Medicine*. New York: D Appleton and Company, pp. 656, 668, 1892.

Pedley, T.J. Flow in collapsible tubes. In: *The Fluid Mechanics of Large Blood Vessels*. Oxford: Cambridge University Press; Chap. 6, pp. 301–368, 1980.

Pentz, W.H. Controlling isolated systolic hypertension. *Post Graduate Medicine, Osler's Maneuver & Pseudo hypertension*, 105(5), May, 1999.

Shapiro, A.H. Steady flow in collapsible tubes. Trans. ASME (ser. K.) *J. Biomech. Eng.* 99:126–147, 1977.

Skalak R., Chien S. *Handbook of Bioengineering*. New York, NY: McGraw-Hill, 1987.

Zuschke, C.A. Pseudo hypertension. *South Medical Journal*. 88(12):1185–1190, 1995.

5

Cardiac Output Measurement

Leslie A. Geddes
Purdue University

5.1 Introduction

Cardiac output is the amount of blood pumped by the right or left ventricle per unit of time. It is expressed in liters per minute (L/min) and normalized by division by body surface area in square meters (m^2). The resulting quantity is called the cardiac index. Cardiac output is sometimes normalized to body weight, being expressed as mL/min per kilogram. A typical resting value for a wide variety of mammals is 70 mL/min per kg.

With exercise, cardiac output increases. In well-trained athletes, cardiac output can increase fivefold with maximum exercise. During exercise, heart rate increases, venous return increases, and the ejection fraction increases. Parenthetically, physically fit subjects have a low resting heart rate, and the time for the heart rate to return to the resting value after exercise is less than that for subjects who are not physically fit.

There are many direct and indirect (noninvasive) methods of measuring cardiac output. Of equal importance to the number that represents cardiac output is the left-ventricular ejection fraction (stroke volume divided by diastolic volume), which indicates the ability of the left ventricle to pump blood.

5.2 Indicator–Dilution Method

The principle underlying the indicator–dilution method is based on the upstream injection of a detectable indicator and on measuring the downstream concentration–time curve, which is called a *dilution curve*. The essential requirement is that the indicator mixes with all the blood flowing through the central mixing pool. Although the dilution curves in the outlet branches may be slightly different in shape, they all have the same area.

Figure 5.1a illustrates the injection of m g of indicator into an idealized flowing stream having the same velocity across the diameter of the tube. Figure 5.1b shows the dilution curve recorded downstream. Because of the flow–velocity profile, the cylinder of indicator and fluid becomes teardrop in shape, as shown in Figure 5.1c. The resulting dilution curve has a rapid rise and an exponential fall, as shown in Figure 5.1d. However, the area of the dilution curve is the same as that shown in Figure 5.1a. Derivation of the flow equation is shown in Figure 5.1, and the flow is simply the amount of indicator (m g) divided by the area of the dilution curve (g/mL × s), which provides the flow in mL/s.

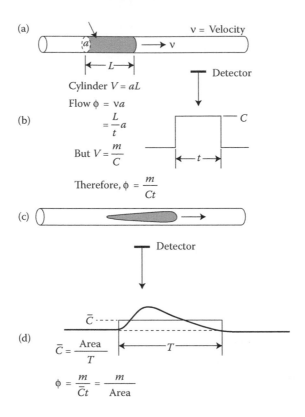

FIGURE 5.1   Genesis of the indicator–dilution curve.

5.2.1 Indicators

Before describing the various indicator–dilution methods, it is useful to recognize that there are two types of indicators, diffusible and nondiffusible. A diffusible indicator will leak out of the capillaries. A nondiffusible indicator is retained in the vascular system for a time that depends on the type of indicator. Whether cardiac output is overestimated with a diffusible indicator depends on the location of the injection and measuring sites. Table 5.1 lists many of the indicators that have been used for measuring cardiac output and the types of detectors used to obtain the dilution curve. It is obvious that the indicator selected must be detectable and not alter the flow being measured. Importantly, the indicator must be nontoxic and sterile.

When a diffusible indicator is injected into the right heart, the dilution curve can be detected in the pulmonary artery, and there is no loss of indicator because there is no capillary bed between these sites; therefore, the cardiac output value will be accurate.

5.2.2 Thermal Dilution Method

Chilled 5% dextrose in water (D5W) or 0.9% NaCl can be used as indicators. The dilution curve represents a transient reduction in pulmonary artery blood temperature following injection of the indicator into the right atrium. Figure 5.2 illustrates the method and a typical thermodilution curve. Note that the indicator is really negative calories. The thermodilution method is based on heat exchange measured in calories, and the flow equation contains terms for the specific heat (C) and the specific gravity (S) of the indicator (i) and blood (b). The expression employed when a #7F thermistor-tipped catheter is used and chilled D5W is injected into the right atrium is as follows:

TABLE 5.1   Indicators

Material	Detector	Retention Data
Evans blue (T1824)	Photoelectric 640 μ	50% loss in 5 days
Indocyanine green	Photoelectric 800 μ	50% loss in 10 min
Coomassie blue	Photoelectric 585–600 μ	50% loss in 15–20 min
Saline (5%)	Conductivity cell	Diffusible[a]
Albumin 1^{131}	Radioactive	50% loss in 8 days
Na^{24}, K^{42}, D_2O, DHO	Radioactive	Diffusible[a]
Hot-cold solutions	Thermodetector	Diffusible[a]

[a] It is estimated that there is about 15% loss of diffusible indicators during the first pass through the lungs.

$$CO = \left[\frac{V(T_b - T_i)60}{A} \right]\left[\frac{S_i C_i}{S_b C_b} \right]F \tag{5.1}$$

where

V = Volume of indicator injected in mL
T_b = Temperature (average of pulmonary artery blood in °C)
T_i = Temperature of the indicator (°C)
60 = Multiplier required to convert mL/s into mL/min
A = Area under the dilution curve in (s×°C)
S = Specific gravity of indicator (i) and blood (b)
C = Specific heat of indicator (i) and blood (b)
($S_i C_i / S_b C_b$ = 1.08 for 5% dextrose and blood of 40% packed-cell volume)
F = Empiric factor employed to correct for heat transfer through the injection catheter (for a #7F catheter, $F = 0.825$ [2]).

(a)

(b)

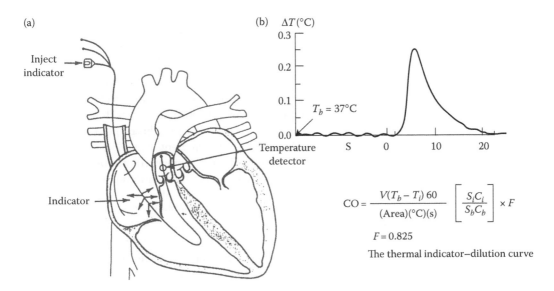

FIGURE 5.2   The thermodilution method (a) and a typical dilution curve (b).

Entering these factors into the expression gives

$$CO = \frac{V(T_b - T_i)53.46}{A} \tag{5.2}$$

where CO = cardiac output in mL/min

$$53.46 = 60 \times 1.08 \times 0.825$$

To illustrate how a thermodilution curve is processed, cardiac output is calculated below using the dilution curve shown in Figure 5.2.

V = 5 mL of 5% dextrose in water
T_b = 37°C
T_i = 0°C
A = 1.59°C s

$$CO = \frac{5(37 - 0)53.46}{1.59} = 6220\,mL/min$$

Although the thermodilution method is *the standard in clinical medicine*, it has a few disadvantages. Because of the heat loss through the catheter wall, several series 5-mL injections of indicator are needed to obtain a consistent value for cardiac output. If cardiac output is low, that is, the dilution curve is very broad, it is difficult to obtain an accurate value for cardiac output. There are respiratory-induced variations in PA blood temperature that confound the dilution curve when it is of low amplitude. Although room-temperature D5W can be used, chilled D5W provides a better dilution curve and a more reliable cardiac output value. Furthermore, it should be obvious that if the temperature of the indicator is the same as that of blood, there will be no dilution curve.

5.2.3 Indicator Recirculation

An ideal dilution curve shown in Figure 5.2 consists of a steep rise and an exponential decrease in indicator concentration. Algorithms that measure the dilution-curve area have no difficulty with such a curve. However, when cardiac output is low, the dilution curve is typically low in amplitude and very broad. Often the descending limb of the curve is obscured by recirculation of the indicator or by low-amplitude artifacts. Figure 5.3a is a dilution curve in which the descending limb is obscured by recirculation of the indicator. Obviously it is difficult to determine the practical end of the curve, which is often specified as the time when the indicator concentration has fallen to a chosen percentage (e.g., 1%) of the maximum amplitude (C_{max}). Because the descending limb represents a good approximation of a decaying exponential curve (e^{-kt}), fitting the descending limb to an exponential allows reconstruction of the curve without a recirculation error, thereby providing a means for identifying the end for what is called the *first pass of the indicator*.

In Figure 5.3b, the amplitude of the descending limb of the curve in Figure 5.3a has been plotted on semilogarithmic paper, and the exponential part represents a straight line. When recirculation appears, the data points deviate from the straight line and therefore can be ignored, and the linear part (representing the exponential) can be extrapolated to the desired percentage of the maximum concentration, say 1% of C_{max}. The data points representing the extrapolated part were replotted in Figure 5.3a to reveal the dilution curve undistorted by recirculation.

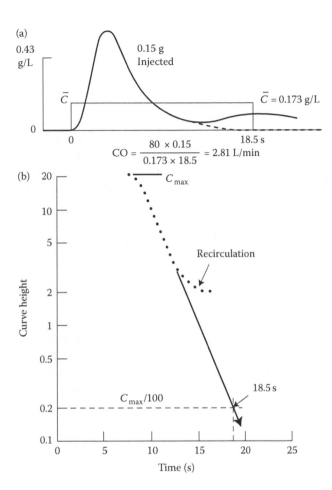

FIGURE 5.3   Dilution curve obscured by recirculation (a) and a semilogarithmic plot of the descending limb (b).

Commercially available indicator–dilution instruments employ digitization of the dilution curve. Often the data beyond about 30% of C_{max} are ignored, and the exponential is computed on digitally extrapolated data.

5.3 Fick Method

The Fick method *employs oxygen as the indicator* and the increase in oxygen content of venous blood as it passes through the lungs, along with the respiratory oxygen uptake, as the quantities that are needed to determine cardiac output (CO = O_2 uptake/$A − V\, O_2$ difference). Oxygen uptake (mL/min) is measured at the airway, usually with an oxygen-filled spirometer containing a CO_2 absorber. The $A − V\, O_2$ difference is determined from the oxygen content (mL/100 mL blood) from any arterial sample and the oxygen content (mL/100 mL) of pulmonary arterial blood. The oxygen content of blood used to be difficult to measure. However, the new blood–gas analyzers that measure, pH, pO_2, pCO_2, hematocrit, and hemoglobin provide a value for O_2 content by computation using the oxygen-dissociation curve.

There is a slight technicality involved in determining the oxygen uptake because oxygen is consumed at body temperature but measured at room temperature in the spirometer. Consequently, the volume of

O_2 consumed per minute displayed by the spirometer must be multiplied by a factor, *F*. Therefore, the Fick equation is

$$CO = \frac{O_2 \text{ uptake/min}(F)}{A - V \, O_2 \text{ difference}}$$ (5.3)

Figure 5.4 is a spirogram showing a tidal volume riding on a sloping baseline that represents the resting expirating level (REL). The slope identifies the oxygen uptake at room temperature. In this subject, the uncorrected oxygen consumption was 400 mL/min at 26°C in the spirometer. With a barometric pressure of 750 mmHg, the conversion factor *F* to correct this volume to body temperature (37°C) and saturated with water vapor is

$$F = \frac{273 + 37}{273 + T_s} \times \frac{P_b - PH_2O}{P_b - 47}$$ (5.4)

where T_s is the spirometer temperature, P_b is the barometric pressure, and PH_2O at T_s is obtained from the water-vapor table (Table 5.2).

A sample calculation for the correction factor *F* is given in Figure 5.4, which reveals a value for *F* of 1.069. However, it is easier to use Table 5.3 to obtain the correction factor. For example, for a spirometer temperature of 26°C and a barometric pressure of 750 mmHg, $F = 1.0691$.

Note that the correction factor *F* in this case is only 6.9%. The error encountered by not including it may be less than the experimental error in making all other measurements.

(a)

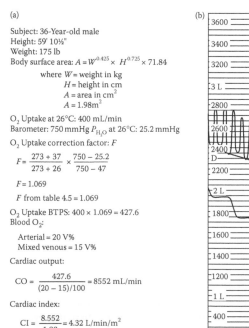

(b)

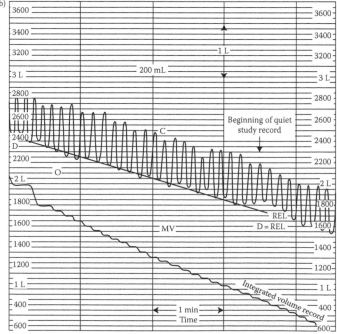

FIGURE 5.4 Measurement of oxygen uptake with a spirometer (b) and the method used to correct the measured volume (a).

TABLE 5.2   Vapor Pressure of Water

Temp. (°C)	0.0	0.2	0.4	0.6	0.8
15	12.788	12.953	13.121	13.290	13.461
16	13.634	13.809	13.987	14.166	14.347
17	14.530	14.715	14.903	15.092	15.284
18	15.477	15.673	15.871	16.071	16.272
19	16.477	16.685	16.894	17.105	17.319
20	17.535	17.753	17.974	18.197	18.422
21	18.650	18.880	19.113	19.349	19.587
22	19.827	20.070	20.316	20.565	20.815
23	21.068	21.324	21.583	21.845	22.110
24	22.377	22.648	22.922	23.198	23.476
25	23.756	24.039	24.326	24.617	24.912
26	25.209	25.509	25.812	26.117	26.426
27	26.739	27.055	27.374	27.696	28.021
28	28.349	28.680	29.015	29.354	29.697
29	30.043	30.392	30.745	31.102	31.461
30	31.825	32.191	32.561	32.934	33.312
31	33.695	34.082	34.471	34.864	35.261
32	35.663	36.068	36.477	36.891	37.308
33	37.729	38.155	38.584	39.018	39.457
34	39.898	40.344	40.796	41.251	41.710
35	42.175	42.644	43.117	43.595	44.078
36	44.563	45.054	45.549	46.050	46.556
37	47.067	47.582	48.102	48.627	49.157
38	49.692	50.231	50.774	51.323	51.879
39	42.442	53.009	53.580	54.156	54.737
40	55.324	55.910	56.510	57.110	57.720
41	58.340	58.960	59.580	60.220	60.860

The example selected shows that the $A–V$ O_2 difference is 20 – 15 mL/100 mL blood and that the corrected O_2 uptake is 400×1.069; therefore the cardiac output is

$$CO = \frac{400 \times 1.069}{(20 - 15)/100} = 8552 \text{ mL/min} \tag{5.5}$$

The Fick method does not require the addition of a fluid to the circulation and may have value in such a circumstance. However, its use requires stable conditions because an average oxygen uptake takes many minutes to obtain.

5.4 Ejection Fraction

The ejection fraction (EF) is one of the most convenient indicators of the ability of the left (or right) ventricle to pump the blood that is presented to it. Let v be the stroke volume (SV) and V be the end-diastolic volume (EDV); the ejection fraction is v/V or SV/EDV.

Measurement of ventricular diastolic and systolic volumes can be achieved radiographically, ultrasonically, and by the use of an indicator that is injected into the left ventricle where the indicator concentration is measured in the aorta on a beat-by-beat basis.

TABLE 5.3   Correction Factor *F* for Standardization of Collected Volume

°C/P_B	640	650	660	670	680	690	700	710	720	730	740	750	760	770	780
15	1.1388	1.1377	1.1367	1.1358	1.1348	1.1339	1.1330	1.1322	1.1314	1.1306	1.1298	1.1290	1.1283	1.1276	1.1269
16	1.1333	1.1323	1.1313	1.1304	1.1295	1.1286	1.1277	1.1269	1.1260	1.1253	1.1245	1.1238	1.1231	1.1224	1.1217
17	1.1277	1.1268	1.1258	1.1249	1.1240	1.1232	1.1224	1.1216	1.1208	1.1200	1.1193	1.1186	1.1179	1.1172	1.1165
18	1.1222	1.1212	1.1203	1.1194	1.1186	1.1178	1.1170	1.1162	1.1154	1.1147	1.1140	1.1133	1.1126	1.1120	1.1113
19	1.1165	1.1156	1.1147	1.1139	1.1131	1.1123	1.1115	1.1107	1.1100	1.1093	1.1086	1.1080	1.1073	1.1067	1.1061
20	1.1108	1.1099	1.1091	1.1083	1.1075	1.1067	1.1060	1.1052	1.1045	1.1039	1.1032	1.1026	1.1019	1.1014	1.1008
21	1.1056	1.1042	1.1034	1.1027	1.1019	1.1011	1.1004	1.0997	1.0990	1.0984	1.0978	1.0971	1.0965	1.0960	1.0954
22	1.0992	1.0984	1.0976	1.0969	1.0962	1.0955	1.0948	1.0941	1.0935	1.0929	1.0923	1.0917	1.0911	1.0905	1.0900
23	1.0932	1.0925	1.0918	1.0911	1.0904	1.0897	1.0891	1.0884	1.0878	1.0872	1.0867	1.0861	1.0856	1.0850	1.0845
24	1.0873	1.0866	1.0859	1.0852	1.0846	1.0839	1.0833	1.0827	1.0822	1.0816	1.0810	1.0805	1.0800	1.0795	1.0790
25	1.0812	1.0806	1.0799	1.0793	1.0787	1.0781	1.0775	1.0769	1.0764	1.0758	1.0753	1.0748	1.0744	1.0739	1.0734
26	1.0751	1.0745	1.0738	1.0732	1.0727	1.0721	1.0716	1.0710	1.0705	1.0700	1.0696	1.0691	1.0686	1.0682	1.0678
27	1.0688	1.0682	1.0677	1.0671	1.0666	1.0661	1.0656	1.0651	1.0646	1.0641	1.0637	1.0633	1.0629	1.0624	1.0621
28	1.0625	1.0619	1.0614	1.0609	1.0604	1.0599	1.0595	1.0591	1.0586	1.0582	1.0578	1.0574	1.0570	1.0566	1.0563
29	1.0560	1.0555	1.0550	1.0546	1.0541	1.0537	1.0533	1.0529	1.0525	1.0521	1.0518	1.0514	1.0509	1.0507	1.0504
30	1.0494	1.0490	1.0486	1.0482	1.0478	1.0474	1.0470	1.0467	1.0463	1.0460	1.0457	1.0453	1.0450	1.0447	1.0444

Source: From Kovach J.C., Paulos P., and Arabadjis C. 1955. *J. Thorac. Surg.* **29**: 552.

Note: $V_s = FV_c$, where V_s is the standardized condition and V_c is the collected condition: $V = \dfrac{1+37/273}{1+t\,°C/273} \times \dfrac{P_B - P_{H_2O}}{P_B - 47}$ $V_c = FV_c$

5.4.1 Indicator–Dilution Method for Ejection Fraction

Holt [1] described the method of injecting an indicator into the left ventricular during diastole and measuring the stepwise decrease in aortic concentration with successive beats (Figure 5.5). From this concentration–time record, end-diastolic volume, stroke volume, and ejection fraction can be calculated. No assumption need be made about the geometric shape of the ventricle. The following describes the theory of this fundamental method.

Let V be the end-diastolic ventricular volume. Inject m g of indicator into this volume during diastole. The concentration (C_1) of indicator in the aorta for the first beat is m/V. By knowing the amount of indicator (m) injected and the calibration for the aortic detector, C_1 is established, and ventricular end-diastolic volume $V = m/C_1$.

After the first beat, the ventricle fills, and the amount of indicator left in the left ventricle is $m - mv/V$. The aortic concentration (C_2) for the second beat is therefore $m - mV/V = m(1 - v/V)$. Therefore, the aortic concentration (C_2) for the second beat is

$$C_2 = \frac{m}{V}\left[1 - \frac{v}{V}\right] \tag{5.6}$$

By continuing the process, it is easily shown that the aortic concentration (C_n) for the nth beat is

$$C_n = \frac{m}{V}\left[1 - \frac{v}{V}\right]^{n-1} \tag{5.7}$$

Figure 5.6 illustrates the stepwise decrease in aortic concentration for ejection fractions (v/V) of 0.2 and 0.5, that is, 20% and 50%.

It is possible to determine the ejection fraction from the concentration ratio for two successive beats. For example,

$$C_n = \frac{m}{V}\left[1 - \frac{v}{V}\right]^{n-1} \tag{5.8}$$

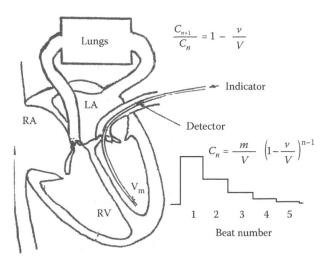

FIGURE 5.5   The saline method of measuring ejection fraction, involving injection of m g of NaCl into the left ventricle and detecting the aortic concentration (C) on a beat-by-beat basis.

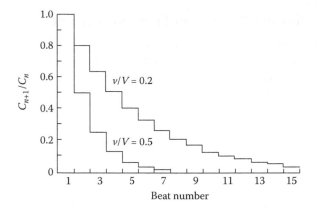

FIGURE 5.6   Stepwise decrease in indicator concentration (*C*) vs. beat number for ejection fraction (*v*/*V*) of 0.5 and 0.2.

$$C_{n+1} = \frac{m}{V}\left[1 - \frac{v}{V}\right]^{n} \tag{5.9}$$

$$\frac{C_{n+1}}{C_n} = 1 - \frac{v}{V} \tag{5.10}$$

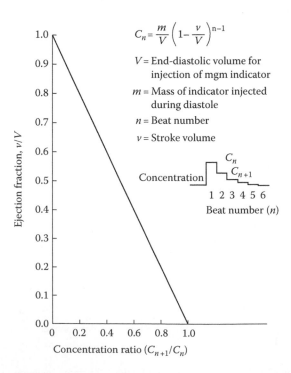

FIGURE 5.7   Ejection fraction (*v*/*V*) vs. the ratio of concentrations for successive beats (*C_{n+1}*/*C_n*).

from which

$$\frac{v}{V} = 1 - \frac{C_{n+1}}{C_n} \tag{5.11}$$

where v/V is the ejection fraction and C_{n+1}/C_n is the concentration ratio for two successive beats, for example, C_2/C_1 or C_3/C_2. Figure 5.7 illustrates the relationship between the ejection fraction v/V and the ratio of C_{n+1}/C_n. Observe that the detector need not be calibrated as long as there is a linear relationship between detector output and indicator concentration in the operating range.

References

1. Holt, J.P. 1956. Estimation of the residual volume of the ventricle of the dog heart by two indicator–dilution techniques. *Circ. Res.* 4: 181.
2. Weissel, R.D., Berger, R.L., and Hechtman, H.B. 1975. Measurement of cardiac output by thermodilution. *N. Engl. J. Med.* 292: 682.

6

External Defibrillators

Willis A. Tacker Jr.
Purdue University

6.1 Introduction

Cardiac defibrillators are electronic devices that have been used for decades to provide a strong electrical shock to a patient in an attempt to convert a *very* rapid (and often chaotic), ineffective heart rhythm to a slower, coordinated, and more effective rhythm. When used to treat ventricular fibrillation (VF) or very rapid ventricular tachycardia the shock may be lifesaving because the heart output is nil or is too low to sustain life. Occurrence of VF is a medical emergency and rapid treatment (within seconds to minutes) is essential for survival.

In the case of a *moderately* accelerated ventricular tachycardia (and impaired heart function), the electrical shock may be useful for slowing the heart rate so that the heart will beat with a more effective rhythm and force. The problem in this other category of patients is that the shortened filling time between contractions does not allow adequate cardiac filling and so blood flow is impaired, but not eliminated. The circuitous pathway that creates the fast heart rate is interrupted by the shock and slowing of the heart rate after the shock corrects this problem. Usually, this non-VF impairment is compatible with life and, therefore, the urgency for treatment is less, because there is less risk of sudden death.

Another use for defibrillators is to shock either atrial flutter or fibrillation, which are abnormally rapid atrial rhythms. These atrial rhythms are much less likely to spontaneously proceed rapidly to death than ventricular arrhythmias. Using electrical shock to treat rapid heart arrhythmias other than VF is usually referred to as "cardioversion" and hence some users refer to the tachycardia treatment devices as cardiovertor—defibrillators. Cardiovertor and defibrillator treatment is different from pacemaker treatment (discussed elsewhere in this book) because a pacemaker stimulates a *slowly* beating heart and uses much weaker shocks. Pacemaking increases the rate of the relatively healthy heart, which increases blood flow.

6.2 Mechanism of Fibrillation

Fibrillation is chaotic electric excitation of the myocardium and results in loss of coordinated mechanical contraction characteristic of normal heart beats. Description of the mechanisms leading to, and maintaining, fibrillation and other rhythm disorders are reviewed elsewhere [1–3] and are beyond the scope of this chapter. In summary, however, these rhythm disorders are commonly held to be a result of reentrant excitation pathways within the heart. The underlying abnormality that leads to the mechanism is the combination of an area of conduction block of cardiac excitation, plus rapidly recurring depolarization of the membranes of the cardiac cells. This leads to rapid repetitive propagation of a single excitation wave or multiple excitatory waves throughout the heart. If the waves are multiple, the rhythm may degrade into total loss of synchronization of cardiac fiber contraction. Without synchronized contraction, the chamber affected will not contract, and this is fatal in the situation of VF. The most common cause of these conditions, and therefore of these rhythm disorders, is cardiac ischemia or infarction as a complication of atherosclerosis. Additional relatively common causes include other cardiac disorders, drug toxicity, electrolyte imbalances in the blood, hypothermia, and electric shocks (especially from alternating current).

6.3 Mechanism of Defibrillation

The corrective measure is to extinguish the rapidly occurring waves of excitation by simultaneously depolarizing all or most of the cardiac cells with a strong electric shock. The cells can then simultaneously repolarize themselves, and this will put them back in phase with each other.

Despite years of intensive research there is still no single theory for the mechanism of defibrillation that explains all the phenomena observed. However, it is generally held that the defibrillating shock must be adequately strong and have adequate duration to affect most of the heart cells. In general, longer duration shocks require less current than shorter duration shocks. This relationship is called the strength–duration relationship and is demonstrated by the curve shown in Figure 6.1. Shocks of strength and duration above and to the right of the current curve (or above the energy curve) have adequate strength to defibrillate, whereas shocks below and to the left do not. From the exponentially decaying current curve an energy curve can also be determined (also shown in Figure 6.1), which is high at very short durations because of high current requirements at short durations, but which is also high at longer durations owing to additional energy being delivered as the pulse duration is lengthened at nearly constant current. Thus, for most electrical waveforms there is a minimum energy for defibrillation at

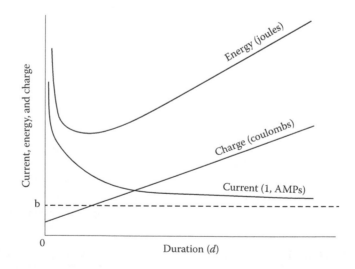

FIGURE 6.1 Strength–duration curves for current, energy, and charge. Adequate current shocks are above and to the right of the current curve. (Modified from Tacker WA, Geddes LA. 1980. *Electrical Defibrillation*, Boca Raton, FL, CRC Press. With permission.)

approximate pulse durations of 3–10 ms. A strength–duration charge curve can also be determined as shown in Figure 6.1, which demonstrates that the minimum charge for defibrillation occurs at the shortest pulse duration tested. Very short duration pulses are not used, however, because the high current and voltage required is damaging to the myocardium. It is also important to note that excessively strong or long shocks may cause damage that leads to immediate refibrillation, thus failing to restore the heart function.

In practice, for a shock applied to the electrodes on the skin surface of the patient's chest, durations are on the order of 3–10 ms and deliver 10s of amperes. The energy delivered to the subject by these shocks is selectable by the operator and for adults is on the order of 50–360 J. The exact shock intensity required at a given duration of electric pulse depends on several variables, including the intrinsic characteristics of the patient (such as body size, the underlying disease problem or the presence of certain drugs, and the length of time the arrhythmia has been present), the techniques for electrode application, and the particular rhythm disorder being treated (highly organized rhythms usually require less energy than extremely disorganized rhythms).

6.4 Clinical Defibrillators

Defibrillator design has evolved through the years, based on technologic improvements in waveform shaping, combined with studies of the effectiveness of different waveforms to defibrillate or cardiovert the various rhythm disorders. Also, decreased time to diagnose the exact rhythm problem is paramount for success under emergency VF conditions and automated signal processing is important to speed up rhythm identification and treatment using the best shock strength. Most defibrillators have automated diagnosis and treatment operating modes and many have manual, nonautomated controls available for specific uses. The optimal amount of automation depends on how the unit will be used. For example, highly automatic external defibrillators (AEDs) are optimal for use by lay persons who may have no training, such as in an airport. The important goal is to prevent sudden death from VF and quick response to simple instructions on the defibrillator is desirable. Another use is for home defibrillation if a defibrillator is kept in the home of a patient who is at high risk for VF. Depending on how, where, and by whom they will be operated, AEDs may be considered automatic or semiautomatic. Figure 6.2 shows an AED and Figure 6.3 shows a wearable defibrillator.

However, a defibrillator intended for use in a hospital electrophysiology laboratory, or perhaps in an ambulance, or a hospital crash cart would have multiple, controllable variables for use by the physician

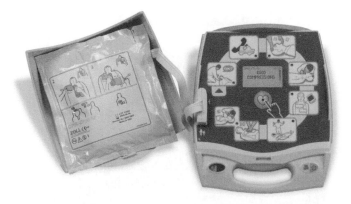

FIGURE 6.2 AED, showing packaged electrodes in the pouch on the left and the electrical shock generator on the right. Drawings and text provide visual instructions and audible voice instructions are provided by speakers in the defibrillator case.

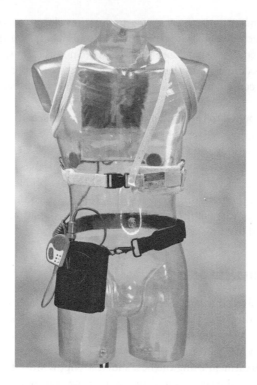

FIGURE 6.3   Wearable defibrillator for high risk patients.

or EMT who is testing or monitoring for arrhythmias and who may have to diagnose and treat the full spectrum of cardiac rhythm disorders, sometimes with great urgency. Hence, most defibrillators routinely used by medical personnel have a built-in control panel, monitor, and synchronizer. Figure 6.4 shows a hospital defibrillator.

Improved defibrillator waveforms have been developed and been advocated during the years from [1] multiple pulse sine waveform to [2] simple capacitor discharge waveform to [3] damped sine (RLC) waveform, to [4] monophasic truncated exponential decay waveform, to [5] a pair of truncated exponential waveforms, to [6] paired, biphasic truncated exponential decay waveforms. It is evident that the

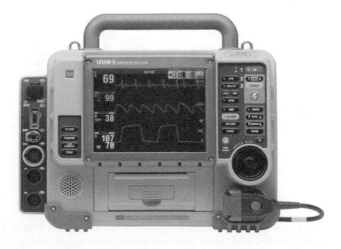

FIGURE 6.4   Defibrillator with monitor and control panel for us by trained medical personnel.

sine waveform and capacitor discharge are less effective and more damaging to the heart than the other waveforms, but there is still controversy about the benefits and limitations of the other waveforms. All of them defibrillate reliably but long-term patient survival with low morbidity is often low. (Of course, many variables other than waveform affect the final outcome.) At present, the biphasic truncated exponential decay waveform is the most widely used.

Optimal *shock intensity* for defibrillation is also controversial because in adult patients stronger shocks have a modestly higher success rate, but probably are more likely to damage the myocardium. Accordingly, experts and users take the position that a weaker first shock should be used for cardioversion, with gradual increase until success occurs. However, for the emergency situation of ventricular defibrillation, the best sequence (strength of first shock and extent of increases with subsequent shocks) has not yet been determined.

6.5 Electrodes

Electrodes for external defibrillation are connected to the defibrillator and are of two types; hand held and self-adhesive. The hand-held ones, shown in Figure 6.5, are most often used by medical personnel and have a metal surface area between 70 and 100 cm²in. They must be coupled to the skin with an electrically conductive gel material that is specifically formulated for defibrillation to achieve low impedance across the electrode–patient interface. Hand-held electrodes are reusable.

The self-adhesive electrodes are patches wired to the patient through conductive flexible adhesive which holds the electrode in place, tightly against the skin. Adhesive electrodes are shown in Figure 6.6. They are disposable and are applied to the chest before the delivery of shock. Adhesive electrodes are left in place for reuse in case subsequent shocks are needed. Electrodes are usually applied with both electrodes on the anterior chest as shown in Figure 6.7, or in an anterior-to-posterior position, as shown in Figure 6.8.

6.6 Synchronization

Most defibrillators for use by medical personnel have the feature of synchronization, which is an electronic sensing and triggering mechanism for application of shock during the QRS complex of the ECG. This is required when treating arrhythmias other than VF (i.e., cardioverting), because when a patient does not have VF, inadvertent application of a shock during the T wave of the ECG often produces VF. Selection by the operator of the synchronized mode of defibrillator operation will cause the defibrillator to automatically sense the QRS complex and apply the shock during the QRS complex. Furthermore, on the ECG display, the timing of the shock on the QRS is graphically displayed so that the operator can be certain that the shock will not fall during the T wave (see Figure 6.9). This prevents production of VF by the defibrillator.

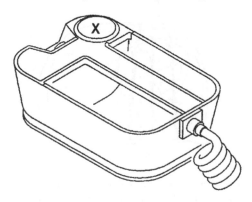

FIGURE 6.5   Hand held electrodes for external use.

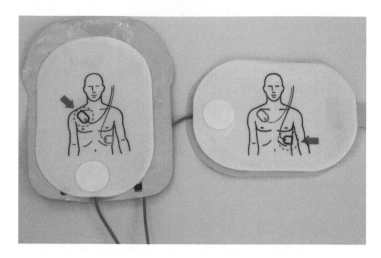

FIGURE 6.6   Disposable adhesive electrodes for external defibrillation.

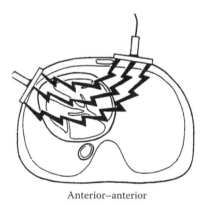

Anterior–anterior

FIGURE 6.7   Cross-sectional view of the chest showing position for standard anterior wall (precordial) electrode placement. Lines of presumed current flow are shown between the electrodes on the skin surface. (Modified from Tacker WA (ed). 1994. *Defibrillation of the Heart: ICDs, AEDs and Manual*, St. Louis, Mosby-Year Book. With permission.)

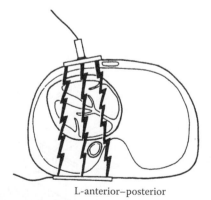

L-anterior–posterior

FIGURE 6.8   Cross-sectional view of the chest showing position for front-to-back electrode placement. Lines of presumed current flow are shown between the electrodes on the skin surface. (Modified from Tacker WA (ed). 1994. *Defibrillation of the Heart: ICDs, AEDs and Manual*, St. Louis, Mosby-Year Book. With permission.)

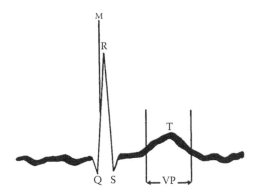

FIGURE 6.9 Timing mark (M) as shown on a synchronized defibrillator monitor. The M designates when in the cardiac cycle a shock will be applied. The T wave must be avoided, since a shock during the vulnerable period (VP) may fibrillate the ventricles. This tracing shows atrial fibrillation as identified by the irregular wavy baseline of the ECG. (Modified from Fein berg B. 1980. *Handbook Series in Clinical Laboratory Science*, vol. 2, Boca Raton, FL, CRC Press. With permission.)

6.7 Defibrillator Safety

Defibrillators are potentially dangerous devices because of their high electrical output. The danger to the patient is that of delivering unsynchronized shocks to a beating heart, a situation which can cause VF. Other problems include inadvertent shocking of the operator or others in the vicinity of use. Proper training and careful use are required for safety. Another risk is injuring the patient by applying excessively strong and/or excessive number of shocks. Failure of a defibrillator to operate correctly is a safety issue because a patient may die of his/her VF.

References

1. Tacker, W. A. Jr. (ed), 1994. *Defibrillation of the Heart: ICDs, AEDs, and Manual*. St. Louis, Mosby-Year Book.
2. Tacker, W. A. Jr. and Geddes, L. A. 1980. *Electrical Defibrillation*. Boca Raton, FL, CRC Press.
3. Paradis, N. A. (ed), 2007. *Cardiac Arrest: The Science and Practice of Resuscitation Medicine*. Cambridge CB2 8RU, United Kingdom, Cambridge University Press.
4. American National Standard ANSI/AAMI DF2, 1989. (second edition, revision of ANSI/AAMI DF2-1981) Safety and performance standard: Cardiac defibrillator devices.
5. Canadian National Standard CAN/CSA C22.2 No. 601.2.4-M90, 1990. Medical electrical equipment, part 2: Particular requirements for the safety of cardiac defibrillators and cardiac defibrillator/monitors.
6. International Standard IEC 601-2-4, 1983. Medical electrical equipment, part 2: Particular requirements for the safety of cardiac defibrillators and cardiac defibrillator/monitors.

Further Information

Detailed presentation of material on defibrillator waveforms, algorithms for ECG analysis, and automatic defibrillation using AEDs, electrodes, design, clinical use, effects of drugs on shock strength required to defibrillate, damage because of defibrillator shocks, and use of defibrillators during open-thorax surgical procedures or trans-esophageal defibrillation are beyond the scope of this chapter. Also, the historical aspects of defibrillation are not presented here. For more information, the reader is referred to the publications at the end of the chapter [1–3]. For American, Canadian, and European defibrillator standards, the reader is referred to the published standards [3–6].

7

Implantable Defibrillators

Paul A. Belk
St. Jude Medical

Thomas J. Mullen
Medtronic

7.1 Introduction

The heart is an electromechanical system, in which mechanical pumping function is initiated and coordinated by automatic rhythmic cardiac electrical activity. Transient electrical disturbances in this activity (cardiac arrhythmias) can immediately cause death. The implantable cardioverter defibrillator (ICD) is a medical device that can be implanted in a human body and will automatically detect and treat cardiac arrhythmias. Mirowski et al. [1] first reported on a demonstration of a functioning ICD in 1970. In his demonstration, he induced a fatal ventricular tachyarrhythmia in a dog. The dog was then successfully and dramatically rescued by the automatic operation of a previously implanted ICD. The first report of successful ICD implantation in humans soon followed [2]. In subsequent decades, advances in ICD technology have reduced ICD size from more than 200 cm^3, originally, to as little as 25 cm^3, while markedly improving functionality, reliability, and longevity. ICDs are now considered as standard of care for patients at risk for ventricular arrhythmia and are implanted in more than 150,000 patients per year in the United States alone [3].

Sudden cardiac death (SCD) is defined as abrupt loss of consciousness caused by failure of cardiac pumping function, generally because of an electrical problem. In certain cases, cardiac activity ceases completely because cardiac electrical impulse generation fails (bradycardic sudden death). Most commonly, however, cardiac electrical activity is present, but is either too rapid for effective mechanical response or too disorganized for coordinated mechanical response (tachycardic sudden death). Despite the term, resuscitation from SCD is possible, but lack of prompt treatment is almost invariably fatal. SCD is responsible for at least 160,000 deaths each year in the United States alone [4].

For most patients, treatment of SCD requires using an external defibrillator, but given the typical delay between identification of SCD and application of an external device, the chance of surviving SCD is less than 7% [4]. In contrast to external defibrillators, ICDs virtually guarantee prompt electrical therapy and one study showed that patients who receive ICD therapy for a lethal ventricular arrhythmia have greater than 75% chance of surviving for at least a year following the episode [5].

However, the expense of the device and associated complications and side effects limit ICD therapy to identifiable high-risk groups. Large numbers of patients in lower-risk groups, in fact, make up the majority of SCD victims and are currently not indicated or eligible to receive a device. As devices become less expensive and as therapy improves, more people become eligible. Improvement of device function would, therefore, potentially save lives of patients not currently indicated and reduce unpleasant side effects in patients who are.

7.2 Hardware

An ICD system consists of the "generator," which contains all the circuitry and energy storage and the "leads" that provide electrical connection to the heart (Figure 7.1).

7.2.1 Generator

To understand the construction of the ICD generator, it would be useful to review its required functions. The generator is implanted subcutaneously, usually in the left upper chest (Figure 7.1), but sometimes in other locations (abdominally or right chest). It normally remains implanted for between 4 and 10 years, until it reaches end of service life (through battery depletion). During this time, it must operate without fail and therefore must be built to the highest standards of quality and reliability. To survive for years implanted within the human body, the generator must be encased in a hermetically sealed casing that can withstand the harsh conditions of the human body. The casing is normally constructed of titanium because of its durability and biocompatibility. Attached to the casing is a "header" that provides ports into which the leads are inserted. The header provides externalization of the electrical connections without compromising the hermetic seal of the casing. Figure 7.2 shows typical components of a generator.

7.2.1.1 Low-Voltage Requirements

The ICD continuously monitors electrical activity in the heart. It may monitor one or more locations usually by analyzing the voltage across a bipolar electrode which is in intimate contact with cardiac tissue. Potentials across this electrode are generally between 1 and 20 mV. They are low-pass filtered with cutoff frequency between 30 and 100 Hz. Electrode impedances vary between 200 and 3000 Ω. In addition to providing therapy for tachyarrhythmias, almost all modern ICDs are capable of providing constant

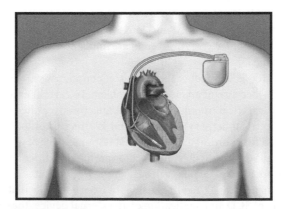

FIGURE 7.1 Schematic representation of a dual-chamber ICD. The generator is implanted in the pectoral region. The defibrillation lead (lower) is in the right ventricle, where it is fixed by a helix at the distal (far) end of the lead. The atrial lead (upper) is secured by flexible tines in the right atrial appendage. (Reproduced with permission of Medtronic, Inc.)

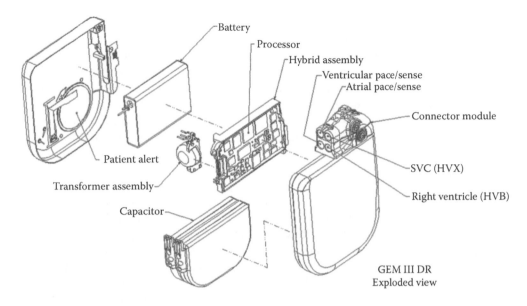

Battery
Processor
Hybrid assembly
Ventricular pace/sense
Atrial pace/sense
Connector module
Patient alert
SVC (HVX)
Transformer assembly
Right ventricle (HVB)
Capacitor

GEM III DR
Exploded view

FIGURE 7.2 Exploded view of ICD generator components. (Reproduced with permission of Medtronic, Inc.)

low-voltage pacing (at rates of 40–80 beats per minute) in the event of unacceptably slow heart rates (bradycardia). Pacing outputs are on the order of 1–5 V into an impedance of roughly 1 kΩ.

7.2.1.2 High-Voltage Requirements

Cardioversion or defibrillation is the electrical termination of arrhythmias using field stimulation. Unlike pacing, in which cardiac excitation is initiated in and propagates from a small region of tissue near the electrode, cardioversion must arrest electrical activity by simultaneous stimulation of most of the heart. In practice, this means establishing a "critical field" across a "critical mass" of cardiac tissue. This requires a compromise between the electrical response of the tissue and the electrical capabilities of the device. The electrical response of cardiac cells is complex, but stimulation mostly depends on the first-order properties of the membrane [6]. Theoretical and experimental studies have shown that the optimum voltage waveform for stimulation of cardiac tissue is a waveform with a characteristic rise time comparable to the cell membrane time constant [7,8].

The easiest waveform to deliver from an implantable device, however, is an exponentially decaying, capacitive discharge waveform because the capacitor is the natural high-voltage storage device. Optimum energy transfer occurs when the time constant of the waveform is similar to the first-order time constant of the cardiac tissue [6], and the polarity of the pulse is reversed at a prespecified voltage and then truncated [9,10]. The resulting pulse rises to as much as 750 V, with a duration of several milliseconds, into an impedance of 30–80 Ω. The need for phase reversal and truncation requires multiple high-voltage switches, usually arranged as an "H-bridge." Typical cardioversion energies are approximately 30 J, although completely subcutaneous systems (in which the leads are outside the chest cavity) may require twice that. Modern ICDs are designed for longevities of 4–9 years under the assumption that they will deliver up to four cardioversion shocks per year or about 500 J of high-voltage output.

7.2.1.3 Battery

Most of the volume of an ICD is required for the long- and short-term energy-storage devices: the battery and high-voltage capacitor. There is a minimum power, the quiescent energy drain, required for continuous function of the device; generally about 1 μW, which the battery must deliver continuously for many years, but it must also be able to deliver more than 4 W for 10 s necessary to charge the high-voltage capacitors for a 30–40 J cardioversion. The voltage characteristics of the battery must also be predictable, so that monitoring battery voltage gives adequate warning of end of battery life.

In modern ICDs, the battery chemistry is based on a lithium anode and a silver vanadium oxide cathode, giving relatively high-energy density and a predictable discharge curve. There are many ways of using this chemistry, and there are trade-offs between energy density and internal resistance. Internal battery resistance limits instantaneous power; therefore, it is often useful to sacrifice available energy density to control internal resistance. Some battery designers choose to make one of the battery electrodes larger than necessary, which limits the increase in internal resistance as the battery depletes, although at the cost of energy storage.

7.2.1.4 High-Voltage Capacitor

A cardioversion shock is usually a pulse of duration approximately 5 ms, delivered into a resistive load of approximately 50 Ω (3.2 kW). Because no miniature battery is even nearly capable of that voltage or that power, ICD generators require high-voltage capacitors. Originally, the capacitors were commodity electronic parts, such as those used for camera flashes, but modern ICD capacitors are designed specifically for that purpose and are optimized for volume, shape, and resistance. Because energy density at high voltage is the key design criterion, high-density technologies such as wet electrolytics are chosen despite their tendency to be leaky and to require periodic recharges to maintain their performance. Typical high-voltage capacitors have a capacitance of approximately 75 μF and a rating of at least 750 V.

7.2.1.5 High-Voltage Hybrid Circuitry

The high-voltage circuitry in an ICD controls high-voltage pulse duration and polarity, as well as charging the capacitors. The need to reverse the polarity of the pulse during delivery necessitates an H-bridge of high-voltage switching components. The need to charge the capacitors from a miniature battery requires high-voltage DC-to-DC conversion using, for example, a fly-back transformer. In addition to miniaturization and very high reliability, efficiency is a critical consideration, not only because of device longevity but also because all components are sealed inside the body, and excessive heat dissipation would result in tissue damage near the device.

7.2.1.6 Low-Voltage Analog Circuitry

Analog ICD circuitry continuously processes the voltage across the bipolar sensing electrode in contact with the cardiac tissue. This circuitry filters and rectifies the voltage waveform and provides a time series of cardiac depolarizations by comparing the amplitude of the processed voltage signal to a continuously adapting threshold. When the resulting time series is sufficiently fast, the signal is sampled for digital processing and storage. Depending on the configuration of the signal processing path, some of these operations are now performed by digital signal processing (DSP) hardware, in which case the analog components provide anti-alias filtering and sampling.

Most ICDs also monitor other analog signals. Taking regular measurements of the impedance of the lead systems can give early warning of lead failure. Also, there are signals that can augment ICD function. ICD patients often have diseases that limit the response of their heart rate to physical activity. Because virtually all transvenous ICDs are capable of pacing the heart, many ICDs are capable of modulating the pacing rate in response to external cues of activity, such as signals from an accelerometer or changes in impedance associated with respiration.

7.2.1.7 Digital Circuitry

A modern ICD contains a complete digital computing system, including a microprocessor, random-access memory (RAM), read-only memory (ROM), programmable nonvolatile memory (such as flash), and often low-power DSP chips. The most important requirements of this system are ultrahigh reliability and very low-power consumption; therefore, microprocessor bandwidth is usually very small compared to other systems, but the microprocessor generally handles all high-level tasks, including the analysis of the rhythm (determining whether therapy is needed) and sequencing of therapy. It also handles processing and storage of data records capturing device function and detected arrhythmic episodes and communication with external devices by telemetry. Critical functions of the ICD often use code from ROM, but it is increasingly possible to specify device functions in nonvolatile memory or even RAM, allowing sophisticated modification of ICD behavior and even the temporary implementation of research functionality.

Because of the susceptibility of writable memory to corruption, memory that contains critical instructions always has automatic integrity checks. Any evidence of data or code corruption initiates a "power-on reset (POR)" operation, in which the device returns to a "safe" set of parameters and trusted programs. POR operation is designed to ensure safety while providing only minimal sophistication.

7.2.2 Leads

Although intimate electrical contact with heart tissue is not necessary for defibrillator operation [11], direct electrical contact with cardiac tissue facilitates sensing of cardiac activity, especially by avoiding noise associated with skeletal muscle activity, and also reduces the voltage and energy that must be delivered to achieve therapeutic effects. Currently, all approved ICDs require direct electrical contact with heart muscle. This contact is accomplished with "leads," or insulated conducting systems that connect from a header on the ICD generator to electrodes in contact with the heart or vascular blood pool (Figure 7.3).

Cardiac lead systems are either epicardial or transvenous. Transvenous lead systems are introduced through the peripheral veins and routed to the endocardial surface through the superior vena cava and the atrium, which significantly constrains the geometry of the electrodes and the efficiency of energy delivery. Epicardial systems, in which the electrodes are in contact with the outer surface of the heart, historically required thoracic surgery and were therefore largely replaced by less-invasive transvenous electrodes. Modern epicardial systems can be implanted minimally invasively, but are still not commonly used. Epicardial systems generally provide more surface area than transvenous systems and, therefore, require less energy, and so were used in early ICD systems. They are also often used in pediatric patients because the lead system tends to be less distorted as the patient grows.

High-voltage lead systems consist of several components [12,13]. The proximal end has the connectors that make electrical contact to the header block on the ICD. The lead body is composed of insulators and conductors that link the poles of the connector to the pace-sensing electrodes and the one or two high-voltage coil electrodes near the distal end of the lead (Figure 7.4). Lead connectors and ICD headers are standardized so that leads from one manufacturer are fully compatible with ICDs from any manufacturer. The contemporary low-voltage standard (IS-1) uses a single port for the low-voltage bipolar electrode and the contemporary high-voltage standard (DF-1) uses one port for each high-voltage electrode, necessitating a bulky set of connectors and header ports for a single ICD lead. A new, lower profile standard (DF-4) has been developed by an industry task force, based on a quadrapolar lead connector that incorporates two high-voltage circuits and a pace-sense circuit within one connector.

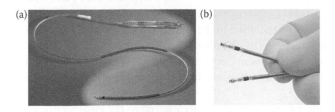

FIGURE 7.3 (a) A dual-coil, true bipolar ICD lead system. (b) Tips of two leads: one active fixation (helix at tip) and one passive fixation (tines at tip). (Reproduced with permission of Medtronic, Inc.)

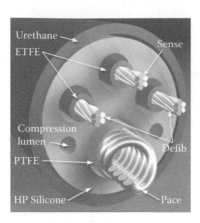

FIGURE 7.4 Transverse section of high-voltage lead body. (Reproduced with permission of Medtronic, Inc.)

The distal end of the lead has electrodes for delivery of defibrillation therapies, delivery of pacing therapies, and sensing of cardiac electrograms (EGMs). The pace-sense electrodes are similar to those in leads for standard implantable pacemakers. "True bipolar" leads have one electrode on the lead tip and a full ring electrode around the circumference of the lead body approximately 1 cm from the tip. "Integrated bipolar" leads have a tip electrode and use the distal high-voltage electrode as the other low-voltage pole. Sensing and pacing can be achieved between the tip and ring electrodes (termed bipolar) or between one of the lead electrodes and the ICD casing (termed unipolar).

Electrodes are constructed of platinum, iridium, titanium, or alloys of these metals. Delivery of high-voltage, high-current defibrillation shocks requires significantly larger surface area; hence, transvenous high-voltage electrodes are designed as exposed coils that spiral along the circumference of the lead and for multiple centimeters of the lead length. The external casing of the ICD itself usually serves as the return electrode in the high-voltage therapy current path, but the return path may also include a second coil electrode on the same lead (dual coil lead), a transvenous coil electrode on an independent lead, or even a nontransvenous, subcutaneous electrode on an independent lead. Although epicardial leads share similar electrode and lead body designs, the electrodes are unconstrained by the requirements for transvenous delivery and typically consist of coil electrodes organized across the surface of a broad patch that can be affixed to the epicardium.

Some older ICD lead bodies were designed with conductors organized as coaxial coils, but in modern ICD leads conductors pass through multiple, parallel lumens enclosed in layers of specialized insulating materials. The conductors are fabricated as cables or multifilar coils or a combination of each, using materials capable of withstanding the continual mechanical stresses without fracture and having low resistance to minimize heating and voltage drops. An alloy of nickel, cobalt, chromium and molybdenum, and MP-35N® is commonly used because of its resistance to fatigue damage, although usually combined with silver to minimize electrical resistance. Modern ICD leads also incorporate materials that slowly release steroid so as to limit the electrical degradation of the lead tissue interface due to inflammatory encapsulation.

Transvenous ICD leads are anchored in the right ventricle by small flexible tines at the lead tip that intertwine in small structures in the chamber ("passive fixation") or by a helix at the lead tip that can be screwed into the myocardial tissue ("active fixation"). The distal defibrillation coil rests within the right ventricle. Dual coil leads are designed such that the proximal coil is positioned in the superior vena cava.

In many ICD systems, pacing and sensing are limited to the right ventricle (single-chamber ICDs), and usually, only a single lead is required. More often, a pace-sense lead is also inserted via the same transvenous route and is fixed in the right atrium (dual-chamber ICD). The right atrial lead provides atrial pacing and sensing and permits the use of more complex dual-chamber tachyarrhythmia sensing, detection, and discrimination algorithms. In triple-chamber or cardiac resynchronization ICDs, a pace-sense lead is also placed in a coronary vein of the left ventricle, to allow independent (though limited) control of left- and right-ventricular depolarization timing.

Although it is tempting to regard them simply as wires, ICD leads are complex medical devices in their own right. The ICD lead must be capable of sensing millivolt-level cardiac electrical activity, delivering low-voltage pacing pulses (occasionally in short-cycle length bursts) and delivering high-voltage, high-current rescue shocks while withstanding the associated thermal and electrical stresses. It must also withstand the significant biochemical stresses to which any implanted medical device is subjected as well as large mechanical stresses imposed by the movement of the arm and upper body and the repetitive mechanical (torsional and bending) stresses associated with implant in or on a beating heart.

7.2.3 Programmer

The automatic behavior of ICDs is controlled by a large number (often more than 100) of adjustable parameters. These parameters allow clinicians to tune arrhythmia detection behaviors, determine the sequences and types of arrhythmia therapies to be delivered, and set the characteristics of brady-cardia pacing. In addition, ICDs often store large amounts of diagnostic data about the device function as well as physiologic parameters such as time-dependent electrical response of the heart and a history of selected arrhythmia episodes. Transfer, modification, and interpretation of this information are traditionally controlled by an external device (a "programmer"), which communicates with the ICD via radio frequency (RF) telemetry (Figure 7.5). Historically, communication between the implanted device and the programmer required placement of a transmitter/receiver unit on the skin in close (a few centimeters) proximity to the location of the implanted device. More recently, with the definition of a dedicated medical devices frequency band, long distance (multiple meters) or "non-contact" telemetry is becoming more widely available. In this way, a clinician can program the function of the device or retrieve diagnostic information from a programmer located in the same room with the patient.

Telemetry communication to and from the implanted device can also be used in the home. In fact, home monitors are available for most ICDs. The home monitor can interrogate a device and provide valuable diagnostic data to clinicians via telephone or Internet uplinks. Although the technology already

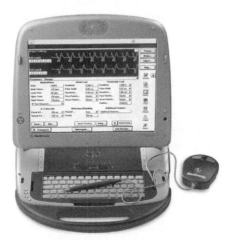

FIGURE 7.5 Programmer with transmitter/receiver unit that is placed in the vicinity of the implanted ICD. Long-range telemetry now eliminates the need for the transmitter/receiver in many ICD systems. (Reproduced with permission of Medtronic, Inc.)

exists to allow it, at this time, due in part to safety concerns, there is limited remote programmability of device parameters permitted.

7.3 Arrhythmia Detection

Arrhythmia detection is and has been a critical area of development for modern ICDs. All ICDs are designed with a bias for overtreatment because the consequence of undertreatment may be death. This was initially relatively unimportant because patients indicated for ICD therapy had already survived multiple episodes of SCD. As indications expand to lower risk groups, however, the risk of overtreatment increases substantially and overtreatment is often unacceptable to otherwise healthy patients at risk for SCD. More sophisticated detection is the primary means for addressing this problem.

The steps that lead from analysis of cardiac rhythm to delivery of ICD therapy can be considered as three distinct subprocesses: sensing, detection, and discrimination. Although the technology is evolving, it is useful to think of *sensing* as primarily a problem in analog signal processing and *detection* as the digital processing of the sensed information. Given that a potentially dangerous tachyarrhythmia is *detected*, the *discrimination* subsystem analyzes aspects of the rhythm to determine whether it can be reliably classified as benign, usually meaning that the arrhythmia is the result of rapid atrial depolarization, and therefore does not significantly degrade cardiac pumping function. The discrimination subsystem can then *withhold* therapy for as long as the rhythm can be classified as benign, although many ICDs include a "high-rate timeout" feature that guarantees therapy delivery (i.e., overrides the discrimination subsystem), after a fixed period of time. Yet, despite advances in detection, the basis of ICD therapy delivery is ventricular rate and duration, just as was the case for the first commercial ICD systems.

7.3.1 Sensing

ICDs continuously monitor the voltage across a bipolar electrode (the near-field EGM). The signal is affected by any nearby electrical activity, including local and distant cardiac activity, activity of skeletal muscles, and external fields such as household power and alternating current motors. In practice, the only aspect of the EGM that is of interest for initial detection of ventricular arrhythmia is associated with local tissue depolarization. This part of the EGM is called the *R-wave*, in analogy to a similar signal on the surface of the electrocardiogram. (Note that dual-chamber ICDs perform similar operations on the atrial EGM.) The purpose of sensing is to reliably identify the timing of the *R*-wave, without being affected by other deflections in the EGM. This has generally been an analog operation, although the incorporation of low-power DSP components has steadily grown and digital operation will soon become the dominant implementation.

Sensing is accomplished through filtering, rectifying, and then thresholding. Filtering effectively isolates the *R*-waves from the other components in the EGM signals. The other cardiac signals, including Ventricular repolarization (*T*-wave), are lower in frequency than the *R*-wave; therefore, most devices use high-pass filtering with cutoff between 10 and 20 Hz. External signals, including skeletal muscle depolarizations and electrical interference are largely common-mode signals, although they are diminished by low-pass filtering. Many ICDs, therefore, use low-pass cutoffs of less than 50 Hz, and most filter below 100 Hz.

After filtering, *R*-waves may be identified by rectification and comparison to a threshold, although a static threshold would be inadequate because the amplitude of filtered *R*-waves is unpredictable. In particular, pathological *R*-waves, which the device must detect to deliver therapy, can change substantially as a result of the pathology. In ventricular fibrillation (VF), the most lethal of ventricular arrhythmias, the *R*-waves can become much smaller than normal and often exhibit high variability.

In practice, this problem is solved by continuous adaptation of either the threshold or the signal gain. The detection sensitivity is lowest (highest threshold) immediately after identification of an *R*-wave, and generally set to a level that would only identify features of similar magnitude. In the absence of further identified activity, the sensitivity increases continuously toward a predefined maximum, ensuring that the largest features in a time-varying signal will be identified.

7.3.2 Detection

ICD detection algorithms primarily rely on the time sequence of *R*-waves determined by the sensing subsystem. It is fundamentally rate based. When the rate of identified *R*-waves is higher than a prespecified threshold, and for a prespecified duration, therapy is presumed to be required unless secondary considerations classify the tachycardia as benign.

7.3.3 Discrimination

Tachycardias are generally classified as ventricular or supraventricular. Ventricular tachycardia (VT) is due to primary ventricular dysfunction and is often acutely dangerous. Supraventricular tachycardia (SVT) is almost never immediately dangerous and does not necessarily respond to ICD therapy; hence, the treatment of SVT by an ICD is generally considered undesirable. The discrimination subsystem identifies rhythms that are sufficiently fast to treat (tachycardia), but are not ventricular in origin (SVT). Again, the bias of the device is to overtreat because the erroneous treatment of SVT is considered preferable to failure to treat a potentially lethal Ventricular.

Discrimination can be pattern based, morphology based, or a combination of the two approaches. In pattern-based discrimination, specific features of the time sequence of events are used to classify the rhythm as SVT. The patterns indicative of SVT include timing irregularity (unless all R-R intervals are shorter than a fixed cutoff), gradual acceleration of the R-R intervals, or, in dual-chamber ICDs, certain specific relationships between the timing of atrial and ventricular events.

Morphology-based discrimination uses the shape of the *R*-wave to identify SVT. SVT, like normal cardiac rhythm, uses the specialized cardiac conduction system to depolarize the ventricle. Therefore, there is a characteristic *R*-wave morphology that is preserved in SVT but not in Ventricular. Morphology analysis is most informative when it samples large regions of the heart; therefore, it usually makes use of the vector between the high-voltage electrodes, unlike sensing, which uses the low-voltage electrodes. It also requires a method for storing the characteristics of the normal morphology. The storage system can be as simple as a characteristic *R*-wave width or may include many components of the morphology using a system such as wavelet decomposition.

7.4 Arrhythmia Therapy

Modern ICDs provide low- and high-voltage therapy that can support the cardiac rhythm when the heart is beating too slowly (bradycardia) or when the electrical rhythm becomes uncontrolled and too fast (tachycardia).

7.4.1 Bradycardia Therapy

Bradycardia therapy in a modern ICD is virtually indistinguishable from that in a modern pacemaker. All ICDs are capable of ventricular demand pacing at adjustable rates and many are capable of rate-responsive pacing, in which the rate of pacing is modulated by external activity cues such as accelerometer signals or measured respiration rate. Dual-chamber ICDs have the same pacing capabilities as dual-chamber pacemakers, providing rate-responsive pacing in the atrium and ventricle, as well as coordinated AV pacing. Triple-chamber or cardiac resynchronization therapy ICDs can stimulate the ventricles independently to improve pumping function when the specialized ventricular conduction system is damaged.

7.4.2 High-Voltage Antitachycardia Therapy

Ventricular tachycardia (VT) is the result of uncontrolled electrical activity in the ventricle. This activity may be coordinated or uncoordinated. The definitive therapy for Ventricular is external stimulation by an electric field sufficiently large to reset the electrical activity of most ventricular cells. This ends the previous (uncontrolled) electrical activity and allows the reestablishment of normal cardiac activity. As explained earlier, this requires depolarization of a "critical mass" of tissue by a high-voltage discharge. When high-voltage therapy is delivered, an attempt is made to synchronize the delivery with a detected *R*-wave. A synchronized shock is termed "cardioversion," whereas an unsynchronized shock is termed "defibrillation" because VF has no coherent electrical activity, and therefore no basis for synchronization (Figure 7.6).

7.4.3 Low-Voltage Antitachycardia Therapy

Although high-voltage therapy is highly effective, it can be an unpleasant experience to the patient and also requires significant energy from the battery. Studies have shown that most Ventricular occurring in patients with ICDs is monomorphic, meaning that ventricular electrical activity, although uncontrolled, is still coordinated [14,15]. The same studies have shown that as many as 75% of these episodes can be terminated by overdrive pacing, termed "antitachycardia pacing (ATP)" (Figure 7.7). The exact timing of the ATP pulses seems to be a significant factor in ATP efficacy and many timing algorithms are available in ICDs. The most commonly used algorithms are "burst" ATP, in which a fixed number of pacing pulses are delivered at a constant fraction of the Ventricular cycle length, and "ramp," or "scan" ATP, in which the interval between pulses is decreased by a specified amount for each pulse. More complex algorithms for ATP have been studied, including combinations of burst and ramp, and methods for choosing the ideal ATP parameters automatically. As yet, nothing has proven to be superior to the delivery of eight pulses at 88% of the Ventricular cycle length [16].

7.5 Diagnostics and Monitoring

Due to memory and energy limitations, early ICDs had limited capability for recording diagnostic data. Today, all ICDs provide some capability for recording of cardiac EGMs and of counters that provide a history of ventricular arrhythmic events and therapies delivered. These data are clinically valuable for determining the appropriateness of device detection and therapy settings. The devices typically supplement the EGM data with simultaneous information about beat-to-beat device function in a "marker channel" (Figures 7.6 and 7.7). Devices also report on battery status to provide early warning for elective device replacement and continuously monitor lead integrity.

An implanted device also offers a unique opportunity for continuous ambulatory collection and trending of physiologic information. Today's devices can provide a history of the incidence and duration of atrial arrhythmias, track heart rate 24 hours/day, and provide estimates of heart rate variability on a daily basis (Figure 7.8). In addition, many devices are equipped with accelerometers that can be used to estimate and track patient activity [17,18]. Other devices track the impedance between electrodes and the ICD housing as a measure of fluid volume in the chest that can be useful in the management of patients with heart failure [19,20]. The addition of implanted sensors to ICDs promises to offer new opportunities for providing important clinical information.

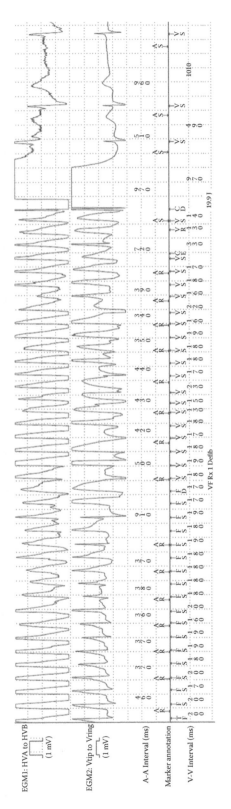

FIGURE 7.6   Record stored by an ICD of successful delivery of a defibrillation. An atrial EGM, (top tracing), ventricular electrogram (middle tracing), and ICD marker channel are shown. Markers include ventricular sense (VS), atrial sense (AS), ventricular pace (VP), atrial pace (AP), end of ICD capacitor charge (CE), and delivery of shock (CD). (Reproduced with permission of Medtronic, Inc.)

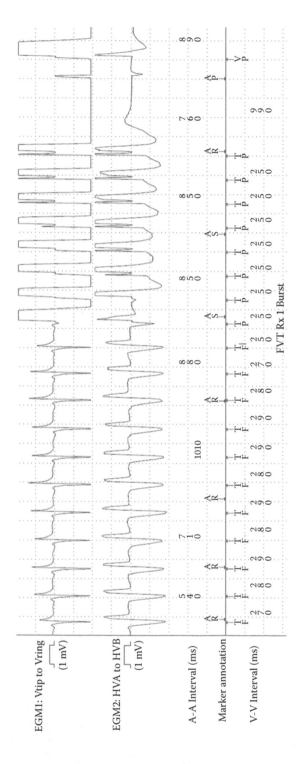

FIGURE 7.7 Stored record of successful delivery of ATP. An atrial EGM (top tracing), ventricular electrogram (middle tracing), and ICD marker channel are shown. TS markers indicate sensing of tachyarrhythmia beats, TP markers indicate delivery of ATP, and VS marker indicates sensing of a normally timed ventricular beat. (Reproduced with permission of Medtronic, Inc.)

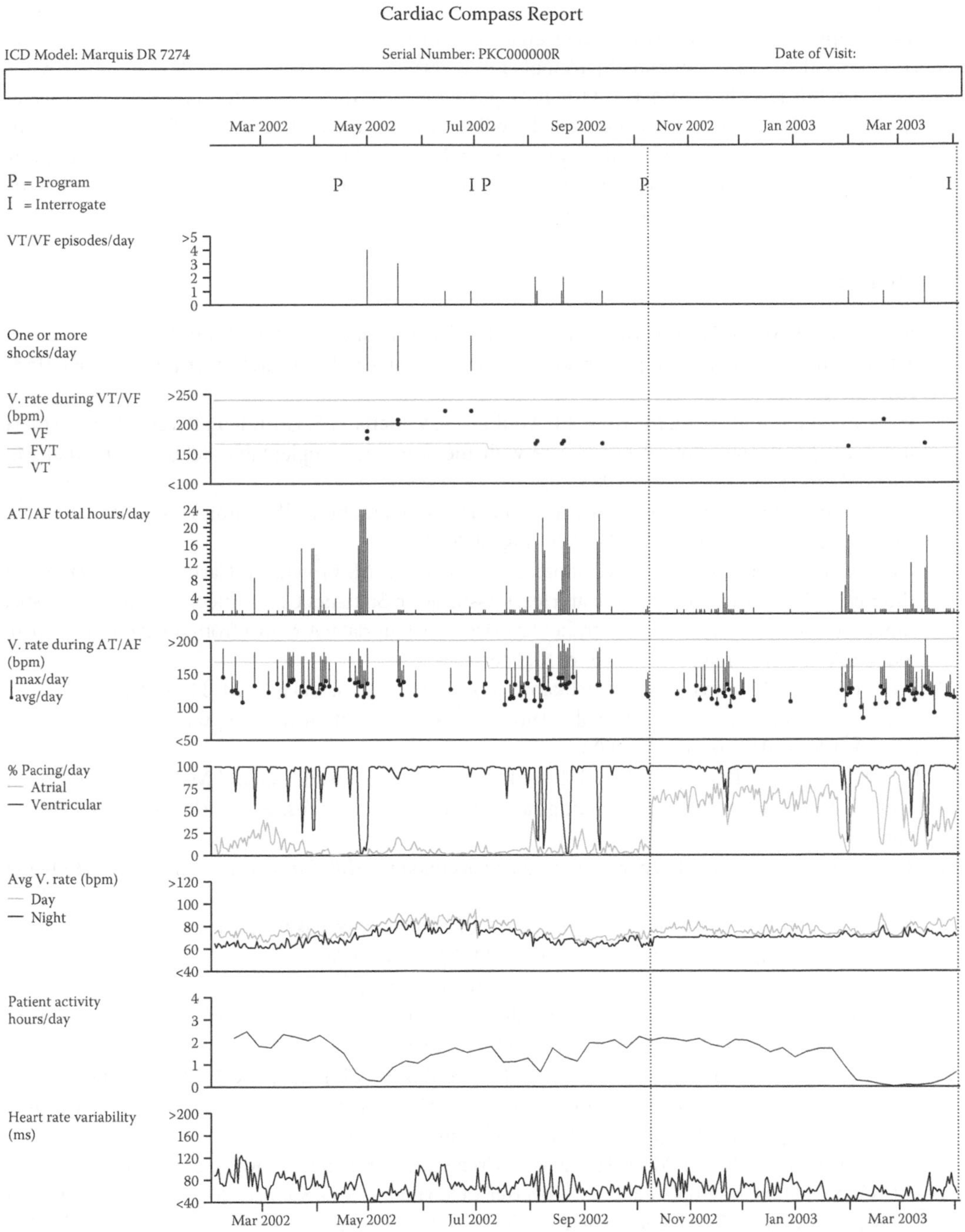

FIGURE 7.8 A diagnostics report issued from an ICD based on stored data. (Reproduced with permission of Medtronic, Inc.)

7.6 Conclusion

The ICD is an established therapy for patients at risk of life-threatening ventricular arrhythmias. It is a complex medical device that incorporates many advances in low-energy electronics and biomaterials.

To date, it is one of the few therapies proven to extend life in patients at risk of SCD and is the only effective therapy for patients who experience an episode of SCD. Beyond this fundamental therapy, the modern ICD is also a fully functional pacemaker and cardiac resynchronization device and provides diagnostic capabilities. The future use of the ICD, particularly in the large fraction of patients who currently do not survive their first episode of SCD will depend on reducing the cost of manufacture and implantation, increasing reliability and longevity, reducing undesirable device side effects such as painful or inappropriate high-voltage therapy, and extending diagnostic capabilities to increase the usefulness of the ICD in the management of patients.

References

1. M. Mirowski, M. M. Mower, W. S. Staewen, B. Tabatznik, and A. I. Mendeloff. Standby automatic defibrillator. An approach to prevention of sudden coronary death. *Arch Intern Med*, 126(1):158–161, July 1970.
2. M. Mirowski, P. R. Reid, M. M. Mower, L. Watkins, E. V. Platia, L. S. Griffith, E. P. Veltri, T. Guarnieri, and J. M. Juanteguy. Clinical experience with the automatic implantable defibrillator. *Arch Mal Coeur Vaiss*, 78:39–42, October 1985.
3. A. J. Camm and S. Nisam. European utilization of the implantable defibrillator: Has 10 years changed the enigma? *Europace*, 12(8):1063–1069, August 2010.
4. Writing Group Members, D. Lloyd-Jones, R. J. Adams, T. M. Brown, M. Carnethon, S. Dai, G. D. Simone, T. B. Ferguson et al. American Heart Association Statistics Committee, and Stroke Statistics Subcommittee. Heart disease and stroke statistics—2010 update: A report from the American Heart Association. *Circulation*, 121(7):e46–e215, February 2010.
5. J. E. Poole, G. W. Johnson, A. S. Hellkamp, J. Anderson, D. J. Callans, M. H. Raitt, R. K. Reddy et al. Prognostic importance of defibrillator shocks in patients with heart failure. *N Engl J Med*, 359(10):1009–1017, September 2008.
6. S. R. Shorofsky, E. Rashba, W. Havel, P. Belk, P. Degroot, C. Swerdlow, and M. R. Gold. Improved defibrillation efficacy with an ascending ramp waveform in humans. *Heart Rhythm*, 2(4):388–394, April 2005.
7. R. D. Klafter. An optimally energized cardiac pacemaker. *IEEE Trans Biomed Eng*, 20(5):350–356, September 1973.
8. R. D. Klafter and L. Hrebien. An *in vivo* study of cardiac pacemaker optimization by pulse shape modification. *IEEE Trans Biomed Eng*, 23(3):233–239, May 1976.
9. S. Saksena, H. An, R. Mehra, P. DeGroot, R. B. Krol, E. Burkhardt, D. Mehta, and T. John. Prospective comparison of biphasic and monophasic shocks for implantable cardioverter-defibrillators using endocardial leads. *Am J Cardiol*, 70(3):304–310, August 1992.
10. M. O. Sweeney, A. Natale, K. J. Volosin, C. D. Swerdlow, J. H. Baker, and P. Degroot. Prospective randomized comparison of 50%/50% versus 65%/65% tilt biphasic waveform on defibrillation in humans. *Pacing Clin Electrophysiol*, 24(1):60–65, January 2001.
11. G. H. Bardy, W. M. Smith, M. A. Hood, I. G. Crozier, I. C. Melton, L. Jordaens, D. Theuns et al. An entirely subcutaneous implantable cardioverter-defibrillator. *N Engl J Med*, 363(1):36–44, May 2010.
12. G. Kalahasty and K. A. Ellenbogen. *ICD Lead Design*, pp. 239–263. Cardiotext Publishing, Minneapolis, MN, 2010.
13. H. M. Haqqani and H. G. Mond. The implantable cardioverter-defibrillator lead: Principles, progress, and promises. *Pacing Clin Electrophysiol*, 32(10):1336–1353, October 2009.
14. M. S. Wathen, P. J. DeGroot, M. O. Sweeney, A. J. Stark, M. F. Otterness, W. O. Adkisson, R. C. Canby et al. Rx II investigators. Prospective randomized multicenter trial of empirical antitachycardia pacing versus shocks for spontaneous rapid ventricular tachycardia in patients with implantable cardioverter-defibrillators: Pacing fast ventricular tachycardia reduces shock therapies (pain-free Rx II) trial results. *Circulation*, 110(17):2591–2596, October 2004.

15. M. S. Wathen, M. O. Sweeney, P. J. DeGroot, A. J. Stark, J. L. Koehler, M. B. Chisner, C. Machado, and W. O. Adkisson. Shock reduction using antitachycardia pacing for spontaneous rapid ventricular tachycardia in patients with coronary artery disease. *Circulation*, 104(7):796–801, August 2001.

16. B. L. Wilkoff, K. T. Ousdigian, L. D. Sterns, Z. J. Wang, R. D. Wilson, and J. M. Morgan. A comparison of empiric to physician-tailored programming of implantable cardioverter-defibrillators: Results from the prospective randomized multicenter empiric trial. *J Am Coll Cardiol*, 48(2):330–339, 2006.

17. R. Germany and C. Murray. Use of device diagnostics in the outpatient management of heart failure. *Am J Cardiol*, 99(10A):11G–16G, May 2007.

18. A. Gardini, P. Lupo, E. Zanelli, S. Bisetti, and R. Cappato. Diagnostic capabilities of devices for cardiac resynchronization therapy. *J Cardiovasc Med (Hagerstown)*, 11(3):186–189, March 2010.

19. R. Germany. The use of device-based diagnostics to manage patients with heart failure. *Congest Heart Fail*, 14(5 Suppl 2):19–24, 2008.

20. D. J. Whellan, K. T. Ousdigian, S. M. Al-Khatib, W. Pu, S. Sarkar, C. B. Porter, B. B. Pavri, C. M. O'Connor, and Partners study investigators. Combined heart failure device diagnostics identify patients at higher risk of subsequent heart failure hospitalizations: Results from partners HF (program to access and review trending information and evaluate correlation to symptoms in patients with heart failure) study. *J Am Coll Cardiol*, 55(17):1803–1810, April 2010.

8

Implantable Stimulators for Neuromuscular Control

Primoz Strojnik
Case Western Reserve University

P. Hunter Peckham
Case Western Reserve University

8.1 Functional Electrical Stimulation

Implantable stimulators for neuromuscular control are the technologically most advanced versions of functional electrical stimulators. Their function is to generate contraction of muscles, which cannot be controlled volitionally because of the damage or dysfunction in the neural paths of the central nervous system (CNS). Their operation is based on the electrical nature of conducting information within nerve fibers, from the neuron cell body (soma), along the axon, where a traveling action potential is the carrier of excitation. While the action potential is naturally generated chemically in the head of the axon, it may also be generated artificially by depolarizing the neuron membrane with an electrical pulse. A train of electrical impulses with certain amplitude, width, and repetition rate, applied to a muscle innervating nerve (a motor neuron) will cause the muscle to contract, very much like in natural excitation. Similarly, a train of electrical pulses applied to the muscular tissue close to the motor point will cause muscle contraction by stimulating the muscle through the neural structures at the motor point.

8.2 Technology for Delivering Stimulation Pulses to Excitable Tissue

A practical system used to stimulate a nerve consists of three components (1) a *pulse generator* to generate a train of pulses capable of depolarizing the nerve, (2) a *lead wire*, the function of which is to deliver the pulses to the stimulation site, and (3) an *electrode*, which delivers the stimulation pulses to the excitable tissue in a safe and efficient manner.

In terms of location of the above three components of an electrical stimulator, stimulation technology can be described in the following terms:

Surface or transcutaneous stimulation, where all three components are outside the body and the electrodes are placed on the skin above or near the motor point of the muscle to be stimulated. This method has been used extensively in medical rehabilitation of nerve and muscle. Therapeutically, it has been used to prevent atrophy of paralyzed muscles, to condition paralyzed muscles before the application of functional stimulation, and to generally increase the muscle bulk. As a functional tool, it has been used in rehabilitation of plegic and paretic patients. Surface systems for functional stimulation have been developed to correct drop-foot condition in hemiplegic individuals (Liberson et al., 1961), for hand control (Rebersek and Vodovnik, 1973), and for standing and stepping in individuals with *paralysis* of the lower extremities (Kralj and Bajd, 1989). This fundamental technology was commercialized by Sigmedics, Inc. (Graupe and Kohn, 1998). The inability of surface stimulation to reliably excite the underlying tissue in a repeatable manner and to selectively stimulate deep muscles has limited the clinical applicability of surface stimulation.

Percutaneous stimulation employs electrodes which are positioned inside the body close to the structures to be stimulated. Their lead wires permanently penetrate the skin to be connected to the external pulse generator. State of the art embodiments of percutaneous electrodes utilize a small-diameter insulated stainless steel lead that is passed through the skin. The electrode structure is formed by removal of the insulation from the lead and subsequent modification to ensure stability within the tissue. This modification includes forming barbs or similar anchoring mechanisms. The percutaneous electrode is implanted using a hypodermic needle as a trochar for introduction. As the needle is withdrawn, the anchor at the electrode tip is engaged into the surrounding tissue and remains in the tissue. A connector at the skin surface, next to the skin penetration point, joins the percutaneous electrode lead to the hardwired external stimulator. The penetration site has to be maintained and care must be taken to avoid physical damage of the lead wires. In the past, this technology has helped develop the existing implantable systems, and it may be used for short and long term, albeit not permanent, stimulation applications (Marsolais and Kobetic, 1986; Memberg et al., 1993).

The term *implantable stimulation* refers to stimulation systems in which all three components, pulse generator, lead wires, and electrodes, are permanently surgically implanted into the body and the skin is solidly closed after the implantation procedure. Any interaction between the implantable part and the outside world is performed using telemetry principles in a contact-less fashion. This chapter is focused on implantable neuromuscular stimulators, which will be discussed in more detail.

8.3 Stimulation Parameters

In functional *electrical stimulation*, the typical stimulation waveform is a train of rectangular pulses. This shape is used because of its effectiveness as well as relative ease of generation. All three parameters of a stimulation train, that is, frequency, amplitude, and pulse-width, have effect on muscle contraction. Generally, the stimulation frequency is kept as low as possible, to prevent muscle fatigue and to conserve stimulation energy. The determining factor is the muscle fusion frequency at which a smooth muscle response is obtained. This frequency varies; however, it can be as low as 12–14 Hz and as high as 50 Hz. In most cases, the stimulation frequency is kept constant for a certain application. This is true both for surface as well as implanted electrodes.

With surface electrodes, the common way of modulating muscle force is by varying the stimulation pulse amplitude at a constant frequency and pulse-width. The stimulation amplitudes may be as low as 25 V at 200 μs for the stimulation of the peroneal nerve and as high as 120 V or more at 300 μs for activation of large muscles such as the gluteus maximus.

In implantable stimulators and electrodes, the stimulation parameters greatly depend on the implantation site. When the electrodes are positioned on or around the target nerve, the stimulation amplitudes are on the order of a few milliamperes or less. Electrodes positioned on the muscle surface (epimysial electrodes) or in the muscle itself (intramuscular electrodes), employ up to ten times higher amplitudes. For muscle force control, implantable stimulators rely either on pulse-width modulation or amplitude modulation. For example, in upper extremity applications, the current amplitude is usually a fixed parameter set to 16 or 20 mA, while the muscle force is modulated with pulse widths within 0–200 μs.

8.4 Implantable Neuromuscular Stimulators

Implantable stimulation systems use an encapsulated pulse generator that is surgically implanted and has subcutaneous leads that terminate at electrodes on or near the desired nerves. In low power consumption applications such as the cardiac pacemaker, a primary battery power source is included in the pulse generator case. When the battery is close to depletion, the pulse generator has to be surgically replaced.

Most implantable systems for neuromuscular application consist of an external and an implanted component. Between the two, an inductive radio-frequency link is established, consisting of two tightly coupled resonant coils. The link allows transmission of power and information, through the skin, from the external device to the implanted pulse generator. In more advanced systems, a back-telemetry link is also established, allowing transmission of data outwards, from the implanted to the external component.

Ideally, implantable stimulators for neuromuscular control would be stand alone, totally implanted devices with an internal power source and integrated sensors detecting desired movements from the motor cortex and delivering stimulation sequences to appropriate muscles, thus bypassing the neural damage. At the present developmental stage, they still need a control source and an external controller to provide power and stimulation information. The control source may be either operator driven, controlled by the user, or triggered by an event such as the heel-strike phase of the gait cycle. Figure 8.1 depicts a neuromuscular prosthesis developed at the Case Western Reserve University (CWRU) and Cleveland Veterans Affairs Medical Center for the restoration of hand functions using an implantable

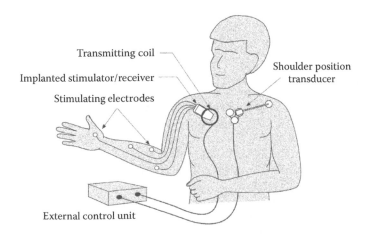

Transmitting coil

Implanted stimulator/receiver

Stimulating electrodes

Shoulder position transducer

External control unit

FIGURE 8.1 Implanted FES hand grasp system.

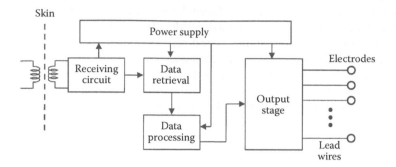

FIGURE 8.2   Block diagram of an implantable neuromuscular stimulator.

neuromuscular stimulator. In this application, the patient uses the shoulder motion to control opening and closing of the hand.

The internal electronic structure of an implantable neuromuscular stimulator is shown in Figure 8.2. It consists of receiving and data retrieval circuits, power supply, data processing circuits, and output stages.

8.4.1 Receiving Circuit

The stimulator's receiving circuit is an LC circuit tuned to the resonating frequency of the external transmitter, followed by a rectifier. Its task is to provide the raw DC power from the received rf signal and at the same time allow extraction of stimulation information embedded in the rf carrier. There are various encoding schemes allowing simultaneous transmission of power and information into an implantable electronic device. They include amplitude and frequency modulation with different modulation indexes as well as different versions of digital encoding such as Manchester encoding where the information is hidden in a logic value transition position rather than the logic value itself. Synchronous and asynchronous clock signals may be extracted from the modulated carrier to drive the implant's logic circuits.

The use of radiofrequency transmission for medical devices is regulated and in most countries limited to certain frequencies and radiation powers. (In the United States, the use of the rf space is regulated by the Federal Communication Commission [FCC].) Limited rf transmission powers as well as conservation of power in battery operated external controllers dictate high coupling efficiencies between the transmitting and receiving antennas. Optimal coupling parameters cannot be uniformly defined; they depend on application particularities and design strategies.

8.4.2 Power Supply

The amount of power delivered into an implanted electronic package depends on the coupling between the transmitting and the receiving coil. The coupling is dependent on the distance as well as the alignment between the coils. The power supply circuits must compensate for the variations in distance for different users as well as for the alignment variations due to skin movements and consequent changes in relative coil-to-coil position during daily usage. The power dissipated on power supply circuits must not raise the overall implant case temperature.

In implantable stimulators that require stimulation voltages in excess of the electronics power supply voltages (20–30 V), the stimulation voltage can be provided directly through the receiving coil. In that case, voltage regulators must be used to provide the electronics supply voltage (usually 5 V), which heavily taxes the external power transmitter and increases the implant internal power dissipation.

8.4.3 Data Retrieval

Data retrieval technique depends on the data-encoding scheme and is closely related to power supply circuits and implant power consumption. Most commonly, amplitude modulation is used to encode the in-going data stream. As the high quality factor of resonant LC circuits increases the efficiency of power transmission, it also effectively reduces the transmission bandwidth and therefore the transmission data rate. Also, high quality circuits are difficult to amplitude modulate since they tend to continue oscillating even with power removed. This has to be taken into account when designing the communication link in particular for the start-up situation when the implanted device does not use the power for stimulation and therefore loads the transmitter side less heavily, resulting in narrower and higher resonant curves. The load on the receiving coil may also affect the low pass filtering of the received rf signal.

Modulation index (m) or depth of modulation affects the overall energy transfer into the implant. At a given rf signal amplitude, less energy is transferred into the implanted device when 100% modulation is used ($m = 1$) as compared to 10% modulation ($m = 0.053$). However, retrieval of 100% modulated signal is much easier than retrieval of a 10% modulated signal.

8.4.4 Data Processing

Once the information signal has been satisfactorily retrieved and reconstructed into logic voltage levels, it is ready for logic processing. For synchronous data processing a clock signal is required. It can be generated locally within the implant device, reconstructed from the incoming data stream, or can be derived from the rf carrier. A crystal has to be used with a local oscillator to assure stable clock frequency. Local oscillator allows for asynchronous data transmission. Synchronous transmission is best achieved using Manchester data encoding. Decoding of Manchester encoded data recovers the original clock signal, which was used during data encoding. Another method is using the downscaled rf carrier signal as the clock source. In this case, the information signal has to be synchronized with the rf carrier. Of course, 100% modulation scheme cannot be used with carrier-based clock signal. Complex command structure used in multichannel stimulators requires intensive data decoding and processing and consequently extensive electronic circuitry. Custom-made, application specific circuits (ASIC) are commonly used to minimize the space requirements and optimize the circuit performance.

8.4.5 Output Stage

The output stage forms stimulation pulses and defines their electrical characteristics. Even though a mere rectangular pulse can depolarize a nervous membrane, such pulses are not used in clinical practice due to their noxious effect on the tissue and *stimulating electrodes*. These effects can be significantly reduced by charge balanced stimulating pulses where the cathodic stimulation pulse is followed by an anodic pulse containing the same electrical charge, which reverses the electrochemical effects of the cathodic pulse. Charge balanced waveforms can be assured by capacitive coupling between the pulse generator and stimulation electrodes. Charge balanced stimulation pulses include symmetrical and asymmetrical waveforms with anodic phase immediately following the cathodic pulse or being delayed by a short, 20–60 μs interval.

The output stages of most implantable neuromuscular stimulators have constant current characteristics, meaning that the output current is independent on the electrode or tissue impedance. Practically, the constant current characteristics ensure that the same current flows through the excitable tissues regardless of the changes that may occur on the electrode–tissue interface, such as the growth of fibrous tissue around the electrodes. Constant current output stage can deliver constant current only within the supply voltage–compliance voltage. In neuromuscular stimulation, with the electrode impedance being on the order of 1 kΩ, and the stimulating currents in the order of 20 mA, the compliance voltage must be above 20 V. Considering the voltage drops and losses across electronic components, the compliance voltage of the output stage may have to be as high as 33 V.

The stimulus may be applied through either monopolar or bipolar electrodes. The monopolar electrode is one in which a single active electrode is placed near the excitable nerve and the return electrode is placed remotely, generally at the implantable unit itself. Bipolar electrodes are placed at the stimulation site, thus limiting the current paths to the area between the electrodes. Generally, in monopolar stimulation the active electrode is much smaller than the return electrode, while bipolar electrodes are the same size.

8.5 Packaging of Implantable Electronics

Electronic circuits must be protected from the harsh environment of the human body. The packaging of implantable electronics uses various materials, including polymers, metals, and ceramics. The encapsulation method depends somewhat on the electronic circuit technology. Older devices may still use discrete components in a classical form, such as leaded transistors and resistors. The newer designs, depending on the sophistication of the implanted device, may employ application-specific integrated circuits (ASICs) and thick film hybrid circuitry for their implementation. Such circuits place considerable requirements for hermeticity and protection on the implanted circuit packaging.

Epoxy encapsulation was the original choice of designers of implantable neuromuscular stimulators. It has been successfully used with relatively simple circuits using discrete, low impedance components. With epoxy encapsulation, the receiving coil is placed around the circuitry to be "potted" in a mold, which gives the implant the final shape. Additionally, the epoxy body is coated with silicone rubber that improves the *biocompatibility* of the package. Polymers do not provide an impermeable barrier and therefore cannot be used for encapsulation of high density, high impedance electronic circuits. The moisture ingress ultimately will reach the electronic components, and surface ions can allow electric shorting and degradation of leakage-sensitive circuitry and subsequent failure.

Hermetic packaging provides the implant electronic circuitry with a long-term protection from the ingress of body fluids. Materials that provide hermetic barriers are metals, ceramics, and glasses. Metallic packaging generally uses a titanium capsule machined from a solid piece of metal or deep-drawn from a piece of sheet metal. Electrical signals, such as power and stimulation, enter and exit the package through hermetic feedthroughs, which are hermetically welded onto the package walls. The *feedthrough* assembly utilizes a ceramic or glass insulator to allow one or more wires to exit the package without contact with the package itself. During the assembly procedures, the electronic circuitry is placed in the package and connected internally to the feedthroughs, and the package is then welded closed. Tungsten Inert Gas (TIG), electron beam, or laser welding equipment is used for the final closure. Assuming integrity of all components, hermeticity with this package is ensured. This integrity can be checked by detecting gas leakage from the capsule. Metallic packaging requires that the receiving coil be placed outside the package to avoid significant loss of rf signal or power, thus requiring additional space within the body to accommodate the volume of the entire implant. Generally, the hermetic package and the receiving antenna are jointly embedded in an epoxy encapsulant, which provides electric isolation for the metallic antenna and stabilizes the entire implant assembly. Figure 8.3 shows such an implantable stimulator designed and made by the CWRU/Veterans Administration Program. The hermetic package is open, displaying the electronic *hybrid circuit*. More recently, alumina-based ceramic packages have been developed that allow hermetic sealing of the electronic circuitry together with enclosure of the receiving coil (Strojnik et al., 1994). This is possible due to the rf transparency of ceramics. The impact of this type of enclosure is still not fully investigated. The advantage of this approach is that the volume of the implant can be reduced, thus minimizing the biologic response, which is a function of volume. Yet, an unexplored issue of this packaging method is the effect of powerful electromagnetic fields on the implant circuits, lacking the protection of the metal enclosure. This is a particular concern with high gain (EMG, ENG, or EKG sensing) amplifiers, which in the future may be included in the implant

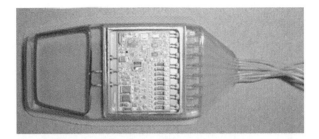

FIGURE 8.3 Photograph of a multichannel implantable stimulator telemeter. Hybrid circuit in titanium package is shown exposed. Receiving coil (left) is embedded in epoxy resin together with titanium case. Double feedthroughs are seen penetrating titanium capsule wall on the right.

package as part of back-telemetry circuits. Physical strength of ceramic packages and their resistance to impact will also require future investigation.

8.6 Leads and Electrodes

Leads connect the pulse generator to the electrodes. They must be sufficiently flexible to move across the joints while at the same time sufficiently sturdy to last for the decades of the intended life of the device. They must also be stretchable to allow change of distance between the pulse generator and the electrodes, associated with body movements. Ability to flex and to stretch is achieved by coiling the lead conductor into a helix and inserting the helix into a small-diameter silicone tubing. This way, both flexing movements and stretching forces exerted on the lead are attenuated, while translated into torsion movements and forces exerted on the coiled conductor. Using multi-strand rather than solid conductors further enhances the longevity. Several individually insulated multi-strand conductors can be coiled together, thus forming a multiple conductor lead wire. Most lead configurations include a connector at some point between the implant and the terminal electrode, allowing for replacement of the implanted receiver or leads in the event of failure. The connectors used have been either single pin in-line connectors located somewhere along the lead length or a multiport/multilead connector at the implant itself. Materials used for lead wires are stainless steels, MP35N (Co, Cr, Ni alloy), and noble metals and their alloys.

Electrodes deliver electrical charge to the stimulated tissues. Those placed on the muscle surface are called epimysial, while those inserted into the muscles are called intramuscular. Nerve stimulating electrodes are called epineural when placed against the nerve, or cuff electrodes when they encircle the nerve. Nerve electrodes may embrace the nerve in a spiral manner individually, or in an array configuration. Some implantable stimulation systems merely use exposed lead-wire conductor sutured to the epineurium as the electrode. Generally, nerve electrodes require approximately one-tenth of the energy for muscle activation as compared to muscle electrodes. However, they require more extensive surgery and may be less selective, but the potential for neural damage is greater than, for example, nerve encircling electrodes.

Electrodes are made of corrosion resistant materials, such as noble metals (platinum or iridium) and their alloys. For example, a platinum–iridium alloy consisting of 10% iridium and 90% platinum is commonly used as an electrode material. Epimysial electrodes developed at CWRU use Ø4 mm Pt90Ir10 discs placed on Dacron reinforced silicone backing. CWRU intramuscular electrodes employ a stainless steel lead-wire with the distal end de-insulated and configured into an electrode tip. A small, umbrella-like anchoring barb is attached to it. With this arrangement, the diameter of the electrode tip does not differ much from the lead wire diameter and this electrode can be introduced into a deep muscle with a trochar-like insertion tool. Figure 8.4 shows enlarged views of these electrodes.

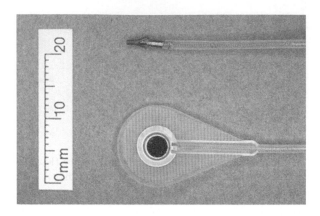

FIGURE 8.4 Implantable electrodes with attached lead wires. Intramuscular electrode (top) has stainless steel tip and anchoring barbs. Epimysial electrode has PtIr disk in the center and is backed by silicone-impregnated Dacron mesh.

8.7 Safety Issues of Implantable Stimulators

The targeted lifetime of implantable stimulators for neuromuscular control is the lifetime of their users, which is measured in tens of years. Resistance to premature failure must be assured by manufacturing processes and testing procedures. Appropriate materials must be selected that will withstand the working environment. Protection against mechanical and electrical hazards that may be encountered during the device lifetime must be incorporated in the design. Various procedures are followed and rigorous tests must be performed during and after its manufacturing to assure the quality and reliability of the device.

- *Manufacturing and testing*—Production of implantable electronic circuits and their encapsulation in many instances falls under the standards governing production and encapsulation of integrated circuits. To minimize the possibility of failure, the implantable electronic devices are manufactured in controlled clean-room environments, using high quality components and strictly defined manufacturing procedures. Finished devices are submitted to rigorous testing before being released for implantation. Also, many tests are carried out during the manufacturing process itself. To assure maximum reliability and product confidence, methods, tests, and procedures defined by military standards, such as MILSTD-883, are followed.
- *Bio-compatibility*—Since the implantable stimulators are surgically implanted in living tissue, an important part of their design has to be dedicated to biocompatibility, that is, their ability to dwell in living tissue without disrupting the tissue in its functions, creating adverse tissue response, or changing its own properties due to the tissue environment. Elements of biocompatibility include tissue reaction to materials, shape, and size, as well as electrochemical reactions on stimulation electrodes. There are known biomaterials used in the making of implantable stimulators. They include stainless steels, titanium and tantalum, noble metals such as platinum and iridium, as well as implantable grades of selected epoxy and silicone-based materials.
- *Susceptibility to electromagnetic interference (EMI) and electrostatic discharge (ESD)*—Electromagnetic fields can disrupt the operation of electronic devices, which may be lethal in situations with life support systems, but they may also impose risk and danger to users of neuromuscular stimulators. Emissions of EMI may come from outside sources; however, the external control unit is also a source of electromagnetic radiation. Electrostatic discharge shocks are not uncommon during the dry winter season. These shocks may reach voltages as high as 15 kV and more. Sensitive electronic components can easily be damaged by these shocks unless protective

design measures are taken. The electronic circuitry in implantable stimulators is generally protected by the metal case. However, the circuitry can be damaged through the feedthroughs either by handling or during the implantation procedure by the electrocautery equipment. ESD damage may happen even after implantation when long lead-wires are utilized. There are no standards directed specifically towards implantable electronic devices. The general standards put in place for electromedical equipment by the International Electrotechnical Commission provide guidance. The specifications require survival after 3 and 8 kV ESD discharges on all conductive and nonconductive accessible parts, respectively.

8.8 Implantable Stimulators in Clinical Use

8.8.1 Peripheral Nerve Stimulators

- *Manipulation*—Control of complex functions for movement, such as hand control, requires the use of many channels of stimulation. At the Case Western Reserve University and Cleveland VAMC, an eight-channel stimulator has been developed for grasp and release (Smith et al., 1987). This system uses eight channels of stimulation and a titanium-packaged, thick-film hybrid circuit as the pulse generator. The implant is distributed by the Neurocontrol Corporation (Cleveland, OH) under the name of Freehand®. It has been implanted in approximately 150 patients in the United States, Europe, Asia, and Australia. The implant is controlled by a dual-microprocessor external unit carried by the patient with an input control signal provided by the user's remaining volitional movement. Activation of the muscles provides two primary grasp patterns and allows the person to achieve functional performance that exceeds his or her capabilities without the use of the implanted system. This system received pre-market approval from the FDA in 1998.
- *Locomotion*—The first implantable stimulators were designed and implanted for the correction of the foot drop condition in hemiplegic patients. Medtronic's Neuromuscular Assist (NMA) device consisted of an rf receiver implanted in the inner thigh and connected to a cuff electrode embracing the peroneal nerve just beneath the head of fibula at the knee (McNeal et al., 1977; Waters et al., 1984). The Ljubljana peroneal implant had two versions (Vavken and Jeglic, 1976; Strojnik et al., 1987) with the common feature that the implant–rf receiver was small enough to be implanted next to the peroneal nerve in the fossa poplitea region. Epineural stimulating electrodes were an integral part of the implant. This feature and the comparatively small size make the Ljubljana implant a precursor of the microstimulators described in Section 8.9. Both NMA and the Ljubljana implants were triggered and synchronized with gait by a heel switch.

The same implant used for hand control and developed by the CWRU has also been implanted in the lower extremity musculature to assist incomplete quadriplegics in standing and transfer operations (Triolo et al., 1996). Since the design of the implant is completely transparent, it can generate any stimulation sequence requested by the external controller. For locomotion and transfer-related tasks, stimulation sequences are preprogrammed for individual users and activated by the user by means of pushbuttons. The implant (two in some applications) is surgically positioned in the lower abdominal region. Locomotion application uses the same electrodes as the manipulation system; however, the lead wires have to be somewhat longer.

- *Respiration*—Respiratory control systems involve a two-channel implantable stimulator with electrodes applied bilaterally to the phrenic nerve. Most of the devices in clinical use were developed by Avery Laboratories (Dobelle Institute) and employed discrete circuitry with epoxy encapsulation of the implant and a nerve cuff electrode. Approximately 1000 of these devices have been implanted in patients with respiratory disorders such as high-level tetraplegia (Glenn et al.,

1986). Activation of the phrenic nerve results in contraction of each hemidiaphragm in response to electrical stimulation. In order to minimize damage to the diaphragms during chronic use, alternation of the diaphragms has been employed, in which one hemidiaphragm will be activated for several hours followed by the second. A review of existing systems was given by Creasy et al. (1996). Astrotech of Finland also recently introduced a phrenic stimulator. More recently, DiMarco et al. (1997) have investigated use of CNS activation of a respiratory center to provide augmented breathing.

- *Urinary control*—Urinary control systems have been developed for persons with spinal cord injury. The most successful of these devices has been developed by Brindley et al. (1982) and is manufactured by Finetech, Ltd. (England). The implanted receiver consists of three separate stimulator devices, each with its own coil and circuitry, encapsulated within a single package. The sacral roots (S2, S3, and S4) are placed within a type of encircling electrode, and stimulation of the proper roots will generate contraction of both the bladder and the external sphincter. Cessation of stimulation results in faster relaxation of the external sphincter than of the bladder wall, which then results in voiding. Repeated trains of pulses applied in this manner will eliminate most urine, with only small residual amounts remaining. Approximately 1500 of these devices have been implanted around the world. This technology also has received FDA pre-market approval and is currently distributed by NeuroControl Corporation.
- *Scoliosis treatment*—Progressive lateral curvature of the adolescent vertebral column with simultaneous rotation is known as idiopathic scoliosis. Electrical stimulation applied to the convex side of the curvature has been used to stop or reduce its progression. Initially rf powered stimulators have been replaced by battery powered totally implanted devices (Bobechko et al., 1979; Herbert and Bobechko, 1989). Stimulation is applied intermittently, stimulation amplitudes are under 10.5 V (510 Ω), and frequency and pulsewidth are within usual FES parameter values.

8.8.2 Stimulators of Central Nervous System

Some stimulation systems have electrodes implanted on the surface of the central nervous system or in its deep areas. They do not produce functional movements; however, they "modulate" a pathological motor brain behavior and by that stop unwanted motor activity or abnormality. Therefore, they can be regarded as stimulators for neuromuscular control.

- *Cerebellar stimulation*—Among the earliest stimulators from this category are cerebellar stimulators for control of reduction of effects of cerebral palsy in children. Electrodes are placed on the cerebellar surface with the leads penetrating cranium and dura. The pulse generator is located subcutaneously in the chest area and produces intermittent stimulation bursts. There are about 600 patients using these devices (Davis, 1997).
- *Vagal stimulation*—Intermittent stimulation of the vagus nerve with 30 s on and 5 min off has been shown to reduce frequency of epileptic seizures. A pacemaker-like device, developed by Cyberonics, is implanted in the chest area with a bipolar helical electrode wrapped around the left vagus nerve in the neck. The stimulation sequence is programmed (most often parameter settings are 30 Hz, 500 μs, 1.75 mA); however, patients have some control over the device using a hand-held magnet (Terry et al., 1991). More than 3000 patients have been implanted with this device, which received the pre-marketing approval (PMA) from the FDA in 1997.
- *Deep brain stimulation*—Recently, in 1998, an implantable stimulation device (Activa by Medtronic) was approved by the FDA that can dramatically reduce uncontrollable tremor in patients with Parkinson's disease or essential tremor (Koller et al., 1997). With this device, an electrode array is placed stereotactically into the ventral intermediate nucleus of thalamic region of

the brain. Lead wires again connect the electrodes to a programmable pulse generator implanted in the chest area. Application of high frequency stimulation (130 Hz, 60–210 μs, 0.25–2.75 V) can immediately suppress the patient's tremor.

8.9 Future of Implantable Electrical Stimulators

8.9.1 Distributed Stimulators

One of the major concerns with multichannel implantable neuromuscular stimulators is the multitude of leads that exit the pulse generator and their management during surgical implantation. Routing of multiple leads virtually increases the implant size and by that the burden that an implant imposes on the tissue. A solution to that may be distributed stimulation systems with a single outside controller and multiple single-channel implantable devices implanted throughout the structures to be stimulated. This concept has been pursued both by the Alfred E. Mann Foundation (Strojnik et al., 1992; Cameron et al., 1997) and the University of Michigan (Ziaie et al., 1997). Microinjectable stimulator modules have been developed that can be injected into the tissue, into a muscle, or close to a nerve through a lumen of a hypodermic needle. A single external coil can address and activate a number of these devices located within its field, on a pulse-to-pulse basis. A glass-encapsulated microstimulator developed at the AEMF is shown in Figure 8.5.

8.9.2 Sensing of Implantable Transducer-Generated and Physiological Signals

External command sources such as the shoulder-controlled joystick utilized by the Freehand system impose additional constraints on the implantable stimulator users, since they have to be donned by an attendant. Permanently implanted control sources make neuroprosthetic devices much more attractive and easier to use. An implantable joint angle transducer (IJAT) has been developed at the CWRU that consists of a magnet and an array of magnetic sensors implanted in the distal and the proximal end of a joint, respectively (Smith et al., 1998). The sensor is connected to the implantable stimulator package, which provides the power and also transmits the sensor data to the external controller, using a back-telemetry link. Figure 8.6 shows a radiograph of the IJAT implanted in a patient's wrist. Myoelectric signals (MES) from muscles not affected by paralysis are another attractive control source for implantable neuromuscular stimulators. Amplified and bin-integrated EMG signal from uninvolved muscles, such as the sterno-cleido-mastoid muscle, has been shown to contain enough information to control an upper extremity neuroprosthesis (Scott et al., 1996). EMG signal is being utilized by a multichannel stimulator–telemeter developed at the CWRU, containing 12 stimulator channels and 2 MES channels integrated into the same platform (Strojnik et al., 1998).

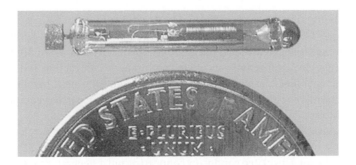

FIGURE 8.5 Microstimulator developed at A.E. Mann Foundation. Dimensions are roughly 2 × 16 mm. Electrodes at the ends are made of tantalum and iridium, respectively.

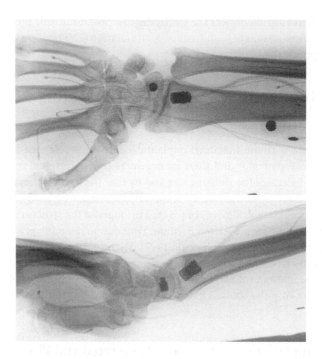

FIGURE 8.6   Radiograph of the joint angle transducer (IJAT) implanted in the wrist. The magnet is implanted in the lunate bone (top) while the magnetic sensor array is implanted in the radius. Leads going to the implant case can be seen as well as intramuscular and epimysial electrodes with their individual lead wires.

8.10 Summary

Implantable stimulators for neuromuscular control are an important tool in rehabilitation of paralyzed individuals with preserved neuromuscular apparatus, as well as in the treatment of some neurological disorders that result in involuntary motor activity. Their impact on rehabilitation is still in its infancy; however, it is expected to increase with further progress in microelectronics technology, development of smaller and better sensors, and with improvements of advanced materials. Advancements in neurophysiological science are also expected to bring forward wider utilization of possibilities offered by implantable neuromuscular stimulators.

Defining Terms

Biocompatibility: Ability of a foreign object to coexist in a living tissue.
Electrical stimulation: Diagnostic, therapeutic, and rehabilitational method used to excite motor nerves with the aim of contracting the appropriate muscles and obtain limb movement.
EMG activity: Muscular electrical activity associated with muscle contraction and production of force.
Feedthrough: Device that allows passage of a conductor through a hermetic barrier.
Hybrid circuit: Electronic circuit combining miniature active and passive components on a single ceramic substrate.
Implantable stimulator: Biocompatible electronic stimulator designed for surgical implantation and operation in a living tissue.
Lead wire: Flexible and strong insulated conductor connecting pulse generator to stimulating electrodes.
Paralysis: Loss of power of voluntary movement in a muscle through injury to or disease to its nerve supply.

rf-radiofrequency: Pertaining to electromagnetic propagation of power and signal in frequencies above those used in electrical power distribution.

Stimulating electrode: Conductive device that transfers stimulating current to a living tissue. On its surface, the electric charge carriers change from electrons to ions or vice versa.

References

Bobechko, W.P., Herbert, M.A., and Friedman, H.G. 1979. Electrospinal instrumentation for scoliosis: Current status. *Orthop. Clin. North. Am.* 10: 927.

Brindley, G.S., Polkey, C.E., and Rushton, D.N. 1982. Sacral anterior root stimulators for bladder control in paraplegia. *Paraplegia* 20: 365.

Cameron, T., Loeb, G.E., Peck, R.A., Schulman, J.H., Strojnik, P., and Troyk, P.R. 1997. Micromodular implants to provide electrical stimulation of paralyzed muscles and limbs. *IEEE Trans. Biomed. Eng.* 44: 781.

Creasey, G., Elefteriades, J., DiMarco, A., Talonen, P., Bijak, M., Girsch, W., and Kantor, C. 1996. Electrical stimulation to restore respiration. *J. Rehab. Res. Dev.* 33: 123.

Davis, R. 1997. Cerebellar stimulation for movement disorders. In P.L. Gildenberg and R.R. Tasker (eds.), *Textbook of Stereotactic and Functional Neurosurgery*, McGraw-Hill, New York.

DiMarco, A.F., Romaniuk, J.R., Kowalski, K.E., and Supinski, G.S. 1997. Efficacy of combined inspiratory intercostal and expiratory muscle pacing to maintain artificial ventilation. *Am. J. Respir. Crit. Care Med.* 156: 122.

Glenn, W.W., Phelps, M.L., Elefteriades, J.A., Dentz, B., and Hogan, J.F. 1986. Twenty years of experience in phrenic nerve stimulation to pace the diaphragm pacing. *Clin. Electrophysiol.* 9: 780.

Graupe, D. and Kohn, K.H. 1998. Functional neuromuscular stimulator for short-distance ambulation by certain thoracic-level spinal-cord-injured paraplegics. *Surg. Neurol.* 50: 202.

Herbert, M.A. and Bobechko, W.P. 1989. Scoliosis treatment in children using a programmable, totally implantable muscle stimulator (ESI). *IEEE Trans. Biomed. Eng.* 36: 801.

Koller, W., Pahwa, R., Busenbark, K., Hubble, J., Wilkinson, S., Lang, A., Tuite, P. et al. 1997. High-frequency unilateral thalamic stimulation in the treatment of essential and parkinsonian tremor. *Ann. Neurol.* 42: 292.

Kralj, A. and Bajd, T. 1989. *Functional Electrical Stimulation: Standing and Walking after Spinal Cord Injury*, CRC Press, Inc., Boca Raton, FL.

Liberson, W.T., Holmquest, H.J., Scot, D., and Dow, M. 1961. Functional electrotherapy: Stimulation of the peroneal nerve synchronized with the swing phase of the gait of hemiplegic patients. *Arch. Phys. Med. Rehab.* 42: 101.

Marsolais, E.B. and Kobetic, R. 1986. Implantation techniques and experience with percutaneous intramuscular electrodes in lower extremities. *J. Rehab. Res. Dev.* 23: 1.

McNeal, D.R., Waters, R., and Reswick, J. 1977. Experience with implanted electrodes. *Neurosurgery* 1: 228.

Memberg, W., Peckham, P.H., Thorpe, G.B., Keith, M.W., and Kicher, T.P. 1993. An analysis of the reliability of percutaneous intramuscular electrodes in upper extremity FNS applications. *IEEE Trans. Biomed. Eng.* 1: 126.

Rebersek, S. and Vodovnik, L. 1973. Proportionally controlled functional electrical stimulation of hand. *Arch. Phys. Med. Rehab.* 54: 378.

Scott, T.R.D., Peckham, P.H., and Kilgore, K.L. 1996. Tri-state myoelectric control of bilateral upper extremity neuroprostheses for tetraplegic individuals. *IEEE Trans. Rehab. Eng.* 2: 251.

Smith, B., Peckham, P.H., Keith, M.W., and Roscoe, D.D. 1987. An externally powered, multichannel, implantable stimulator for versatile control of paralyzed muscle. *IEEE Trans. Biomed. Eng.* 34: 499.

Smith, B., Tang, Z., Johnson, M.W., Pourmehdi, S., Gazdik, M.M., Buckett, J.R., and Peckham, P.H. 1998. An externally powered, multichannel, implantable stimulator–telemeter for control of paralyzed muscle. *IEEE Trans. Biomed. Eng.* 45: 463.

Strojnik, P., Acimovic, R., Vavken, E., Simic, V., and Stanic, U. 1987. Treatment of drop foot using an implantable peroneal underknee stimulator. *Scand. J. Rehab. Med.* 19: 37.

Strojnik, P., Meadows, P., Schulman, J.H., and Whitmoyer, D. 1994. Modification of a cochlear stimulation system for FES applications. *Basic Appl. Myol.* BAM 4: 129.

Strojnik, P., Pourmehdi, S., and Peckham, P. 1998. Incorporating FES control sources into implantable stimulators. *Proceedings of the 6th Vienna International Workshop on Functional Electrostimulation*, Vienna, Austria.

Strojnik, P., Schulman, J., Loeb, G., and Troyk, P. 1992. Multichannel FES system with distributed microstimulators. *Proceedings of the 14th Annual International Conference IEEE*, MBS, Paris, p. 1352.

Terry, R.S., Tarver, W.B., and Zabara, J. 1991. The implantable neurocybernetic prosthesis system. *Pacing Clin. Electrophysiol.* 14: 86.

Triolo, R.J., Bieri, C., Uhlir, J., Kobetic, R., Scheiner, A., and Marsolais, E.B. 1996. Implanted functional neuromuscular stimulation systems for individuals with cervical spinal cord injuries: Clinical case reports. *Arch. Phys. Med. Rehabil.* 77: 1119.

Vavken, E. and Jeglic, A. 1976. Application of an implantable stimulator in the rehabilitation of paraplegic patients. *Int. Surg.* 61: 335–339.

Waters, R.L., McNeal, D.R., and Clifford, B. 1984. Correction of footdrop in stroke patients via surgically implanted peroneal nerve stimulator. *Acta Orthop. Belg.* 50: 285.

Ziaie, B., Nardin, M.D., Coghlan, A.R., and Najafi, K. 1997. A single-channel implantable microstimulator for functional neuromuscular stimulation. *IEEE Trans. Biomed. Eng.* 44: 909.

Further Information

Additional references on early work in FES which augment peer review publications can be found in Proceedings from Conferences in Dubrovnik and Vienna. These are the *External Control of Human Extremities* and *the Vienna International Workshop on Electrostimulation*, respectively.

9

Respiration

Leslie A. Geddes
Purdue University

9.1 Lung Volumes

The amount of air flowing into and out of the lungs with each breath is called the tidal volume (TV). In a typical adult this amounts to about 500 mL during quiet breathing. The respiratory system is capable of moving much more air than the tidal volume. Starting at the *resting expiratory level* (REL in Figure 9.1), it is possible to inhale a volume amounting to about seven times the tidal volume; this volume is called the *inspiratory capacity* (IC). A measure of the ability to inspire more than the tidal volume is the *inspiratory reserve volume* (IRV), which is also shown in Figure 9.1. Starting from REL, it is possible to forcibly exhale a volume amounting to about twice the tidal volume; this volume is called the *expiratory reserve volume* (ERV). However, even with the most forcible expiration, it is not possible to exhale all the air from the lungs; a *residual volume* (RV) about equal to the expiratory reserve volume remains. The sum of the expiratory reserve volume and the residual volume is designated the *functional residual capacity* (FRC). The volume of air exhaled from a maximum inspiration to a maximum expiration is called the *vital capacity* (VC). The *total lung capacity* (TLC) is the total air within the lungs, that is, that which can be moved in a vital-capacity maneuver plus the residual volume. All except the residual volume can be determined with a volume-measuring instrument such as a spirometer connected to the airway.

9.2 Pulmonary Function Tests

In addition to the static lung volumes just identified, there are several time-dependent volumes associated with the respiratory act. The *minute volume* (MV) is the volume of air per breath (tidal volume) multiplied by the respiratory rate (R), that is, $MV = (TV) R$. It is obvious that the same minute volume can be produced by rapid shallow or slow deep breathing. However, the effectiveness is not the same, because not all the respiratory air participates in gas exchange, there being a dead space volume. Therefore the alveolar ventilation is the important quantity which is defined as the tidal volume (TV) minus the dead space (DS) multiplied by the respiratory rate R, that is, alveolar ventilation = (TV–DS) R. In a normal adult subject, the dead space amounts to about 150 mL, or 2 mL/kg.

9.2.1 Dynamic Tests

Several timed respiratory volumes describe the ability of the respiratory system to move air. Among these are *forced vital capacity* (FVC), *forced expiratory volume* in *t* seconds (FEV$_t$), the *maximum ventilatory*

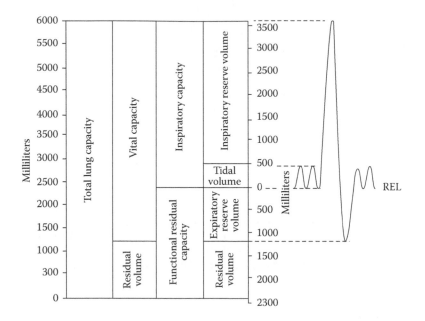

FIGURE 9.1   Lung volumes.

volume (MVV), which was previously designated the *maximum breathing capacity* (MBC), and the *peak flow* (PF). These quantities are measured with a spirometer without valves and CO_2 absorber or with a pneumotachograph coupled to an integrator.

9.2.1.1 Forced Vital Capacity

Forced vital capacity (FVC) is shown in Figure 9.2 and is measured by taking the maximum inspiration and forcing all of the inspired air out as rapidly as possible. Table 9.1 presents normal values for males and females.

9.2.1.2 Forced Expiratory Volume

Forced expiratory volume in t seconds (FEV_t) is shown in Figure 9.2, which identifies $FEV_{0.5}$ and $FEV_{1.0}$, and Table 9.1 presents normal values for $FEV_{1.0}$.

9.2.1.3 Maximum Voluntary Ventilation

Maximum voluntary ventilation (MVV) is the volume of air moved in 1 min when breathing as deeply and rapidly as possible. The test is performed for 20 s and the volume scaled to a 1-min value; Table 9.1 presents normal values.

9.2.1.4 Peak Flow

Peak flow (PF) in L/min is the maximum flow velocity attainable during an FEV maneuver and represents the maximum slope of the expired volume–time curve (Figure 9.2); typical normal values are shown in Table 9.1.

9.2.1.5 The Water-Sealed Spirometer

The water-sealed spirometer was the traditional device used to measure the volume of air moved in respiration. The Latin word *spirare* means to breathe. The most popular type of spirometer consists of a hollow cylinder closed at one end, inverted and suspended in an annular space filled with water to

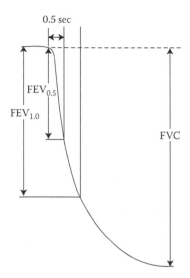

FIGURE 9.2   The measurement of timed forced expiratory volume (FEV_t) and forced vital capacity (FVC).

provide an air-tight seal. Figure 9.3 illustrates the method of suspending the counterbalanced cylinder (bell), which is free to move up and down to accommodate the volume of air under it. Movement of the bell, which is proportional to volume, is usually recorded by an inking pen applied to a graphic record which is caused to move with a constant speed. Below the cylinder, in the space that accommodates the volume of air, are inlet and outlet breathing tubes. At the end of one or both of these tubes is a check valve designed to maintain a unidirectional flow of air through the spirometer. Outside the spirometer the two breathing tubes are brought to a Y tube which is connected to a mouthpiece. With a pinch clamp placed on the nose, inspiration diminishes the volume of air under the bell, which descends, causing the stylus to rise on the graphic record. Expiration produces the reverse effect. Thus, starting with the spirometer half-filled, quiet respiration causes the bell to rise and fall. By knowing the "bell factor," the volume of air moved per centimeter excursion of the bell, the volume change can be quantitated. Although a variety of flowmeters are now used to measure respiratory volumes, the spirometer with a CO_2 absorber is ideally suited to measure oxygen uptake.

TABLE 9.1   Dynamic Volumes

Males
  FVC (L) = 0.133H − 0.022A − 3.60(SEE = 0.58)[a]
  FEV1 (L) = 0.094H − 0.028A − 1.59(SEE = 0.52)[a]
  MVV (L/min) = 3.39H − 1.26A − 21.4(SEE = 29)[a]
  PF (L/min) = (10.03 − 0.038A)H[b]
Females
  FVC (L) = 0.111H − 0.015A − 3.16(SD = 0.42)[c]
  FEV1 (L) = 0.068H − 0.023A − 0.92(SD = 0.37)[c]
  MVV (L/min) = 2.05H − 0.57A − 5.5(SD = 10.7)[c]
  PF (L/min) = (7.44 − 0.0183A) H[c]

Note: H = height in inches, A = age in years, L = liters, L/min = liters per minute, SEE = standard error of estimate, SD = standard deviation.
  [a] Kory et al. 1961. *Am. J. Med.* 30: 243.
  [b] Leiner et al. 1963. *Am. Rev. Resp. Dis.* 88: 644.
  [c] Lindall, Medina, and Grismer. 1967. *Am. Rev. Resp. Dis.* 95: 1061.

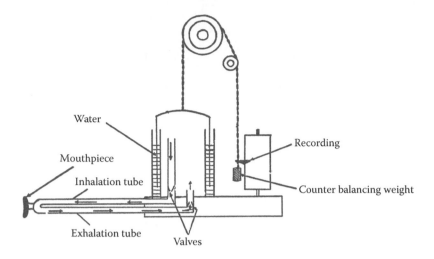

FIGURE 9.3 The simple spirometer.

9.2.1.6 Oxygen Uptake

A second and very important use for the water-filled spirometer is measurement of oxygen used per unit of time, designated the O_2 *uptake*. This measurement is accomplished by incorporating a soda-lime, carbon-dioxide absorber into the spirometer as shown in Figure 9.4. Soda-lime is a mixture of calcium hydroxide, sodium hydroxide, and silicates of sodium and calcium. The exhaled carbon dioxide combines with the soda-lime and becomes solid carbonates. A small amount of heat is liberated by this reaction.

Starting with a spirometer filled with oxygen and connected to a subject, respiration causes the bell to move up and down (indicating tidal volume) as shown in Figure 9.5. With continued respiration the baseline of the recording rises, reflecting disappearance of oxygen from under the bell. By measuring the slope of the baseline on the spirogram, the volume of oxygen consumed per minute can be determined. Figure 9.5 presents a typical example along with calculation.

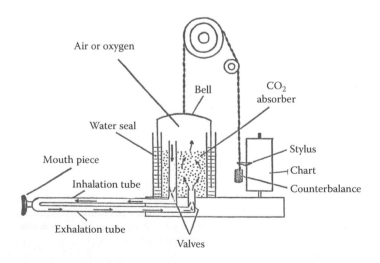

FIGURE 9.4 The spirometer with CO_2 absorber and a record of oxygen uptake.

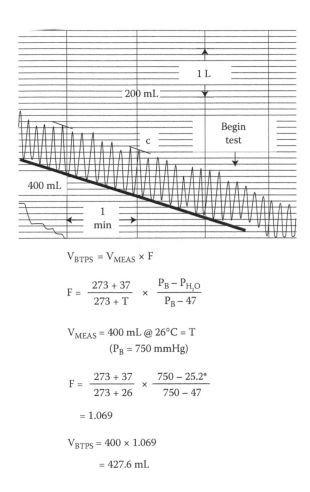

$$V_{BTPS} = V_{MEAS} \times F$$

$$F = \frac{273 + 37}{273 + T} \times \frac{P_B - P_{H_2O}}{P_B - 47}$$

$$V_{MEAS} = 400 \text{ mL @ } 26°C = T$$
$$(P_B = 750 \text{ mmHg})$$

$$F = \frac{273 + 37}{273 + 26} \times \frac{750 - 25.2^*}{750 - 47}$$

$$= 1.069$$

$$V_{BTPS} = 400 \times 1.069$$

$$= 427.6 \text{ mL}$$

FIGURE 9.5 Oxygen consumption.

9.2.1.7 The Dry Spirometer

The water-sealed spirometer was the most popular device for measuring the volumes of respiratory gases; however, it is not without its inconveniences. The presence of water causes corrosion of the metal parts. Maintenance is required to keep the device in good working order over prolonged periods. To eliminate these problems, manufacturers have developed dry spirometers. The most common type employs a collapsible rubber or plastic bellows, the expansion of which is recorded during breathing. The earlier rubber models had a decidedly undesirable characteristic which caused their abandonment. When the bellows were in its mid-position, the resistance to breathing was a minimum; when fully collapsed, it imposed a slight negative resistance; and when fully extended it imposed a slight positive resistance to breathing. Newer units with compliant plastic bellows minimize this defect.

9.2.2 The Pneumotachograph

The pneumotachograph is a device which is placed directly in the airway to measure the velocity of air flow. The volume per breath is therefore the integral of the velocity–time record during inspiration or expiration. Planimetric integration of the record, or electronic integration of the velocity–time signal, yields the tidal volume. Although tidal volume is perhaps more easily recorded with the spirometer, the

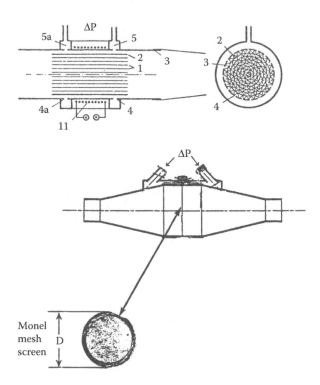

FIGURE 9.6   Pneumotachographs.

dynamics of respiration are better displayed by the pneumotachograph, which offers less resistance to the air stream and exhibits a much shorter response time—so short in most instruments that cardiac impulses are often clearly identifiable in the velocity–time record.

If a specially designed resistor is placed in a tube in which the respiratory gases flow, a pressure drop will appear across it. Below the point of turbulent flow, the pressure drop is linearly related to air-flow velocity. The resistance may consist of a wire screen or a series of capillary tubes; Figure 9.6 illustrates both types. Detection and recording of this pressure differential constitutes a pneumotachogram; Figure 9.7 presents a typical air–velocity record, along with the spirogram, which is the integral of the flow signal. The small-amplitude artifacts in the pneumotachogram are cardiac impulses.

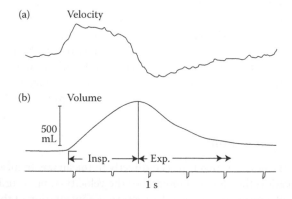

FIGURE 9.7   Velocity (a) and volume changes (b) during normal, quiet breathing; b is the integral of a.

For human application, linear flow rates up to 200 L/min should be recordable with fidelity. The resistance to breathing depends upon the flow rate, and it is difficult to establish an upper limit of tolerable resistance. Silverman and Whittenberger (1950) stated that a resistance of 6 mm H_2O is perceptible to human subjects. Many of the high-fidelity pneumotachographs offer 5–10 mm H_2O resistance at 100 and 200 L/min. It would appear that such resistances are acceptable in practice.

Response times of 15–40 ms seem to be currently in use. Fry et al. (1957) analyzed the dynamic characteristics of three types of commercially available, differential-pressure pneumotachographs which employed concentric cylinders, screen mesh, and parallel plates for the air resistors. Using a high-quality, differential-pressure transducer with each, they measured total flow resistance ranging from 5 to 15 cm H_2O. Frequency response curves taken on one model showed fairly uniform response to 40 Hz; the second model showed a slight increase in response at 50 Hz, and the third exhibited a slight drop in response at this frequency.

9.2.3 The Nitrogen-Washout Method for Measuring FRC

The *functional residual capacity* (FRC) and the *residual volume* (RV) are the only lung compartments that cannot be measured with a volume-measuring device. Measuring these requires use of the nitrogen analyzer and application of the dilution method.

Because nitrogen does not participate in respiration, it can be called a *diluent*. Inspired and expired air contains about 80% nitrogen. Between breaths, the FRC of the lungs contains the same concentration of nitrogen as in environmental air, that is, 80%. By causing a subject to inspire from a spirometer filled with 100% oxygen and to exhale into a second collecting spirometer, all the nitrogen in the FRC is replaced by oxygen, that is, the nitrogen is "washed out" into the second spirometer. Measurement of the concentration of nitrogen in the collecting spirometer, along with a knowledge of its volume, permits calculation of the amount of nitrogen originally in the functional residual capacity and hence allows calculation of the FRC, as now will be shown.

Figure 9.8 illustrates the arrangement of equipment for the nitrogen-washout test. Note that two check valves, (I, EX) are on both sides of the subject's breathing tube, and the nitrogen meter is connected to the mouthpiece. Valve V is used to switch the subject from breathing environmental air to the measuring system. The left-hand spirometer contains 100% oxygen, which is inhaled by the subject via valve I. Of course, a nose clip must be applied so that all the respired gases flow through the breathing tube connected to the mouthpiece. It is in this tube that the sampling inlet for the nitrogen analyzer is located. Starting at the resting expiratory level, inhalation of pure oxygen causes the nitrogen analyzer

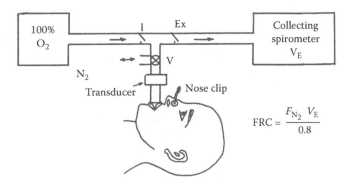

FIGURE 9.8 Arrangement of equipment for the nitrogen-washout technique. Valve V allows the subject to breathe room air until the test is started. The test is started by operating valve V at the end of a normal breath, that is, the subject starts breathing 100% O_2 through the inspiratory valve (I) and exhales the N_2 and O_2 mixture into a collecting spirometer via the expiratory valve EX.

to indicate zero. Expiration closes valve I and opens valve EX. The first expired breath contains nitrogen derived from the FRC (diluted by the oxygen which was inspired); the nitrogen analyzer indicates this percentage. The exhaled gases are collected in the right-hand spirometer. The collecting spirometer and all the interconnecting tubing was first flushed with oxygen to eliminate all nitrogen. This simple procedure eliminates the need for applying corrections and facilitates calculation of the FRC. With continued breathing, the nitrogen analyzer indicates less and less nitrogen because it is being washed out of the FRC and is replaced by oxygen. Figure 9.9 presents a typical record of the diminishing concentration of expired nitrogen throughout the test. In most laboratories, the test is continued until the concentration of nitrogen falls to about 1%. The nitrogen analyzer output permits identification of this concentration. In normal subjects, virtually all the nitrogen can be washed out of the FRC in about 5 min.

If the peaks on the nitrogen-washout record are joined, a smooth exponential decay curve is obtained in normal subjects. A semilog of N_2 vs. time provides a straight line. In subjects with trapped air, or poorly ventilated alveoli, the nitrogen-washout curve consists of several exponentials as the multiple poorly ventilated regions give up their nitrogen. In such subjects, the time taken to wash out all the nitrogen usually exceeds 10 min. Thus, the nitrogen concentration–time curve provides useful diagnostic information on ventilation of the alveoli.

If it is assumed that all the collected (washed-out) nitrogen was uniformly distributed within the lungs, it is easy to calculate the FRC. If the environmental air contains 80% nitrogen, then the volume of nitrogen in the functional residual capacity is 0.8 (FRC). Because the volume of expired gas in the collecting spirometer is known, it is merely necessary to determine the concentration of nitrogen in this volume. To do so requires admitting some of this gas to the inlet valve of the nitrogen analyzer. Note that this concentration of nitrogen (F_{N2}) exists in a volume which includes the volume of air expired (V_E) plus the original volume of oxygen in the collecting spirometer (V_0) at the start of the test and the volume of the tubing (V_t) leading from the expiratory collecting valve. It is therefore advisable to start with an empty collecting spirometer ($V_0 = 0$). Usually the tubing volume (V_t) is negligible with respect to the volume of expired gas collected in a typical washout test. In this situation the volume of nitrogen collected is $V_E F_{N_2}$, where F_{N_2} is the fraction of nitrogen within the collected gas. Thus, 0.80 (FRC) = $F_{N_2}(V_E)$. Therefore,

$$\text{FRC} = \frac{F_{N_2} V_E}{0.80} \tag{9.1}$$

It is important to note that the value for FRC so obtained is at ambient temperature and pressure and is saturated with water vapor (ATPS). In respiratory studies, this value is converted to body temperature and saturated with water vapor (BTPS).

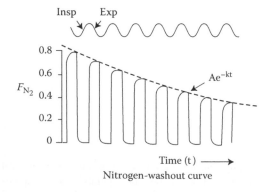

FIGURE 9.9　The nitrogen-washout curve.

In the example shown in Figure 9.9, the washout to 1% took about 44 breaths. With a breathing rate of 12/min, the washout time was 220 s. The volume collected (V_E) was 22 L and the concentration of nitrogen in this volume was 0.085 (F_{N_2}); therefore,

$$\text{FRC} = \frac{0.085 \times 22,000}{0.80} = 2,337 \text{ mL} \tag{9.2}$$

9.3 Physiologic Dead Space

The volume of ventilated lung that does not participate in gas exchange is the physiologic dead space (V_d). It is obvious that the physiologic dead space includes anatomic dead space, as well as the volume of any alveoli that are not perfused. In the lung, there are theoretically four types of alveoli, as shown in Figure 9.10. The normal alveolus (A) is both ventilated and perfused with blood. There are alveoli that are ventilated but not perfused (B); such alveoli contribute significantly to the physiologic dead space. There are alveoli that are not ventilated but perfused (C); such alveoli do not provide the exchange of respiratory gases. Finally, there are alveoli that are both poorly ventilated and poorly perfused (D); such alveoli contain high CO_2 and N_2 and low O_2. These alveoli are the last to expel their CO_2 and N_2 in washout tests.

Measurement of physiologic dead space is based on the assumption that there is almost complete equilibrium between alveolar pCO_2 and pulmonary capillary blood. Therefore, the arterial pCO_2 represents mean alveolar pCO_2 over many breaths when an arterial blood sample is drawn for analysis of pCO_2. The Bohr equation for physiologic dead space is

$$V_d = \left[\frac{\text{paCO}_2 - \text{pECO}_2}{\text{paCO}_2} \right] V_E \tag{9.3}$$

In this expression, $paCO_2$ is the partial pressure in the arterial blood sample which is withdrawn slowly during the test; $pECO_2$ is the partial pressure of CO_2 in the volume of expired air; V_E is the volume of expired air per breath (tidal volume).

In a typical test, the subject would breathe in room air and exhale into a collapsed (Douglas) bag. The test is continued for 3 min or more, and the number of breaths is counted in that period. An arterial blood sample is withdrawn during the collection period. The pCO_2 in the expired gas is measured, and

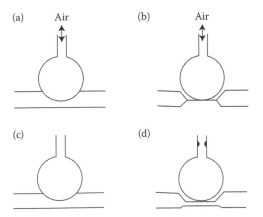

FIGURE 9.10 The four types of alveoli. (a) Ventilated and perfused. (b) Ventilated and not perfused. (c) Perfused and not ventilated. (d) Poorly perfused poorly ventilated.

then the volume of expired gas is measured by causing it to flow into a spirometer or flowmeter by collapsing the collecting bag.

In a typical 3-min test, the collected volume is 33 L, and the pCO_2 in the expired gas is 14.5 mm Hg. During the test, the pCO_2 in the arterial blood sample was 40 mm Hg. The number of breaths was 60; therefore, the average tidal volume was 33,000/60 = 550 mL. The physiologic dead space (V_d) is

$$V_d = \left[\frac{40 - 14.5}{40}\right]550 = 350 \text{ mL} \tag{9.4}$$

It is obvious that an elevated physiological dead space indicates lung tissue that is not perfused with blood.

References

Fry D.I., Hyatt R.E., and McCall C.B. 1957. Evaluation of three types of respiratory flowmeters. *Appl. Physiol.* 10: 210.

Silverman L. and Whittenberger J. 1950. Clinical pneumotachograph. *Meth. Med. Res.* 2: 104.

10

Mechanical Ventilation

Khosrow Behbehani
University of Texas

10.1 Introduction

This chapter provides an overview of the structure and function of mechanical ventilators. Mechanical ventilators, which are often also called respirators, are used to artificially ventilate the lungs of patients who are unable to breathe naturally from the atmosphere. In almost 105 years of development, many mechanical ventilators with different designs have been manufactured (Macintyre and Branson, 2009). Very early devices used bellows that were manually operated to inflate the lungs. Today's respirators employ an array of sophisticated components, such as microprocessors, fast-response servo valves, and precision transducers to mechanically ventilate the incapacitated patients. Large varieties of ventilators are now available for short-term treatment of acute respiratory dysfunction as well as long-term therapy for chronic respiratory conditions.

It is reasonable to broadly classify today's ventilators into two groups. The first and indeed the largest class is the critical care respirators used primarily in hospitals to treat patients for acute pulmonary disorders or following certain surgical procedures. The second class of mechanical ventilators includes less complicated machines that are primarily used at home to treat patients with chronic respiratory disorders.

The level of design complexity and engineering needed for the critical care ventilators is higher than the ventilators used for chronic treatment. However, many of the engineering concepts employed in designing critical care ventilators can also be applied in the simpler chronic care units. Therefore, this chapter focuses on the design of intensive care ventilators. Hence, the terms respirator, mechanical ventilator, or ventilator will be used from this point to refer to the intensive care unit respirators.

From the beginning, the designers of mechanical ventilators realized that in the vast majority of cases, the main task of a respirator is to ventilate the lungs in a manner as close to natural respiration

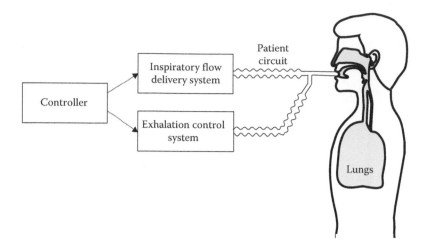

FIGURE 10.1   A simplified diagram of the functional blocks of a positive-pressure ventilator.

as possible. Since natural inspiration is a result of negative pressure in the pleural cavity generated by the distention of the diaphragm, designers initially developed ventilators that created the same effect. These ventilators are called negative-pressure ventilators. However, almost all modern ventilators use pressures greater than atmospheric pressures to ventilate the lungs and therefore they are known as positive-pressure ventilators. Owing to the overwhelming prevalence of positive-pressure ventilators in treating patients, this chapter describes only the positive-pressure ventilators.

10.2 Positive-Pressure Ventilators

Positive-pressure ventilators generate the inspiratory flow by applying a positive pressure (greater than the atmospheric pressure) to the airways. Figure 10.1 shows a simplified block diagram of a positive-pressure ventilator. During inspiration, the inspiratory flow delivery system creates a positive pressure in the tubes connected to the patient's airway, called *patient circuit*, and the exhalation control system closes a valve at the outlet of the tubing to the atmosphere. When the ventilator switches to exhalation, the inspiratory flow delivery system stops the positive pressure and the exhalation valve opens to the atmosphere. The use of a positive pressure gradient in creating the flow allows treating patients with high lung resistance and low compliance. As a result, positive-pressure ventilators have been very successful in treating a variety of breathing disorders, such as chronic obstructive pulmonary disorder, lung edema, and obstructed airways.

Positive-pressure ventilators have been employed to treat patients of all ages ranging from neonates to the elderly. Owing to anatomical differences between various patient populations, the ventilators and their modes of treating infants are different from those for adults. Nonetheless, their fundamental engineering design principles are similar. Adult ventilators comprise a larger percentage of ventilators manufactured and used in clinics. Therefore, the emphasis here is on the description of adult positive-pressure ventilators. Specifically, the concepts presented will be illustrated using a microprocessor-based design example, as almost all modern ventilators use microprocessor for the control of breath delivery.

10.3 Ventilation Modes

Since the advent of respirators, clinicians have devised various strategies to ventilate the lungs based on patient's conditions. As a result, two main categories of ventilation modes have been defined:

mandatory and spontaneous. *Mandatory mode* refers to the strategy for treating patients who need the respirator to completely take over the task of ventilating their lungs. However, some patients are able to exert the respiratory effort needed to breathe on their own, but may need to remain on the ventilator to receive oxygen-enriched air flow or slightly elevated airway pressure. When a ventilator delivers a breath to the patient according to the level of effort exerted by the patient, it is said that the ventilator operates in *spontaneous mode*. In many cases, it is necessary to first treat the patient with mandatory ventilation and as the patient's condition improves, spontaneous ventilation is introduced to wean the patient from mandatory breathing and restore natural breathing. For this purpose, several schemes for combining mandatory and spontaneous breathing have been established. For instance, when a patient is able to generate the needed effort for few breaths, but not sufficient for completely proper ventilation, mandatory breaths are added intermittently to supplement the patient's spontaneous breathing. Such a scheme is simply referred to as *synchronized intermittent mandatory ventilation* (SIMV).

10.3.1 Mandatory Ventilation

Responding to the clinicians' needs, biomedical engineers have employed two rather distinct approaches for delivering mandatory breaths: *volume-* and *pressure-controlled ventilation*. Volume-controlled ventilation refers to delivering a specified tidal volume to the patient during the inspiratory phase. Pressure-controlled ventilation refers to raising the airway pressure to a desired level (set by the therapist) during the inspiratory phase of each breath. Regardless of the type, a ventilator operating in mandatory mode must control all aspects of breathing, such as tidal volume, respiration rate, inspiratory flow pattern, and oxygen concentration of the breath. This is often labeled as *controlled mandatory ventilation* (CMV), a term that encompasses both volume- as well as pressure-controlled ventilation.

Figure 10.2 shows the flow and pressure waveforms for volume-controlled ventilation. In this illustration, the inspiratory flow waveform is chosen to be a half sine wave. In Figure 10.2a, t_i is the inspiration duration, t_e the exhalation period, and Q_i the amplitude of inspiratory flow. The ventilator delivers a tidal volume equal to the area under the flow waveform in Figure 10.2a at regular intervals ($t_i + t_e$) set by the therapist. The resulting pressure waveform is shown in Figure 10.2b. It is noted that during volume-controlled ventilation, the ventilator attempts to deliver the desired volume of breath, irrespective of the patient's respiratory mechanics. However, the resulting pressure waveform, such as the one shown in Figure 10.2b, will be different depending on the patient's respiratory mechanics. Of course, for safety

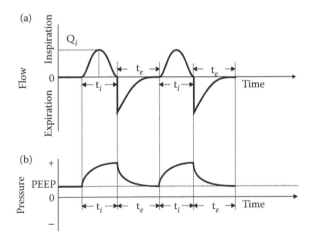

FIGURE 10.2 (a) Inspiratory flow for a mandatory volume-controlled ventilation breath and (b) airway pressure resulting from the breath delivery with a nonzero PEEP.

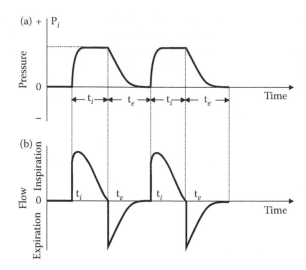

FIGURE 10.3   (a) Inspiratory pressure pattern for a mandatory pressure-controlled ventilation breath and (b) airway flow pattern resulting from the breath delivery. Note that PEEP is zero.

purposes, the ventilator must limit the maximum applied airway pressure according to the therapist's setting.

As can be seen in Figure 10.2b, the airway pressure at the end of exhalation may not end at atmospheric pressure (zero gauge). The *positive end expiratory pressure* or PEEP is sometimes used to prevent the alveoli from collapsing during expiration (Pierce, 2007). In other cases, the expiration pressure is allowed to return to the atmospheric level.

Figure 10.3 shows a plot of the pressure and flow during a mandatory pressure-controlled ventilation. In this case, the respirator raises the airway pressure and maintains it at the desired level, P_i, which is set by the therapist, independent of the patient's respiratory mechanics. Although the ventilator maintains the same pressure trajectory for patients with different respiratory mechanics, the resulting flow trajectory, shown in Figure 10.3b, will depend on the respiratory mechanics of each patient. As in the case of mandatory volume-controlled ventilation, the total volume of delivered breaths is monitored to ensure that patients receive adequate ventilation.

Owing to the need for monitoring both pressure and volume, in more recent years, new modes that combine several aspects of the volume- and pressure-controlled ventilation are devised. These modes are generally referred to as dual-control modes. Although these modes are relatively new and not all of their clinical outcomes are known, they utilize more of the power and flexibility that new ventilator hardware and software offer (Lellouche and Brochard, 2009). Two dual-control modes are described below.

10.3.2 Adaptive Pressure Control

This new mode is a form of pressure-controlled ventilation that simultaneously keeps track of the delivered tidal volume. Figure 10.4 shows characteristic changes of pressure, volume, and flow of inspiratory flow in this mode. As shown in the top panel of Figure 10.4, for each breath, (a) through (e), the ventilator controls the inspiratory pressure to a level that may vary from breath to breath. Specifically, the ventilator controls the pressure, but also monitors the delivered tidal volume and compares it with the desired tidal volume. If the actual delivered tidal volume matches the desired level, such as in (a), then the level of controlled pressure for the next breath will be the same. However, if the next breath produced a larger than desired tidal volume, such as in (b), then the controlled pressure will be reduced in the next breath (c). Similarly, if the tidal volume falls short, such as in (d), then the controlled pressure in the next breath, (e), will be raised to

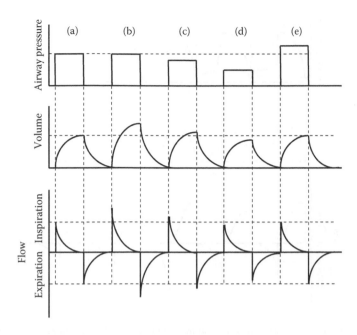

FIGURE 10.4 Patterns respiratory desired pressure and resulting volume and flow for adaptive pressure control ventilation mode. Breath illustration (a) through (e) shows how the applied inspiratory pressure is automatically adjusted to achieve the desired tidal volume.

a higher level to achieve the desired volume. Hence, the ventilator seeks delivering the desired tidal volume at fixed pressures that are adjusted from breath to breath. It is noted that in this mode of ventilation, while the pressure remains constant within the inspiratory interval, the level of inspiratory pressure is varied from one breath to the next by the ventilator to achieve the desired level of tidal volume.

10.3.3 Adaptive Support Ventilation

This new mode of ventilation aims to minimize the work of breathing as was proposed by Otis in 1950 (Otis et al., 1950), while accommodating changes in the patient's respiratory mechanics (Brunner and Iotti, 2002). A major point of distinction for this mode of ventilation is that it takes into account the respiratory mechanics of the patient (i.e., resistance and elastance of the combined airway and air-delivery system). Hence, it may be considered as one of the first closed-loop ventilators that adapts to the patient's condition. Adaptive support ventilation (ASV) can be applied as both a mandatory ventilation and a spontaneous ventilation. In this chapter, we describe only the mandatory ventilation form of ASV. A description of ASV in spontaneous breathing may be found in Wu et al. (2010) and Mireles-Cabodevila et al. (2009). When ASV is used to ventilate the patient in mandatory ventilation mode, the clinician inputs the ideal body weight (IBW) for the patient (based on height, gender, age, etc.). Using IBW, an (assumed) ideal minute volume is obtained by multiplying the IBW by 100 mL/min/kg. As the name implies, *minute volume* refers to the total inspiratory volume that a patient receives in 1 min. Additionally, the clinician needs to enter another parameter called percent of minute volume (PMV). The PMV indicates how the desired minute volume for the patient compares with the minute volume computed from IBW. For instance, a PMV of 100% means that the desired minute volume for the patient is the same as the minute volume computed from IBW. Alternatively, a PMV of 110% indicates that the desired minute volume is 10% above what is computed from the IBW. Once, the operator enters the IBW and PMV, the ASV algorithm determines an optimized respiration rate and tidal volume to minimize the work of breathing according to the principles proposed by Otis (Brunner and Iotti, 2002).

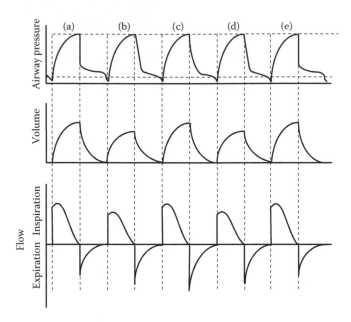

FIGURE 10.5   Patterns of respiratory pressure, volume, and flow for adaptive support ventilation mode. Breath illustrations (a) through (d) demonstrate how the respiratory frequency and volume are adjusted to minimize the work of breathing.

Figure 10.5 shows an illustration of the ASV breath delivery. In this illustration, the ventilator attempts to maintain the same airway pressure and PMV while respiratory mechanics vary. Specifically, breath (b) in Figure 10.5 has the same peak airway pressure as in (a), but a reduced peak inspiratory flow and lower respiration rate. This typifies the response of ASV to an increase in the respiratory impedance resulting in a lower peak flow to achieve the same peak airway pressure. Breath (c) in Figure 10.5 illustrates the ASV's ability to restore the flow and rate to the level of breath (a) if the patient's airway impedance goes back to the level equal to the one for breath (a). Breath (d) illustrates that if the impedance rises to the level of (b), the ASV algorithm will again adjust the flow and respiration rate accordingly.

10.3.4 Spontaneous Ventilation

An important phase in providing respiratory care to a recovering pulmonary patient is weaning the patient from the respirator. As the patient recovers and regains the ability to breathe independently, the spontaneous mode of ventilation allows the patient to initiate a breath and control the breath rate, flow rate, and the tidal volume. Ideally, when a respirator is functioning in the spontaneous mode, it should allow the patient take breaths with the same ease as breathing from the atmosphere. This, however, is difficult to achieve because the respirator does not have an infinite gas supply or an instantaneous response. In practice, the patient generally has to exert more effort to breathe in spontaneous mode than from the atmosphere. However, patient's effort is reduced as the ventilator response speed increases (Chatburn, 2004). Spontaneous ventilation is often used in conjunction with mandatory ventilation because the patient may still need breaths that are delivered entirely by the ventilator. Alternatively, when a patient can completely breathe on his own but needs oxygen-enriched breath or elevated airway pressure, spontaneous ventilation alone may be used.

As in the case of mandatory ventilation, several modes of spontaneous ventilation have been devised by therapists. Two of the most important and popular spontaneous breath delivery modes are described below.

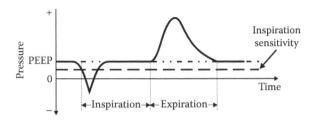

FIGURE 10.6 Airway pressure during a CPAP spontaneous breath delivery.

10.3.5 Continuous Positive Airway Pressure in Spontaneous Mode

In this mode, the ventilator maintains a positive pressure at the airway as the patient attempts to inspire. Figure 10.6 illustrates a typical airway pressure waveform during continuous positive airway pressure (CPAP) breath delivery. The therapist sets the sensitivity level lower than PEEP. The sensitivity is the pressure level that the patient has to attain by making an effort to breathe. This, in turn, triggers the ventilator to deliver a spontaneous breath by supplying air (or a mixture of air and oxygen) to raise the pressure back to the PEEP level. Typically, the PEEP and sensitivity levels are selected such that the patient will be impelled to exert effort to breathe independently. As in the case of the mandatory mode, when the patient exhales, the ventilator shuts off the flow of gas and opens the exhalation valve to allow the patient to exhale into the atmosphere.

10.3.6 Pressure Support in Spontaneous Mode

This mode is similar to the CPAP mode with the exception that during the inspiration the ventilator attempts to maintain the patient's airway pressure at a level above PEEP, called pressure support level. In fact, CPAP may be considered a special case of pressure support ventilation in which the support level is fixed at the atmospheric level.

Figure 10.7 shows a typical airway pressure waveform during the delivery of a *pressure support* breath. In this mode, when the patient's airway pressure drops below the therapist-set sensitivity line, the breath delivery system raises the airway pressure to the pressure support level (>PEEP), selected by the therapist. The ventilator stops the inspiratory gas flow when the patient starts to exhale and controls the exhalation valve to achieve the set PEEP level.

10.3.7 Breath Delivery Control

In a microprocessor-based ventilator, the mechanisms for delivering mandatory volume- and pressure-controlled ventilation have mostly common components. The primary difference lies in the control algorithms governing the delivery of breaths to the patient.

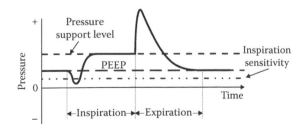

FIGURE 10.7 Airway pressure during a pressure support spontaneous breath delivery.

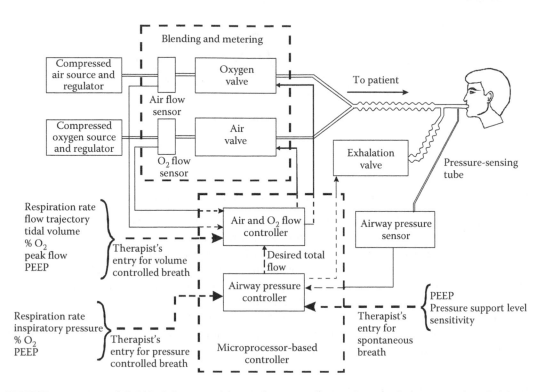

FIGURE 10.8   A simplified block diagram of a control structure for mandatory and spontaneous breath delivery.

Figure 10.8 shows a simplified block diagram for delivering mandatory and spontaneous ventilation. Compressed air and oxygen are normally stored in high pressure tanks ($\cong 1400$ kPa) that are attached to the inlets of the ventilator. In some ventilators, an air compressor is used in place of a compressed air tank. Manufacturers of mechanical respirators have designed a variety of blending and metering devices (Chatburn, 2004). The primary purpose of the device is to enrich the inspiratory air flow with proper levels of oxygen and deliver a tidal volume according to the therapist's specifications. Since nearly two decades, the microprocessors are used to control the metering and blending of the breath delivery (Puritan-Bennett, 1990). In Figure 10.8, the air and oxygen valves are placed in closed feedback loops with the air and oxygen flow sensors. The microprocessor controls the valves to deliver the desired inspiratory air and oxygen flows for mandatory and spontaneous ventilation. During inhalation, the exhalation valve is closed to direct all of the delivered flows to the lungs. When exhalation begins, the microprocessor actuates the exhalation valve to achieve the desired PEEP level. The airway pressure sensor, shown on the right side of Figure 10.8, generates the feedback signal necessary for maintaining the desired PEEP (in both mandatory and spontaneous modes) and airway pressure during inspiratory breath delivery.

10.3.8 Mandatory Volume-Controlled Inspiratory Flow Delivery

In a microprocessor-controlled ventilator (Figure 10.8), the electronically actuated valves open from a closed position to allow the flow of blended gases to the patient. The control of flow through each valve depends on the therapist's specification for the mandatory breath. That is, the clinician must specify the following parameters for the delivery of volume-controlled mandatory ventilation breaths: (1) respiration rate; (2) flow waveform; (3) tidal volume; (4) oxygen concentration (of the delivered breath); (5) peak flow; and (6) PEEP, as shown in the lower left side of Figure 10.8. It is noted that the PEEP selected by the therapist in the mandatory mode is only used for the control of exhalation flow; this will be described later in this chapter. The microprocessor uses the first five of the above parameters to compute the total desired inspiratory flow trajectory. To illustrate this point, consider the delivery of a tidal volume using a half sine wave as shown in Figure 10.3. If the therapist selects a tidal volume of V_t (L), a respiration rate of n breaths per minute (bpm), the amplitude of the respirator flow, Q_i (L/s), then the total desired inspiratory flow, $Q_d(t)$, for a single breath, can be computed from the following equation:

$$Q_d(t) = \begin{cases} Q_i \sin\left(\dfrac{\pi t}{t_i}\right) & 0 \leq t < t_i \\ 0 & t < t \leq t_e \end{cases} \tag{10.1}$$

where t_i signifies the duration of inspiration and is computed from the following relationship:

$$t_i = \frac{\pi V_t}{2Q_i} \tag{10.2}$$

The duration of expiration in seconds is obtained from

$$t_e = \frac{60}{n} - t_i \tag{10.3}$$

The ratio of the inspiratory to expiratory period of a mandatory breath is often used for adjusting the respiration rate. This ratio is represented by *I:E (ratio)* and computed as follows. First, the inspiratory and expiratory periods are normalized with respect to t_i. Hence, the normalized inspiratory period becomes unity and the normalized expiratory period is given by $R = (t_e/t_i)$. Then, I:E ratio is simply expressed as 1:R.

To obtain the desired oxygen concentration in the delivered breath, the microprocessor computes the discrete form of $Q_d(t)$ as $Q_d(k)$, where k signifies the sample interval. Then, the total desired flow, $Q_d(k)$, is partitioned using the following relationships:

$$Q_{da}(k) = \frac{(1 - m)Q_d(k)}{(1 - c)} \tag{10.4}$$

and

$$Q_{dx}(k) = \frac{(m - c)Q_d(k)}{(1 - c)} \tag{10.5}$$

where $Q_{da}(k)$ is the desired air flow (the subscript *da* stands for desired air), $Q_{dx}(k)$ is the desired oxygen flow (the subscript *dx* stands for desired oxygen), m is the desired oxygen concentration, and c is the oxygen concentration of the ventilator air supply.

Several control design strategies may be appropriate for the control of air and oxygen flow delivery valves. A simple controller is the proportional plus integral controller that can be readily implemented in a microprocessor. For example, the controller for the air valve has the following form:

$$I(k) = K_p E(k) + K_i A(k) \tag{10.6}$$

where $E(k)$ and $A(k)$ are given by

$$E(k) = Q_{da}(k) - Q_{sa}(k) \tag{10.7}$$

$$A(k) = A(k-1) + E(k) \tag{10.8}$$

where $I(k)$ is the input (voltage or current) to the air valve at the kth sampling interval, $E(k)$ the error in the delivered flow, $Q_{da}(k)$ the desired air flow, $Q_{sa}(k)$ the sensed or actual air flow (the subscript sa stands for sensed air flow), $A(k)$ the integral (rectangular integration) part of the controller, and Kp and Ki are the controller design parameters. It is noted that Equations 10.6 through 10.8 are applicable to the control of either air or oxygen valve. For the control of oxygen flow valve, $Q_{dx}(k)$ replaces $Q_{da}(k)$ and $Q_{sx}(k)$ replaces $Q_{sa}(k)$, where $Q_{sx}(k)$ represents the sensed oxygen flow (the subscript sx stands for sensed oxygen flow).

The control structure shown in Figure 10.8 provides the flexibility of quickly adjusting the percent oxygen in the enriched breath gases. That is, the controller can regulate both the total flow and the percent oxygen delivered to the patient. Because the internal volume of the flow control valve is usually small (<50 mL), the desired change in the oxygen concentration of the delivered flow can be achieved within one inspiratory period. In actual clinical applications, rapid change of percent oxygen from one breath to another is often desirable, as it reduces the waiting time for the delivery of the desired oxygen concentration. A design similar to the one shown in Figure 10.8 has been successfully implemented in a microprocessor-based ventilator (Behbehani, 1984) and deployed in hospitals around the world.

10.3.9 Pressure-Controlled Inspiratory Flow Delivery

The therapist entry for pressure-controlled ventilation is shown in Figure 10.8 (lower left-hand side). In contrast to the volume-controlled ventilation, where $Q_d(t)$ was computed directly from operators' entry (Equations 10.1 through 10.3), the total desired flow is generated by the closed-loop airway pressure controller shown in Figure 10.8. This controller uses the therapist-selected inspiratory pressure, respiration rate, and the I:E ratio to compute the desired inspiratory pressure trajectory. The trajectory serves as the controller reference input. The controller then computes the flow necessary to make the actual airway pressure track the reference input. Assuming a proportional-plus-integral controller, the governing equations are

$$Q_d(k) = C_p E_p(k) + C_i A_p(k) \tag{10.9}$$

where Q_d is the computed desired flow, C_p and C_i are the controller design parameters, k represents the sample interval, and $E_p(k)$ and $A_p(k)$ are computed using the following equations:

$$E_p(k) = P_d(k) - P_s(k) \tag{10.10}$$

$$A_p(k) = A_p(k-1) + E_p(k) \tag{10.11}$$

where $E_p(k)$ is the difference between the desired pressure trajectory, $P_d(k)$, and the sensed airway pressure, $P_s(k)$, the parameter $A_p(k)$ represents the integral portion of the controller. Using Q_d from Equation 10.9, the control of air and O_2 valves is accomplished in the same manner as in the case of volume-controlled ventilation described earlier (Equations 10.4 through 10.8).

10.3.10 Expiratory Pressure Control in Mandatory Mode

It is often desirable to keep the patient's lungs inflated at the end of expiration at a pressure greater than the atmospheric level (Pierce, 2007). That is, rather than allowing the lungs to deflate during the exhalation, the controller closes the exhalation valve when the airway pressure reaches the PEEP level. When expiration begins, the ventilator terminates flow to the lungs. Hence, the regulation of the airway pressure is achieved by controlling the flow of patient-exhaled gases through the exhalation valve.

In a microprocessor-based ventilator, an electronically actuated valve can be employed that has adequate dynamic response ($\approx$20 ms rise time) to regulate PEEP. For this purpose, the pressure in the patient's breath delivery circuit is measured using a pressure transducer (Figure 10.8). The microprocessor initially opens the exhalation valve completely to minimize resistance to expiratory flow. At the same time, it samples the pressure transducer's output and begins to close the exhalation valve as the pressure begins to approach the desired PEEP level. Because the patient's exhaled flow is the only source of pressure, if the airway pressure drops below PEEP, it cannot be brought back up until the next inspiratory period. Hence, an overrun (i.e., a drop to a level below PEEP) in the closed-loop control of PEEP should be avoided.

10.3.11 Spontaneous Breath Delivery Control

The small diameter ($\cong$5 mm) pressure sensing tube, shown on the right side of Figure 10.8, pneumatically transmits the pneumatic pressure signal from the patient's airway to a pressure transducer placed in the ventilator. The output of the pressure transducer is amplified, filtered, and then sampled by the microprocessor. The controller receives the therapist's inputs regarding the spontaneous breath characteristics, such as the PEEP, sensitivity, and oxygen concentration, as shown in the lower right-hand side of Figure 10.8. The desired airway pressure is computed from the therapist entries of PEEP, pressure support level, and sensitivity. The multiple-loop control structure shown in Figure 10.8 is used to deliver a CPAP or a pressure support breath. The sensed proximal airway pressure is compared with the desired airway pressure. The airway pressure controller computes the total inspiratory flow level required to raise the airway pressure to the desired level. This flow level serves as the reference input or total desired flow for the flow control loop. Hence, in general, the desired total flow trajectory for the spontaneous breath delivery may be different for each inspiratory cycle. If the operator has specified oxygen concentration greater than 21.6% (the oxygen concentration of the ventilator air supply), the controller will partition the total required flow into the air and oxygen flow rates using Equations 10.4 and 10.5. The flow controller then uses the feedback signals from air and oxygen flow sensors and actuates the air and oxygen valves to deliver the desired flows.

For a microprocessor-based ventilator, the control algorithm for regulating the airway pressure can also be a proportional plus integral controller (Behbehani, 1984; Behbehani and Watanabe, 1986). In this case, the governing equations are identical to Equations 10.9 through 10.11.

10.4 Summary

Modern positive-pressure mechanical ventilators have been quite successful in treating patients with pulmonary disorders. Two major categories of breath delivery modes for these ventilators are mandatory and spontaneous. The volume- and pressure-controlled mandatory breath delivery and the governing control equations for these modes are presented in this chapter. Similarly, CPAP and support pressure modes of spontaneous breath delivery are described. Recent development of dual control modes that allow simultaneous monitoring and control of airway pressure and minute volume are also presented.

Defining Terms

Continuous positive airway pressure (CPAP): A spontaneous ventilation mode in which the ventilator maintains a constant positive pressure, near or below PEEP level, in the patient's airway while the patient breathes at will.

Controlled mandatory ventilation (CMV): A term that encompasses both pressure- and volume-controlled ventilation modes. It reflects that the ventilator controls all parameters of ventilating the patient.

I:E ratio: The ratio of normalized inspiratory interval to normalized expiratory interval of a mandatory breath. Both intervals are normalized with respect to the inspiratory period. Hence, the normalized inspiratory period is always unity.

Mandatory mode: A mode of mechanically ventilating the lungs, in which the ventilator controls all breath delivery parameters, such as tidal volume, respiration rate, flow waveform, and so on.

Minute volume: Total inspiratory volume delivered to a patient in 1 min.

Patient circuit: A set of tubes connecting the patient's airway to the outlet of a respirator.

Positive end expiratory pressure (PEEP): A therapist-selected patient's airway pressure level that the ventilator maintains at the end of expiration in either mandatory or spontaneous breathing.

Pressure support: A spontaneous breath delivery mode during which the ventilator applies a positive pressure greater than PEEP to the patient's airway during inspiration.

Pressure support level: Refers to the pressure level, above PEEP, that the ventilator maintains during the spontaneous inspiration.

Pressure-controlled ventilation: A mandatory mode of ventilation where during the inspiration phase of each breath a constant pressure is applied to the patient's airway independent of the patient's respiratory mechanics.

Spontaneous mode: A ventilation mode in which the patient initiates and breathes from the ventilator-supplied gas at will.

Synchronized intermittent mandatory ventilation: A mandatory mode of ventilation that is combined with a spontaneous mode and allows the patient to initiate and breathe spontaneously while monitoring the total volume of spontaneously delivered breaths and supplementing with mandatory breaths as needed.

Volume-controlled ventilation: A mandatory mode of ventilation where the volume of each breath is set by the therapist and the ventilator delivers that volume to the patient independent of the patient's respiratory mechanics.

References

Behbehani, K. 1984. PLM-Implementation of a multiple closed-loop control strategy for a microprocessor-controlled respirator. *Proceedings of the ACC Conference*, 574–576.

Behbehani, K. and Watanabe, N.T. 1986. A new application of digital computer simulation in the design of a microprocessor-based respirator. *Summer Simulation Conference*, 415–420.

Brunner, J.X. and Iotti, G.A. 2002. Adaptive support ventilation. *Minerva Anestesiol*, 68(5):365–368.

Chatburn, R.L. 2004. *Mechanical Ventilation*, 1st ed., Mandu Press Ltd., Cleveland Heights, Ohio.

Lellouche, F. and Brochard, L. 2009. Advanced closed loops during mechanical ventilation (PAV, NAVA, ASV, SmartCare). *Best Practice and Research Clinical Anesthesiology* 23:81–93.

MacIntyre, N.R. and Branson, R.D. 2009. *Mechanical Ventilation*, 2nd ed., Saunders Elsevier, St. Louis, Missouri.

Mireles-Cabodevila, E., Diaz-Guzman, E., Heresi, G.A., and Chaburn, R.L. 2009. Alternative modes of mechanical ventilation: A review for the hospitalist. *Cleveland Clinic Journal of Medicine* 76(7): 417–430.

Otis, A.B., Fenn, W.O., and Rahn H. 1950. Mechanics of breathing in man. *Journal of Applied Physiology* 2:592–607.

Pierce, L.N.B. 2007. *Management of the Mechanically Ventilated Patients*, 2nd ed., Saunders Elsevier, St. Louis, Missouri.

Puritan-Bennett 7200 Ventilator System Series. Ventilator, Options and Accessories, Part. No. 22300A, Carlsbad, California, September 1990.

Wu, C., Lin, H., Perng, W., Yang, S., Chen, C., Huang, Y.T., and Huang, K. 2010. Correlation between the % min vol setting and work of breathing during adaptive support ventilation in patients with respiratory failure. *Respiratory Care*, 55(3):334–341.

11

Essentials of Anesthesia Delivery

A. William Paulsen
Quinnipiac University

11.1 Introduction

This chapter will provide an introduction to the practice of anesthesiology and to the technology currently employed. Limitations on the length of this chapter, considering the enormous size of the topic, requires that this chapter relies on other elements within this handbook and other texts cited as general references for many of the details that inquisitive minds desire and deserve. References by Dorsch and Dorsch (2008), Gallagher and Issenberg (2007), Kofke and Nadkarni (2007), Kyle and Murray (2008), and Loeb (1993) give additional information regarding the topics in this chapter.

11.2 Components of Anesthesia Care

Anesthesia care usually begins with preoperative evaluation and assessment of the patient days before they enter the hospital or surgery center for surgery. Preoperative care begins when the patient enters the holding area before surgery where they are evaluated again and their medical history is reviewed as venous access is established and preoperative medication administered. The patient is transported to the operating room and all the monitoring systems are applied. When everyone is ready, anesthesia is induced and the surgery begins. Following the completion of surgery, the patient moves to the recovery room where they are monitored by the postanesthesia recovery unit nurses.

The practice of anesthesia includes more than just providing relief from pain; in fact, pain relief can be considered a secondary facet of the specialty. In actuality, the modern concept of the safe and efficacious delivery of anesthesia requires consideration of three fundamental tenets and is ordered here by relative importance:

1. Maintenance of vital organ function
2. The relief of pain
3. The maintenance of the "internal milieu"

The first, maintenance of vital organ function, is concerned with preventing damage to cells and organ systems that could result from inadequate supply of oxygen and other metabolic substrates. The delivery of blood and cellular substrates is often referred to as perfusion of the cells or tissues. During the delivery of an anesthetic, the patient's "vital signs" are monitored in an attempt to prevent inadequate tissue perfusion. However, the surgery itself, the patient's existing pathophysiology, drugs given for the relief of pain, or even the management of blood pressure may compromise tissue perfusion. There is a great need for a patient monitoring system to provide direct information concerning adequacy of perfusion. Why is adequate perfusion of tissues a higher priority than providing relief of pain for which anesthesia is named? A rather obvious extreme example is that without cerebral perfusion or perfusion of the spinal cord, delivery of an anesthetic is not necessary. Damage to other organ systems may result in a range of complications from delaying the patient's recovery to diminishing their quality of life or to premature death.

In other words, the primary purpose of anesthesia care is to maintain adequate delivery of required substrates to each organ and cell, which will hopefully preserve cellular function throughout the body. Surgical retraction may result in diminished blood flow to organ systems, again demonstrating the need to monitor adequacy of perfusion.

The second principle of anesthesia is to relieve the pain caused by surgery. The first use of ether for surgical anesthesia occurred in March of 1842 in Georgia by a surgeon named Crawford Long. More than 4 years later in October of 1846, there was a public demonstration of ether anesthesia for the relief of pain from a surgical procedure at the Massachusetts General Hospital. The use of ether and chloroform to render a patient unconscious spread quickly to England and Europe.

The field of treating chronic pain and suffering caused by many disease states is now managed by a subspecialty within anesthesia, called pain management. However, many pain services are multidisciplinary relying on neurologists, anesthesiologists, as well as other physician specialists.

The third principle of anesthesia is the maintenance of the internal environment of the body. For example, the regulation of electrolytes (sodium, potassium, chloride, magnesium, calcium, etc.), acid–base balance, and a host of supporting functions on which cellular function and organ system communications rest.

11.3 Who Delivers Anesthesia?

The person delivering anesthesia may be

- An anesthesiologist (physician specializing in anesthesiology)
- An anesthesiology physician assistant (a person trained in a medical school at the masters level to administer anesthesia as a member of the care team led by an anesthesiologist)
- Or a nurse anesthetist (a nurse with intensive care unit experience who has additional training in nurse anesthesia at the master's level)

11.4 Types of Anesthesia

There are three major categories of anesthesia provided to patients: (1) general anesthesia, (2) conduction anesthesia, and (3) monitored anesthesia care. General anesthesia typically includes the intravenous injection of anesthetic drugs (hypnotics such as propofol) that render the patient unconscious, followed by delivery of inhalation anesthetic drugs, intravenous analgesics, and often drugs that paralyze skeletal muscles. Immediately following drug administration, a plastic tube is inserted into the trachea and the patient is connected to an electropneumatic system to maintain ventilation of the lungs. All inhalation anesthetics are provided as liquids that require vaporizers to convert the liquid into a breathable vapor. In some cases, nitrous oxide is also administered along with the inhalation agent or other intravenous anesthetic drugs to maintain anesthesia for surgical procedures. When combinations of inhalation agents and intravenous agents are used together to provide anesthesia, it is called a balanced anesthetic.

Conduction anesthesia refers to blocking the conduction of pain and possibly motor nerve impulses traveling along specific nerves. This is also called regional anesthesia because it affects only a specific region of the body. The common forms of conduction anesthesia include spinal and epidural anesthesia, as well as specific nerve blocks, for example, axillary nerve blocks that are used to facilitate surgery of the forearm and hand. To achieve a successful conduction anesthetic, local anesthetic agents, such as lidocaine are injected into the proximity of specific nerves to block the conduction of electrical impulses. In addition, sedation may be provided intravenously to keep the patient comfortable while they are lying still for the surgery.

Monitored anesthesia care refers to monitoring and managing the patient's vital signs while administering sedatives and analgesics to keep the patient comfortable. Also, the anesthesia team is available to treat complications related to the surgical procedure. Typically, the surgeon administers topical or local anesthetics to alleviate regional pain. Throughout the hospital and in outlying locations, nurses, physician assistants, and others are providing what is called conscious sedation for patients. Conscious sedation can be very helpful in gastrointestinal laboratories, radiology, and other areas where patients need to be sedated but not anesthetized. Unfortunately, sedation is part of a continuum that spans local anesthesia only without much sedation, to general anesthesia. A person who administers a propofol infusion to make the patient comfortable may inadvertently cause the patient to stop breathing from the side effects of propofol. Without proper monitoring, the knowledge to recognize and effectively interpret the monitored data, and the skills required to manage a general anesthetic, the outcomes may be less than desired. There are many patient safety issues here that could benefit from improved technology and better drugs.

To provide the range of support required, from the paralyzed mechanically ventilated patient to the patient receiving monitored anesthesia care, a versatile anesthesia delivery system must be available to the anesthesia care team. Today's anesthesia delivery system comprises six major elements (Figure 11.1):

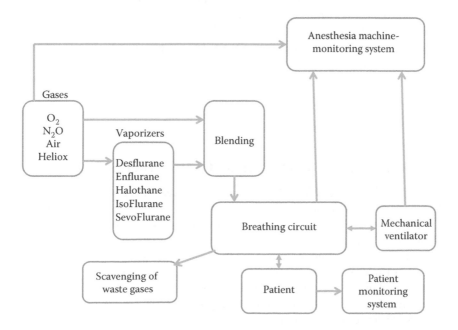

FIGURE 11.1 Block diagram of the basic components of the anesthesia delivery system.

(1) the primary and secondary sources of gases (O_2, air, N_2O, vacuum, gas scavenging, and possibly CO_2 and helium); (2) the gas blending and vaporization system; (3) the breathing circuit (including methods for manual and mechanical ventilation); (4) the excess gas scavenging system that minimizes potential pollution of the operating room by anesthetic gases; (5) instruments and equipment to monitor the function of the anesthesia delivery system; and (6) patient monitoring instrumentation and equipment. Newer additions to the anesthesia machine include the control of infusion pumps for the delivery of total intravenous anesthesia (TIVA), and closed-loop control of the patient's carbon dioxide concentrations and inhalation anesthetic levels (released in Europe, but not yet approved by the Food and Drug Administration (FDA) for use in the United States).

11.5 Gases Used during Anesthesia and Their Sources

Most inhaled anesthetic agents are liquids that are vaporized in a device within the anesthesia delivery system. The exception is xenon that is a naturally occurring gas and worthy of mention because it is an almost perfect inhalational anesthetic—except for one thing, cost. While it can provide general anesthesia, it is prohibitively expensive to produce because its concentration in the atmosphere is only 0.0000087% by volume.

The vaporized agents are then blended with other breathing gases before flowing into the breathing circuit and being administered to the patient. The most commonly administered form of anesthesia is called a balanced general anesthetic and is a combination of inhalation agent plus intravenous analgesic drugs. Intravenous drugs often require electromechanical devices to administer an appropriately controlled flow of drug to the patient.

Gases needed for the delivery of anesthesia are generally limited to oxygen (O_2), air, nitrous oxide (N_2O), and possibly helium (He). Vacuum and gas scavenging systems are also required. There needs to be secondary sources of these gases in the event of primary failure or questionable contamination. Typically, primary sources are those supplied from a hospital distribution system at 345 kPa (50 psig) through gas columns or wall outlets. The secondary sources of gas are cylinders hung on yokes on the anesthesia delivery system.

Oxygen provides an essential metabolic substrate for all human cells, but it is not without dangerous side effects. Prolonged exposure to high concentrations of oxygen may result in toxic effects within the lung that decrease diffusion of gas into and out of the blood. In neonates, the return to breathing air following prolonged exposure to elevated O_2 concentrations may result in a debilitating explosive blood vessel growth.

Oxygen is usually delivered to the hospital in liquid form (boiling point of −183°C), stored in cryogenic tanks, vaporized, and supplied to the hospital piping system as a gas. The reason for liquid storage is efficiency, since 1 L of liquid becomes 860 L of gas at standard temperature and pressure. The secondary source of oxygen within an anesthesia delivery system is usually one or more *E* cylinders filled with gaseous oxygen at a pressure of 15.2 MPa (2200 psig).

11.5.1 Air (78% N_2, 21% O_2, 0.9% Ar, and 0.1% Other Gases)

The primary use of air during anesthesia is as a diluent to decrease the inspired oxygen concentration. The typical primary source of medical air (there is an important distinction between "air" and "medical air" related to the quality and the requirements for periodic testing) is a special compressor that avoids hydrocarbon-based lubricants for purposes of medical air purity. Dryers are employed to rid the compressed air of water before distribution throughout the hospital. Medical facilities with limited need for medical air may use banks of *H* cylinders of dry medical air. A secondary source of air may be available on the anesthesia machine as an *E* cylinder containing dry gas at 15.2 MPa.

Nitrous oxide is a colorless, odorless, and nonirritating gas that does not support human life. Breathing more than 85% N_2O may be fatal. N_2O is not an anesthetic (except under hyperbaric conditions), rather, it is an analgesic and an amnestic. There are many reasons for administering N_2O during the course of

TABLE 11.1 Physical Properties of Gases Used during Anesthesia

Gas	Molecular Wt	Density (g/L)	Viscosity (cp)	Specific Heat (kJ/kg°C)
Oxygen	31.999	1.326	0.0203	0.917
Nitrogen	28.013	1.161	0.0175	1.040
Air	28.975	1.200	0.0181	1.010
Nitrous oxide	44.013	1.836	0.0144	0.839
Carbon dioxide	44.01	1.835	0.0148	0.850
Helium	4.003	0.1657	0.0194	5.190

an anesthetic including enhancing the speed of induction and emergence from anesthesia, decreasing the concentration requirements of potent inhalation anesthetics (i.e., halothane, isoflurane, etc.), and as an essential adjunct to narcotic analgesics. N_2O is supplied to anesthetizing locations from banks of *H* cylinders that are filled with 90% liquid at a pressure of 5.1 MPa (745 psig). Secondary supplies are available on the anesthesia machine in the form of *E* cylinders, again containing 90% liquid. Continual exposure to low levels of N_2O in the workplace has been implicated in several medical problems, including spontaneous abortion, infertility, birth defects, cancer, liver and kidney disease, and others. Although there is no conclusive evidence to support most of these implications, there is a recognized need to scavenge all waste anesthetic gases and periodically sample N_2O levels in the workplace to maintain the lowest possible levels consistent with reasonable risk to the operating room personnel and cost to the institution (Dorsch and Dorsch, 2008).

Carbon dioxide is colorless, odorless, but very irritating to breathe in higher concentrations. CO_2 is a by-product of human cellular metabolism and is not a life-sustaining gas. CO_2 influences many physiologic processes either directly or through the action of hydrogen ions by the reaction $CO_2 + H_2O \leftrightarrow H_2CO_3 \leftrightarrow H^+ + HCO_3^-$. Although not very common in the United States today, in the past, CO_2 was administered during anesthesia to stimulate respiration that was depressed by anesthetic agents and to cause increased blood flow in otherwise compromised vasculature during certain surgical procedures. Like N_2O, CO_2 is supplied as a liquid in *H* cylinders and then vaporized for distribution in pipeline systems or as a liquid in *E* cylinders that are located on the anesthesia machine. CO_2 may be used during cardiopulmonary bypass procedures while artificially oxygenating the blood.

Helium is a colorless, odorless, and nonirritating gas that does not support life. The primary use of helium in anesthesia is to enhance gas flow through small orifices as in asthma, airway trauma, or tracheal stenosis. The viscosity of helium is not different from other anesthetic gases (refer to Table 11.1) and is therefore not beneficial when the airway flow is laminar. However, in the event that ventilation must be performed through abnormally narrow orifices or tubes that create turbulent flow conditions, helium is the preferred carrier gas. Resistance to turbulent flow is proportional to the density rather than viscosity of the gas and helium is an order of magnitude less dense than other gases. A secondary advantage of helium is that it has a large specific heat relative to other anesthetic gases and, therefore, can carry the heat from laser surgery out of the airway more effectively than air, oxygen, or nitrous oxide, although this has never been demonstrated to be clinically significant. Helium is usually supplied as a mixture with oxygen (heliox, 25% O_2, and 75% helium).

11.5.2 Gas Blending and Vaporization System

The basic anesthesia machine utilizes primary low-pressure gas sources of 345 kPa (50 psig) available from wall or ceiling column outlets, and secondary high-pressure gas sources located on the machine. Oxygen may come from either the low-pressure source or from the 15.2 MPa (2200 psig) high-pressure yokes via cylinder pressure regulators. All anesthesia machines are required to have a safety system for limiting the minimum concentration of oxygen that can be delivered to the patient to 25%. Most currently available anesthesia machines are microprocessor based and of varying levels of electronic

TABLE 11.2   Physical Properties of Currently Available Volatile Anesthetic Agents

Agent Generic Name	Boiling Point (°C at 760 mmHg)	Vapor Pressure (mmHg at 20°C)	Liquid Density (g/mL)	MAC[a] (%)
Halothane	50.2	243	1.86	0.75
Enflurane	56.5	175	1.517	1.68
Isoflurane	48.5	238	1.496	1.15
Desflurane	23.5	664	1.45	6.0
Sevoflurane	58.5	160	1.51	2.0

[a] Minimum alveolar concentration is the percent of the agent required to provide surgical anesthesia to 50% of the population in terms of a cumulative dose–response curve. The lower the MAC, the more potent is the agent.

sophistication. Some machines use mechanical needle valves to control gas flows and employ electronic flow sensors for display purposes rather than use rotameter glass flow tubes. Other more sophisticated machines use electronic flow controllers instead of mechanical needle valves. Some machines even use microprocessor control of vaporization managing and measuring the flow of gas flowing through the vaporization chamber and the bypass line.

The physical properties of inhalational anesthetics are provided in Table 11.2. Note that desflurane, compared to other agents, has a boiling point that is close to normal room temperature and a vapor pressure that is close to atmospheric pressure at sea level. These properties dictated a new type of vaporizer that heats the agent to 39°C in order to meter the flow of desflurane vapor into the gas flow stream. The minimum alveolar concentration (MAC) of halothane, from Table 11.2 indicates that the agent is the most potent of the agents available today with desflurane as the least potent.

Microprocessors with their measurement and control functions provide means for integration of monitoring and assuring proper operation of the machine, but not proper use by the clinician. Anesthesia machines are becoming more like automobiles in that the microprocessors that monitor and control the engine performance have now eliminated the ability of the users to identify and locate problems. The machines have become so sophisticated that clinicians are no longer able to troubleshoot or find workarounds for problems that occur during use. Even the factory service personnel have become so specialized that hospitals that own several models of anesthesia delivery systems have different service personnel for different machines. Local service provided by clinical engineering departments to anesthesia equipment is becoming similar to how these departments handle patient monitoring. Clinical engineering departments stock printed circuit boards and modules that can be exchanged rather than troubleshooting to the component level. The advantages of all electronic anesthesia machines are to monitor proper function of complex electronics, integrate alarm functions to create smart alarms, and begin to implement control functions such as closed-loop control of ventilatory parameters. The downside to all electronic machines is the creation of numerous complex catastrophic failure modes.

Currently, most anesthesia machines in the United States use calibrated flow through vaporizers, meaning that all the gases from the various flowmeters are mixed in the manifold before entering the vaporizer. Any given vaporizer has a calibrated control knob that once set to the desired concentration for a specific agent will deliver that concentration to the patient. Some form of interlock system must be provided such that only one vaporizer may be activated at any given time. Figure 11.2 schematically illustrates the operation of a purely mechanical vaporizer with temperature compensation. This simple flow-over design permits a fraction of the total gas flow to pass into the vaporizing chamber where it becomes saturated with vapor before being added back to the total gas flow. Mathematically, this is approximated by

$$F_A = \frac{Q_{VC}{}^*P_A}{P_B{}^*(Q_{VC} + Q_G) - P_A{}^*Q_G}$$

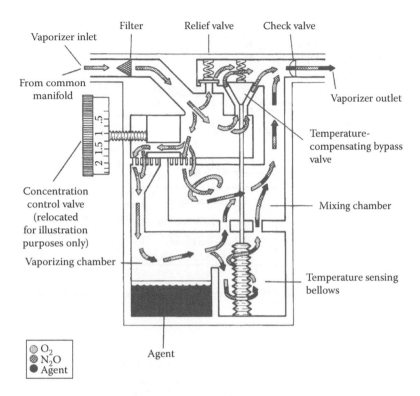

FIGURE 11.2 Schematic diagram of a calibrated in-line vaporizer that uses the flow-over technique for adding anesthetic vapor to the breathing-gas mixture.

where F_A is the fractional concentration of agent at the outlet of the vaporizer, Q_G the total flow of gas entering the vaporizer, Q_{VC} the amount of Q_G that is diverted into the vaporization chamber, P_A the vapor pressure of the agent, and P_B the barometric pressure. From Figure 11.2, the temperature compensator would decrease Q_{VC} as temperature increased because vapor pressure is proportional to temperature. The concentration accuracy over a range of clinically expected gas flows and temperatures is approximately ±15%. Because vaporization is an endothermic process, anesthetic vaporizers must have sufficient thermal mass and conductivity to permit the vaporization process to proceed independently of the rate at which the agent is being used.

The vaporizer for desflurane is in many cases unique in that it is electronic, and as Figure 11.3 illustrates, the liquid agent is heated and injects the desflurane vapor into the breathing gas. The electronics are all analog for safety reasons.

11.5.3 Breathing Circuits

The concept behind an effective breathing circuit is to provide an adequate volume of a controlled concentration of gas to the patient during inspiration and to carry the exhaled gases away from the patient during exhalation. There are several forms of breathing circuits that can be classified into two basic types: (1) open circuit, meaning no rebreathing of any gases and no CO_2 absorber present and (2) closed circuit, indicating the presence of CO_2 absorber and some rebreathing of other gases. Open circuits are rarely used because of the expense of delivering high gas flows as there is a great potential for the patient to rebreathe their own exhaled gases unless the fresh gas inflow is 2–3 times the patient's minute volume. The open circuits do have the advantage that their time constant for changing concentrations of oxygen or anesthetic agents is significantly less than a closed or semiclosed breathing system. Figure 11.4 illustrates the most popular

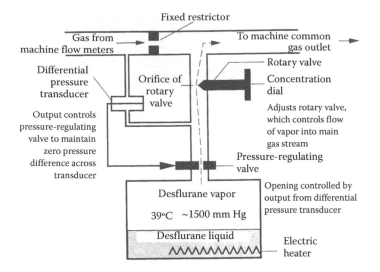

FIGURE 11.3 Schematic diagram of the TEC 6 electronic vaporizer for the administration of desflurane.

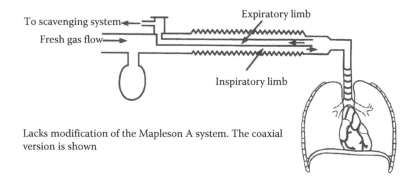

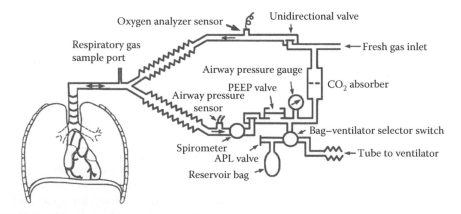

FIGURE 11.4 Diagram of a closed-circuit circle breathing system with unidirectional valves, inspired oxygen sensor, pressure sensor, and CO_2 absorber.

form of breathing circuit, the circle system, with oxygen monitor, circle pressure gage, volume monitor (spirometer), and airway pressure sensor. The circle is a closed system or semiclosed when the fresh gas inflow exceeds the patient's requirements. Excess gas evolves into the scavenging device and some of the exhaled gas is rebreathed after having the CO_2 removed. The inspiratory and expiratory valves in the circle system guarantee that gas flows to the patient from the inspiratory limb and away from the patient through the exhalation limb. In the event of a failure of either or both of these valves, the patients will rebreathe exhaled gas that contains CO_2, which is a potentially dangerous situation.

There are two forms of mechanical ventilation used during anesthesia: volume ventilation where the volume of gas delivered to the patient remains constant regardless of pressure that is required and pressure ventilation where the ventilator provides sufficient volume to the patient that is required to produce some desired pressure in the breathing circuit. Volume ventilation is the most popular because the volume delivered remains theoretically constant despite changes in lung compliance. Pressure ventilation is useful when compliance losses in the breathing circuit are high relative to the volume delivered to the lungs. Pressure ventilation also permits the alveoli with longer time constants ($\tau = R \times C$, R is airway resistance, C is alveolar compliance) to fill more completely.

There are multiple variations in these two methods of ventilation now available on anesthesia delivery systems:

1. Volume-controlled ventilation—the patient receives a specific volume of gas delivered to the lungs at set time intervals with pressure limit.
2. Pressure-controlled ventilation—a constant pressure applied to the airway and the lungs fill according to their compliance and the set pressure (volume = compliance × pressure).
3. Pressure-controlled ventilation with volume guarantee—a set pressure is delivered to the breathing circuit, but that pressure is altered by the ventilator until the set tidal volume is achieved.
4. Pressure-assist ventilation—this mode permits the patient to trigger a breath delivered by the ventilator assisting the patient's breathing.
5. Synchronous intermittent mandatory ventilation (SIMV)—this mode permits the patient to breathe on their own (spontaneous ventilation), but supplements the volume that the patient breathes according to a set breathing rate. For example, the SIMV rate may be set to 4 breaths per minute while the patient is breathing low volumes at a rate of 20 breaths/min. Every 12 s, the ventilator will assist a patient-triggered breath and deliver an adequate tidal volume. If the patient stops breathing, then the ventilator will deliver a set volume of gas 4 times/min.

Humidification is an important adjunct to the breathing circuit because it maintains the integrity of the cilia that line the airways and promote the removal of mucus and particulate matter from the lungs. Humidification of dry breathing gases can be accomplished by simple passive heat and moisture exchangers inserted into the breathing circuit at the level of the endotracheal tube connectors, or by elegant dual-servo electronic humidifiers that heat a reservoir filled with water and also heat a wire in the gas-delivery tube to prevent rainout of the water before it reaches the patient. Electronic safety measures must be included in these active devices because of the potential for burning the patient and the fire hazard.

11.5.4 Gas Scavenging Systems

The purpose of scavenging exhaled and excess anesthetic agents is to reduce or eliminate the potential hazard to employees who work in the environment where anesthetics are administered, including operating rooms, obstetrical areas, special-procedure areas, physician's offices, dentist's offices, and veterinarian's surgical suites. Typically, more gas is administered to the breathing circuit than is required by the patient, resulting in the necessity to remove excess gas from the circuit. The scavenging system must be capable of collecting gas from all components of the breathing circuit, including adjustable pressure level valves, ventilators, and sample-withdrawal type gas monitors, without

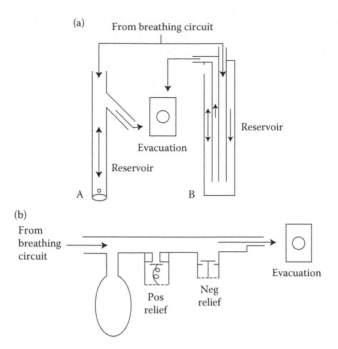

FIGURE 11.5   Examples of open- and closed-gas scavenger interfaces. The closed interface requires relief valves in the event of scavenging flow failure.

altering characteristics of the circuit, such as pressure or gas flow to the patient. There are two broad types of scavenging systems as illustrated in Figure 11.5: the open interface is a simple design that requires a large physical space for the reservoir volume, and the closed interface with an expandable reservoir bag that must include relief valves for handling the cases of no scavenged flow and great excess of scavenged flow.

Trace-gas analysis must be performed to guarantee the efficacy of the scavenging system. The National Institutes of Occupational Safety and Health (NIOSH) recommends that trace levels of nitrous oxide must be maintained at or below 25 ppm time-weighted average and that halogenated anesthetic agents remain below 2 ppm.

11.6 Monitoring the Function of the Anesthesia Delivery System

The anesthesia machine can produce a single or combinations of catastrophic events, any one of which could be fatal to the patient: (1) delivery of a hypoxic gas mixture to the patient; (2) the inability to adequately ventilate the lungs by not producing positive pressure in the patient's lungs, not delivering an adequate volume of gas to the lungs, or by improper breathing circuit connections that permit the patient's lungs to receive only rebreathed gases; and (3) the delivery of an overdose of an inhalational anesthetic agent. The necessary monitoring equipment to guarantee proper function of the anesthesia delivery system includes at least

- Inspired oxygen concentration monitor with absolute low-level alarm of 19%
- Airway pressure monitor with alarms for
  - Low pressure indicative of inadequate breathing volume and possibly a leak
  - Sustained elevated pressures that could compromise cardiovascular function
  - High pressures that could cause pulmonary barotrauma
  - Subatmospheric pressure that could cause collapse of the lungs

- Exhaled gas volume monitor
- Carbon dioxide monitor (capnography)
- Inspired and exhaled concentration of anesthetic agents

Sound monitoring principles require: (1) the earliest possible detection of untoward events (before they result in physiologic derangements) and (2) specificity that results in rapid identification and resolution of the problem. An extremely useful rule to always consider is *"never monitor the anesthesia delivery system performance through the patient's physiologic responses."* That is, never intentionally use a device, such as a pulse oximeter, to detect a breathing circuit disconnection because the warning is very late and there is no specific information provided that leads to rapid resolution of the problem.

11.7 Monitoring the Patient

The anesthetist's responsibilities to the patient include providing relief from pain and preserving all existing normal cellular function of all organ systems. Currently, the latter obligation is fulfilled by monitoring essential physiologic parameters and correcting any substantial derangements that occur before they are translated to permanent cellular damage. The inadequacy of current monitoring methods can be appreciated by realizing that most monitoring modalities only indicate damage after an insult has occurred, at which point the hope is that it is reversible or that further damage can be prevented.

Standards for basic intraoperative monitoring of patients undergoing anesthesia, which were developed and adopted by the American Society of Anesthesiologists, became effective in 1990 and were last revised in 2005. Standard I concerns the responsibilities of anesthesia personnel, whereas standard II requires that the patient's oxygenation, ventilation, circulation, and temperature must be evaluated continually during all anesthetics. The following list includes patient monitoring options that are available to anesthesia providers:

- *Electrocardiogram*
- *Pulse oximetry*
- Urine output
- Cardiac output
- Electroencephalogram (EEG)
- Evoked potentials
- *Noninvasive or invasive blood pressure*
- *Temperature*
- Nerve stimulators
- Mixed venous oxygen saturation
- Transesophageal echo cardiography (TEE)
- Coagulation status
- Blood gases and electrolytes (Po_2, Pco_2, pH, BE, Na^+, K^+, Cl^-, Ca^{2+}, and glucose)
- Capnography and breathing gas analysis (O_2, CO_2, N_2O, anesthetic agents)
- BiSpectral index or entropy monitoring systems

11.7.1 Control of Patient Temperature

Anesthesia alters the thresholds for temperature regulation and the patient becomes unable to maintain normal body temperature. As the patient's temperature falls even a few degrees toward room temperature, several physiologic derangements occur: (1) drug action is prolonged, (2) blood coagulation is impaired, and (3) postoperative infection rate increases. On the positive side, cerebral protection from inadequate perfusion is enhanced by just a few degrees of cooling. Proper monitoring of core body temperature and forced hot air warming of the patient is essential.

11.7.2 Monitoring the Depth of Anesthesia

There are two very unpleasant experiences that patients may have while undergoing an inadequate anesthetic: (1) the patient is paralyzed and unable to communicate their state of discomfort, they are feeling the pain of surgery, and are aware of their surroundings; (2) the patient may be paralyzed, unable to communicate, and is aware of their surroundings, but is not feeling any pain. The ability to monitor the depth of anesthesia would provide a safeguard against these unpleasant experiences; however, despite numerous instruments and approaches to the problem, it remains elusive. Brain stem auditory-evoked responses have come closest to the depth of anesthesia monitoring, but it is difficult to perform, expensive, and not possible to perform during many types of surgery. A promising technology, called bispectral index (BIS monitoring) is purported to measure the level of patient hypnosis through multivariate analysis of a single channel of the EEG.

11.7.3 Anesthesia Computer-Aided Record Keeping

Conceptually, every anesthetist desires an automated anesthesia record-keeping system. Anesthesia care can be improved through the feedback provided by correct record keeping, but today's systems have an enormous overhead associated with their use when compared to standard paper record keeping. No doubt that automated anesthesia record keeping reduces the drudgery of routine recording of vital signs, but to enter drugs and drips and their dosages, fluids administered, urine output, blood loss, and other data require much more time and machine interaction than the current paper system. Despite attempts to use every input/output device ever produced by the computer industry from keyboards to bar codes to voice and handwriting recognition, no solution has been found that meets wide acceptance. The tenants of a successful system must include

1. The concept of a user-transparent system, which is ideally defined as no required communication between the computer and the clinician (far beyond the concept of user friendly), and therefore that is intuitively obvious to use even to the most casual users.
2. Recognition of the fact that educational institutions have very different requirements from private practice institutions.
3. Real-time hard copy of the record produced at the site of anesthetic administration that permits real-time editing and notation.
4. Ability to interface with a great variety of patient and anesthesia delivery system monitors from various suppliers.
5. Ability to interface with a large number of hospital information systems.
6. Inexpensive to purchase and maintain.

11.7.4 Alarms

Vigilance is the key to effective risk management but maintaining a vigilant state is not easy. The practice of anesthesia has been described as moments of shear terror connected by times of intense boredom. Alarms can play a significant role in redirecting one's attention during the boredom to the most important event regarding patient safety but only if false alarms can be eliminated, alarms can be prioritized, and all alarms concerning anesthetic management can be displayed in a single clearly visible location. Alarms should be integrated through multiple monitoring modalities to provide a sensitivity of one and specificity of one. The areas of patient and equipment alarms are a fertile ground for research.

11.7.5 Ergonomics

The study of ergonomics attempts to improve performance by optimizing the relationship between people and their work environment. Ergonomics has been defined as a discipline that investigates and applies information about human requirements, characteristics, abilities, and limitations to the design, development, and testing of equipment, systems, and jobs (Loeb, 1993). This field of study applied to anesthesia is only in its infancy and examples of poor ergonomic design abound in the anesthesia workplace.

11.7.6 Simulation in Anesthesia

Almost all anesthesia academic training institutions have simulators that are used for teaching anesthesia-related skills, critical thinking, assessing knowledge and clinical judgment, and for rehearsing team-based crisis management (Gallagher and Issenberg, 2007; Kofke and Nadkarni, 2007; Kyle and Murray, 2008). Complete patient simulators are hands-on high-fidelity realistic simulators that interface with physiologic monitoring equipment to simulate patient responses to equipment malfunctions, operator errors, and drug therapies. There are also crisis management simulators for coordinating team activities such as cardiac arrest, malignant hyperthermia, and triage following large-scale disasters. Simulators are currently being explored for certification and continued demonstration of qualifications for anesthesiologists and anesthetists. Several commercially available high-fidelity patient simulators dominate the simulation landscape in anesthesia. The best method of training is a combination of simulation and direct patient care. Haptic simulators are useful for teaching skills and specific procedures.

11.7.7 Reliability

The design of an anesthesia delivery system is unlike the design of most other medical devices because it is a life-support system. As such, its core elements deserve all the considerations of the latest fail-safe technologies. Too often, in today's quest to apply microprocessor technology to everything, trade-offs are made among reliability, cost, and engineering elegance. There is an ongoing debate concerning the advantages of microprocessor-based machines with numbers of catastrophic failure modes versus simple ultrareliable mechanical systems with an absolute minimum of catastrophic failure modes. There is a phase in the development cycle in which electronic controls are added with no real advantage over simple ultrareliable machines. The next phase is closing the loop and providing many advantages that make the delivery of anesthesia safer. However, the inclusion of microprocessors can enhance the safety of anesthesia delivery if they are implemented without adding catastrophic failure modes.

References

Dorsch, J.A., Dorsch, S.E. 2008. *Understanding Anesthesia Equipment*, 5th ed. Wolters Kluwer/Lippincott Williams & Wilkins, Philadelphia, PA.

Gallagher, C.J., Issenberg, S.B. 2007. *Simulation in Anesthesia*, Saunders Elsevier, Philadelphia.

Kofke, W.A., Nadkarni, V.M. 2007. New vistas in patient safety and simulation. *Anesthesiology Clinics* 25(2).

Kyle, R.R., Murray, W.B. 2008. *Clinical Simulation; Operations, Engineering and Management*. Academic Press, Elsevier, Inc., Burlington, MA.

Loeb, R. 1993. Ergonomics of the anesthesia workplace. *STA Interface* 4(3):18.

12

Electrosurgical Devices

Jeffrey L. Eggleston
Covidien Energy-Based Devices

Wolf W. von Maltzahn
Rensselaer Polytechnic Institute

12.1 Introduction

An electrosurgical unit (ESU) passes high-frequency electric current through biological tissues to achieve surgical modification of the tissue, such as cutting, coagulation, desiccation, ablation, lesioning, shrinkage, sealing, or fusion. Electrosurgery is also known as high-frequency (HF) surgery or surgical diathermy. The fundamental frequency of electrosurgical waveforms is generally above 200 kHz to minimize the potential for neuromuscular stimulation. Various forms of electrosurgery have been in practice since the 1920s to cut tissue effectively while at the same time controlling the amount of bleeding. Cutting is achieved primarily with a continuous sinusoidal waveform, whereas coagulation is achieved with a series of sinusoidal wave packets. The surgeon selects either one of these waveforms or a blend of them to suit the surgical needs. Electrosurgical current may be delivered using several methods with the most widely used being the monopolar and bipolar modes. The most noticeable difference between these two modes is the manner in which the electrical current enters and leaves the tissue. In the monopolar mode, the current flows from a small active electrode into the surgical site, spreads through the body, and returns to a large dispersive electrode on the skin. The high current density in the vicinity of the active electrode achieves the desired tissue effect, such as cutting or coagulation, whereas the low current density under the dispersive electrode causes no tissue damage. The monopolar mode may be used for cutting, coagulating, ablating, or lesioning tissue. In the bipolar mode, the current flows only through the tissue in contact with the bipolar electrodes. The most common type of bipolar instrument is in the form of forceps. The bipolar mode may be used for coagulation, desiccation, tissue ablation, vessel sealing, or tissue fusion.

The following sections describe in detail the theoretical and technological design details of ESUs, including their modes of operation, typical applications, and potential hazards.

12.2 Theory of Operation

In principle, electrosurgery is based on rapid heating of the tissue. To better understand the thermodynamic events during electrosurgery, it helps to know the general effects of heat on biological tissue.

Consider a tissue volume that experiences a temperature increase from normal body temperature to 45°C within a few seconds. Although the cells in this tissue volume show neither microscopic nor macroscopic changes, some cytochemical changes do in fact occur. However, these changes are reversible and the cells return to their normal function when the temperature returns to normal values. Above 45°C, irreversible changes take place that inhibit normal cell functions and lead to cell death. First, between 45°C and 60°C, the proteins in the cell lose their quaternary configuration and solidify into a glutinous substance that resembles the white of a hard-boiled egg. This process, termed coagulation, is accompanied by tissue blanching. Further, increasing the temperature up to 100°C leads to tissue drying, that is, the aqueous cell contents evaporate. This process is called desiccation. If the temperature is increased beyond 100°C, the solid contents of the tissue reduce to carbon, a process referred to as carbonization. Tissue damage not only depends on temperature, however, but also on the length of exposure to heat. Thus, the overall temperature-induced tissue damage is an integrative effect between temperature and time that is expressed mathematically by the Arrhenius relationship, where an exponential function of temperature is integrated over time [1].

In the monopolar mode, the active electrode either touches the tissue directly or is held a few millimeters above the tissue. When the electrode is held above the tissue, the electric current bridges the air gap by creating an electric discharge arc. A visible arc forms when the electric field strength exceeds 1 kV/mm in the gap and disappears when the field strength drops below a certain threshold level.

When the active electrode touches the tissue and the current flows directly from the electrode into the tissue without forming an arc, the rise in tissue temperature follows the bioheat equation

$$T - T_0 = \frac{1}{\sigma \rho c} J^2 t \tag{12.1}$$

where T and T_0 are the final and initial temperatures (K), σ is the electrical conductivity (S/m), ρ the tissue density (kg/m^3), c the specific heat of the tissue (J/kg K), J the current density (A/m^2), and t the duration (s) of heat application [1]. The bioheat equation is valid for short application times where secondary effects, such as heat transfer to surrounding tissues, blood perfusion, and metabolic heat, can be neglected. According to Equation 12.1, the surgeon has primarily three means of controlling the cutting or coagulation effect during electrosurgery: the contact area between the active electrode and tissue, the electrical current density, and the activation time. In most commercially available electrosurgical generators, the only output variables that can be adjusted are power and waveform (mode). The power setting as well as the type and size of the active electrode allows the surgeon some control over the current. Table 12.1 lists typical output power and mode settings for various surgical procedures. Table 12.2 lists some typical tissue impedance ranges seen during the use of an ESU in surgery. The values are shown as ranges because the impedance increases as the tissue dries out, and at the same time the output power of the ESU decreases.

12.3 Monopolar Mode

A continuous sinusoidal waveform, of sufficient voltage, cuts the tissue with very little hemostasis. This waveform is simply called cut or pure cut. During each positive and negative swing of the sinusoidal waveform, a new discharge arc forms and disappears at essentially the same tissue location. The electric current concentrates at this tissue location causing a sudden increase in temperature because of resistive heating. The rapid rise in temperature then vaporizes intracellular fluids, increases cell pressure, and ruptures the cell membrane, thereby parting the tissue. This chain of events is confined to the vicinity of the arc, because from there the electric current spreads to a much larger tissue volume and the current density is no longer sufficiently high to cause resistive heating damage. Typical output values for ESUs, in cut and other modes, are shown in Table 12.3.

TABLE 12.1   Typical ESU Power Settings for Various Surgical Procedures

Power-Level Range	Procedures
Low power	
<30 W cut	Neurosurgery
<30 W coag	Dermatology
	Plastic surgery
	Oral surgery
	Laparoscopic sterilization
	Vasectomy
Medium power	
30 W–150 W cut	General surgery
30 W–70 W coag	Laparotomies
	Head and neck surgery (ENT)
	Major orthopedic surgery
	Major vascular surgery
	Routine thoracic surgery
	Polypectomy
High power	
>150 W cut	Transurethral resection procedures
>70 W coag	(TURPs)
	Thoracotomies
	Ablative cancer surgery
	Mastectomies

Note: Ranges assume the use of a standard blade-type electrode; The use of a needle electrode, or other small current concentrating electrode, allows lower settings to be used; Users are urged to use the lowest setting that provides the desired clinical results.

TABLE 12.2   Typical Tissue Impedance Ranges during Electrosurgery

	Impedance Range (Ω)
Cut Mode Application	
Prostate tissue	400–1700
Oral cavity	1000–2000
Liver tissue	
Muscle tissue	
Gall bladder	1500–2400
Skin tissue	1700–2500
Bowel tissue	2500–3000
Periosteum	
Mesentery	3000–4200
Omentum	
Adipose tissue	3500– 4500
Scar tissue	
Adhesions	
Coag mode application	
Contact coagulation to stop bleeding	100–1000

TABLE 12.3   Typical Output Characteristics of ESUs

	Output Voltage Range Open Circuit, $V_{peak-peak}$ (V)	Output Power Range (W)	Frequency (kHz)	Crest Factor $\left(\dfrac{V_{peak}}{V_{rms}}\right)$	Duty Cycle (%)
Monopolar Modes					
Cut	200–5000	1–400	300–1750	1.4–2.1	100
Blend	1500–5800	1–300	300–1750	2.1–6.0	25–80
Desiccate	400–6500	1–200	240–800	3.5–6.0	50–100
Fulgurate/spray	6000–12,000	1–200	300–800	6.0–20.0	10–70
Bipolar mode					
Coagulate/ desiccate	200–1000	1–70	300–1050	1.6–12.0	25–100

Experimental observations have increasingly shown that hemostasis is achieved when cutting with an interrupted sinusoidal waveform or amplitude-modulated continuous waveform. These waveforms are typically called blend or blended cut. Some ESUs offer a choice of blend waveforms to allow the surgeon to select the degree of hemostasis desired.

When a continuous or interrupted waveform is used while the electrode is in direct contact with the tissue and the output voltage is too low to cause arcing, desiccation of the tissue occurs. Some ESUs have a distinct mode for this purpose called desiccation or contact coagulation.

In noncontact coagulation, the duty cycle of an interrupted waveform and the crest factor (ratio of peak voltage to rms voltage) influence the degree of hemostasis. Although a continuous waveform reestablishes the arc at essentially the same tissue location concentrating the heat there, an interrupted waveform causes the arc to reestablish itself at different tissue locations. The arc seems to dance from one location to the other, raising the temperature of the top tissue layer to coagulation levels. These noncontact coagulation waveforms are also called fulguration or spray. Because the current inside the tissue spreads very quickly from the point where the arc strikes, the heat concentrates in the top layer, primarily desiccating the tissue and causing some carbonization.

The most widely used monopolar active electrode is a small flat blade with symmetrical leading and trailing edges that is embedded at the tip of an insulated handle. The edges of the blade are shaped to easily initiate discharge arcs and to help the surgeon manipulate the incision; they cannot mechanically cut the tissue. Because the surgeon holds the handle in his hands like a pencil, it is often referred to as the "pencil." Many pencils contain one or more switches in their handle to control the electrosurgical waveform, primarily to switch between cutting and coagulation. Other active electrodes include needle electrodes, loop electrodes, ball electrodes, and laparoscopic electrodes. Needle electrodes are used for coagulating small tissue volumes like in neurosurgery or plastic surgery. Loop electrodes are used to resect nodular structures, such as polyps or to excise tissue samples for pathological analysis. An example would be the large loop excision of the transformation zone (LLETZ) procedure in which the transition zone of the cervix is excised. Electrosurgery at the tip of an endoscope or laparoscope requires yet another set of active electrodes and specialized training of the surgeon.

Besides the traditional uses described above, there are many new applications that use monopolar energy. Tissue may be ablated or lesions created to selectively kill undesired cells. Examples are soft tissue ablation that uses a rigid monopolar electrode introduced into a tumor and cardiac ablation, which uses a flexible catheter to create a lesion in the heart to treat an arrhythmia. The delivery of monopolar energy may also be enhanced by the addition of a controlled column of argon gas in the path between the active electrode and the tissue. The flow of argon gas assists in clearing the surgical site of fluid and improves visibility. When used in the coagulation mode, the argon gas is turned into a plasma, allowing tissue damage and smoke to be reduced, and producing a thinner, more flexible eschar. When used with the cut mode, lower power levels may be used.

12.4 Dispersive Electrodes

Dispersive electrodes are also called plate electrodes, passive electrodes, return electrodes, neutral electrodes, or grounding pads. The main purpose of the dispersive electrode is to return the monopolar high-frequency current to the ESU without causing harm to the patient. This is usually achieved by attaching a large-surface-area electrode to the patient's skin at some point away from the surgical site. The large electrode area and low contact impedance reduce the current density to levels where tissue heating is minimal. Because the ability of a dispersive electrode to avoid tissue heating and burns is of primary importance, dispersive electrodes are often characterized by their "heating factor." The heating factor describes the energy dissipated under the dispersive electrode and is equal to $I^2 t$, where I is the rms current and t the time of exposure in seconds. During surgery, a typical value for the heating factor is 3 A^{2}s, but factors of up to 9 A^{2}s may occur during certain procedures [2].

Two types of dispersive electrodes are in common use today, the resistive type and the capacitive type. In disposable form, both electrodes have a similar structure and appearance. A thin, rectangular metallic foil has an insulating layer on the outside, connects to a gel-like material on the patient side and may be surrounded by adhesive foam. In the resistive type, the gel-like material is made of adhesive conductive gel, whereas in the capacitive type, it is made of dielectric nonconductive material. The adhesive foam and adhesive gel layer ensure that both electrodes maintain good skin contact to the patient, even if the electrode gets stressed mechanically from pulls on the electrode cable or some moisture develops under the electrode pad. Both types have specific advantages and disadvantages. Electrode failures and subsequent patient injury can be attributed mostly to improper application, electrode dislodgment, and electrode defects rather than to electrode design. There also exists a reusable capacitive dispersive electrode with an extra large, nonadhesive surface that is placed between the patient and the operating room table.

12.5 Bipolar Mode

The bipolar mode concentrates the current flow between two electrodes or two groups of electrodes, requiring considerably less power for achieving the same coagulation effect than the monopolar mode. For example, consider coagulating a small blood vessel with 3 mm external diameter and 2 mm internal diameter, a tissue resistivity of 360 Ωcm, a contact area of 2 × 4 mm, and a distance between the forceps tips of 1 mm. The tissue resistance between the forceps is 450 Ω as calculated from $R = \rho L/A$, where ρ is the resistivity, L the distance between the forceps, and A the contact area. Assuming a typical current density of 200 mA/cm^2, a small current of 16 mA, a voltage of 7.2 V, and a power level of 0.12 W suffice to coagulate this small blood vessel. In contrast, during monopolar coagulation, current levels of 200 mA and power levels of 100 W or more are not uncommon to achieve the same surgical effect. The temperature increase in the vessel tissue follows the bioheat Equation 12.1. If the specific heat of the vessel tissue is 4.2 J/kg K and the tissue density is 1 g/cm^3, then the temperature of the tissue between the forceps increases from 37°C to 57°C in 5.83 s. When the active electrode touches the tissue, less tissue damage occurs during coagulation because the charring and carbonization that accompany fulguration are avoided.

Surgeons may select among different sizes and shapes of forceps to further refine the desired clinical result. Fine-tipped forceps are frequently used in neurosurgery where very low power levels result in very small areas of tissue coagulation. Some hardware manufacturers have an autobipolar mode, which automatically turns the bipolar energy on when a tissue is grasped and automatically turns the energy off when a selectable level of coagulation is reached. This gives the surgeon a consistent level of coagulation, reduces tissue sticking, and greatly reduces fatigue in long procedures.

Advanced bipolar technologies include the sealing of blood vessels, fusion of tissue, tissue ablation, and bipolar cutting. Vessel sealing and tissue fusion uses special instruments and control algorithms to fuse the collagen within tissue. The most common use of this technology is to permanently seal blood vessels.

Tissue ablation utilizes bipolar or multipolar electrodes and specialized output waveforms to ablate soft or connective tissue. A tonsillectomy is an example of a procedure that may be performed using this bipolar method. Bipolar cutting does the same job as monopolar cutting but with the active and return electrodes in the same instrument. This allows lower powers to be used and a dispersive electrode is not required.

12.6 ESU Hazards

Improper use of electrosurgery may expose both the patient and the surgical staff to various hazards. By far, the most frequent hazard is an undesired burn. Less frequent are undesired neuromuscular stimulation, interference with pacemakers, or other devices, fires, and gas explosions [1,3].

Monopolar current returns to the ESU through the dispersive electrode. If the contact area of the dispersive electrode is large and the current exposure time short, then the skin temperature under the electrode does not rise above 45°C, which has been shown to be the maximum safe temperature [4]. However, to include a safety margin, the skin temperature should not rise more than 6°C above the normal surface temperature of 29–33°C [5]. The current density at any point under the dispersive electrode has to be significantly below the recognized burn threshold of 100 mA/cm² for 10 s. This means that the contact area between the electrode and the patient is the most important factor in preventing a dispersive electrode burn.

To avoid burns under dispersive electrodes, the IEC Standard for HF Surgical Devices [5] requires that "HF surgical equipment having a rated output power of more than 50 W shall be provided with a continuity monitor or contact quality monitor …." The most common of these is the contact quality monitor. A contact quality monitor consists of a circuit to measure the impedance between the two sides of a split dispersive electrode and the skin. This impedance is inversely proportional to the actual area of contact between the patient and the dispersive electrode. A small high-frequency current flows from one section of the dispersive electrode through the skin to the second section of the dispersive electrode. If the impedance between these two sections exceeds a certain threshold, or increases by a certain percentage, the patient contact area has unacceptably decreased, an audible alarm sounds, and the ESU output is disabled. The cable continuity monitor is less common. Unlike the contact quality monitor, this monitor only checks the continuity of the cable between the ESU and the dispersive electrode and sounds an alarm if the resistance in that conductor is greater than 1 Ω.

There are other sources of undesired burns. Active electrodes become hot when they are used. After use, the active electrode should be placed in a protective holster, if available, or on a suitable surface to isolate it from the patient and surgical staff [6]. The correct placement of an active electrode will also prevent the patient and/or surgeon from being injured, if an inadvertent activation of the ESU occurs (e.g., someone accidentally stepping on a foot pedal). Some surgeons use a practice called "buzzing the hemostat" in which a small bleeding vessel is grasped with a clamp or hemostat and the active electrode touched to the clamp while activating. Because of the high voltages involved and the stray capacitance to ground, the surgeon's glove may be compromised. This results in an instantaneous burn to the surgeon's finger, which feels like an electrical shock. If the surgical staff cannot be convinced to eliminate the practice of buzzing hemostats, the probability of burns can be reduced by using a cut waveform instead of a coagulation waveform (lower voltage), by maximizing contact between the surgeon's hand and the clamp, and by not activating until the active electrode is firmly touching the clamp.

Although it is commonly assumed that neuromuscular stimulation ceases or is insignificant at frequencies above 10 kHz, such stimulation has been observed in anesthetized patients undergoing certain electrosurgical procedures. This undesirable side effect of electrosurgery is generally attributed to nonlinear events that occur during the electric arcing between the active electrode and tissue [1]. These nonlinear events may rectify the high-frequency current leading to both dc and low-frequency ac components. These current components can reach magnitudes that stimulate nerve and muscle cells. To minimize the probability of unwanted neuromuscular stimulation, most ESUs incorporate in their output circuit a high-pass filter that suppresses dc and low-frequency ac components.

The use of electrosurgery means the presence of electric discharge arcs. This presents a potential fire hazard in an operating room where oxygen and flammable gases may be present. These flammable gases may be introduced by the surgical staff (anesthetics or flammable cleaning solutions), or may be generated within the patient themselves (bowel gases). The use of disposable paper drapes and dry surgical gauze also provides a flammable material that may be ignited by sparking or by contact with a hot active electrode. Therefore, prevention of fires and explosions depends primarily on the prudence and judgment of the ESU operator [7].

12.7 ESU Design

Modern ESUs contain building blocks that are also found in other medical devices, such as microprocessors, power supplies, enclosures, cables, indicators, displays, and alarms. The main building blocks unique to ESUs are control input switches, the high-frequency power amplifier, and the safety monitor.

Input control switches include front panel controls, footswitch controls, and handswitch controls. To make operating an ESU more uniform between models and manufacturers, and to reduce the possibility of operator error, the ANSI/AAMI/IEC 60601-2-2 standard [6] makes specific recommendations concerning the physical construction of ESUs and prescribes mechanical and electrical performance standards. For instance, front panel controls need to have their function identified by a permanent label and their output indicated on alphanumeric displays or on graduated scales; the pedals of foot switches need to be labeled and respond to a specified activation force; and if the active electrode handle incorporates two finger switches, their positions have to correspond to specific functions. Additional recommendations can be found in Reference 6.

Currently, three basic high-frequency power amplifiers are in use: the parallel connection of a bank of bipolar power transistors, the hybrid connection of parallel bipolar power transistors cascaded with metal oxide silicon field effect transistors (MOSFETs), and the bridge connection of MOSFETs. Each has unique properties and represents a stage in the evolution of ESUs.

In those devices that use a parallel bank of bipolar power transistors, the transistors are arranged in a Class A configuration. The bases, collectors, and emitters are all connected in parallel, and the collective base node is driven through a current-limiting resistor. A feedback resistor capacitor (RC) network between the base node and the collector node stabilizes the circuit. The collectors are usually fused individually before connecting to the common node, and through the primary coil of the step-up transformer to the high-voltage power supply. A capacitor and resistor in parallel to the primary coil create a resonant tank circuit that generates the output waveform at a specific frequency. Additional elements may be switched in and out of the primary parallel resistor inductor capacitor (RLC) circuit to alter the output power and waveform for various electrosurgical modes. Small-value resistors between the emitters and ground improve the current sharing between transistors. This configuration sometimes requires the use of matched sets of high-voltage power transistors.

A similar arrangement exists in amplifiers using parallel bipolar power transistors cascaded with a power MOSFET. This arrangement is called a hybrid cascode amplifier. In this type of amplifier, the collectors of a group of bipolar transistors are connected, via protection diodes, to one side of the primary of the step-up transformer. The other side of the primary is connected to the high-voltage power supply. The emitters of two or three bipolar transistors are connected, via current-limiting resistors, to the drain of an enhancement mode MOSFET. The source of the MOSFET is connected to ground and the gate of the MOSFET is connected to a voltage-snubbing network driven by a fixed-amplitude pulse created by a high-speed MOS driver circuit. The bases of the bipolar transistors are connected, via current control RC networks, to a common variable base voltage source. Each collector and base is separately fused. In cut modes, the gate drive pulse is at a fixed frequency and the base voltage is varied according to the power setting. In the coagulation modes, the base voltage is fixed, and the pulse width driving the MOSFET is varied. This changes the conduction time of the amplifier and controls the amount of energy imparted to the output transformer and its load. In the coagulation and the high-power cut modes, the bipolar power transistors are saturated and the voltage across the bipolar/MOSFET combination is low. This translates to high efficiency and low power dissipation.

The most common high-frequency power amplifier in use is a bridge connection of MOSFETs. In this configuration, the drains of a series of power MOSFETs are connected, via protection diodes, to one side of the primary of the step-up output transformer. The drain protection diodes protect the MOSFETs against the negative voltage swings of the transformer primary. The other side of the transformer primary is connected to the high-voltage power supply. The sources of the MOSFETs are connected to ground. The gate of each MOSFET has a resistor connected to ground and one to its driver circuitry. The resistor to ground speeds up the discharge of the gate capacitance when the MOSFET is turned on while the gate series resistor eliminates turn off oscillations. Various combinations of capacitors and/or inductor capacitor (LC) networks can be switched across the primary of the step-up output transformer to obtain different waveforms. In cut modes, the output power is controlled by varying the high-voltage power supply. In coagulation modes, the output power is controlled by varying the on time of the gate drive pulse.

Many manufacturers have begun to include sophisticated computer-based systems in their ESUs that not only simplify the use of the device but also increase the safety of patient and operator [8]. Some devices offer a so-called power-peak system that delivers a very short power peak at the beginning of electrosurgical cutting to start the cutting arc. Other modern devices use continuous monitoring of current and voltage levels to make automatic power adjustments and provide a smooth cutting action from the beginning of the incision to its end. Increased computing power, more sophisticated evaluation of voltage and current waveforms, and the addition of miniaturized sensors will continue to make ESUs more user friendly and safer.

Defining Terms

Active electrode: Electrode used for achieving desired surgical effect.
Coagulation: Solidifying proteins through the use of high-frequency currents that elevate the temperature of the tissue and reduce or terminate bleeding.
Desiccation: Drying of the tissue due to evaporation of intracellular fluids.
Dispersive electrode: Return electrode at which no electrosurgical effect is intended.
Fulguration: Random discharge of sparks between active electrode and tissue surface to achieve coagulation and/or desiccation.
Spray: Another term for fulguration. Sometimes, this waveform has a higher crest factor than fulguration.

References

1. Pearce, J.A., *Electrosurgery*, John Wiley & Sons, New York, 1986.
2. Overmyer, K.M., J.A. Pearce, and D.P. DeWitt, Measurements of temperature distributions at electro-surgical dispersive electrode sites, *J. Biomech.*, 101:66–72, 1972.
3. Francis G.G., *Unexplained Patient Burns: Investigating Iatrogenic Injuries*, Quest Publishing, Brea, CA, 1988.
4. Pearce, J.A., L.A. Geddes, J.F. Van Vleet, K. Foster, and J. Allen, Skin burns from electrosurgical current, *Med. Instrum.*, 17(3):225–231, 1983.
5. International Standard, Medical Electrical Equipment, Part 2: Particular requirements for the basic safety and essential performance of high frequency surgical equipment and high frequency surgical accessories, IEC 60601-2-2, 5th ed., 2009, International Electrotechnical Commission, Geneva, Switzerland.
6. Reed, A., Preventing thermal burns from electrosurgical instruments, *Infect. Control Today*, July 2001.

7. Podnos, Y.D. and R.A. Williams, Fires in the operating room, *Bull. Am. Coll. Surg.*, 82:8:14–17, 1997.
8. Haag, R. and A. Cuschieri, Recent advances in high-frequency electrosurgery: Development of automated systems, *J. R. Coll. Surg. Ednb.*, 38:354–364, 1993.

Further Information

American National Standard, Medical Electrical Equipment, Part 1: General requirements for basic safety and essential performance, ANSI/AAMI ES60601-1, 2005, Association for the Advancement of Medical Instrumentation, Arlington, VA.

American National Standard, Medical Electrical Equipment, Part 2: Particular requirements for the basic safety and essential performance of high frequency surgical equipment and high frequency surgical accessories, ANSI/AAMI/IEC 60601-2-2, 5th ed., 2009, Association for the Advancement of Medical Instrumentation, Arlington, VA.

International Standard, Medical Electrical Equipment, Part 1: General requirements for basic safety and essential performance, IEC 601-1, 3rd ed., 2005, International Electrotechnical Commission, Geneva, Switzerland.

13

Biomedical Lasers

Millard M. Judy
Baylor Research Institute

Approximately 20 years ago the CO_2 laser was introduced into surgical practice as a tool to photothermally ablate, and thus to incise and to debulk, soft tissues. Subsequently, three important factors have led to the expanding biomedical use of laser technology, particularly in surgery. These factors are (1) the increasing understanding of the wavelength selective interaction and associated effects of *ultraviolet–infrared (UV–IR) radiation* with biologic tissues, including those of acute damage and long-term healing, (2) the rapidly increasing availability of lasers emitting (essentially monochromatically) at those wavelengths that are strongly absorbed by molecular species within tissues, and (3) the availability of both optical fiber and lens technologies as well as of endoscopic technologies for delivery of the laser radiation to the often remote internal treatment site. Fusion of these factors has led to the development of currently available biomedical laser systems.

This chapter briefly reviews the current status of each of these three factors. In doing so, each of the following topics will be briefly discussed:

1. The physics of the interaction and the associated effects (including clinical efforts) of UV–IR radiation on biologic tissues
2. The fundamental principles that underlie the operations and construction of all lasers
3. The physical properties of the optical delivery systems used with the different biomedical lasers for delivery of the laser beam to the treatment site

4. The essential physical features of those biomedical lasers currently in routine use ranging over a number of clinical specialties, and brief descriptions of their use
5. The biomedical uses of other lasers used surgically in limited scale or which are currently being researched for applications in surgical and diagnostic procedures and the photosensitized inactivation of cancer tumors

In this review, effort is made in the text and in the last section to provide a number of key references and sources of information for each topic that will enable the reader's more in-depth pursuit.

13.1 Interaction and Effects of UV–IR Laser Radiation on Biologic Tissues

Electromagnetic radiation in the UV–IR spectral range propagates within biologic tissues until it is either scattered or absorbed.

13.1.1 Scattering in Biologic Tissue

Scattering in matter occurs only at the boundaries between regions having different optical refractive indices and is a process in which the energy of the radiation is conserved (Van de Hulst, 1957). Since biologic tissue is structurally inhomogeneous at the microscopic scale, for example, both subcellular and cellular dimensions, and at the macroscopic scale, for example, cellular assembly (tissue) dimensions, and predominantly contains water, proteins, lipids, and all different chemical species, it is generally regarded as a scatterer of UV–IR radiation. The general result of scattering is deviation of the direction of propagation of radiation. The deviation is strongest when wavelength and scatterer are comparable in dimension (Mie scattering) and when wavelength greatly exceeds particle size (Rayleigh scattering) (Van de Hulst, 1957). This dimensional relationship results in the deeper penetration into biologic tissues of those longer wavelengths which are not absorbed appreciably by pigments in the tissues. This results in the relative transparency of nonpigmented tissues over the visible and near-IR wavelength ranges.

13.1.2 Absorption in Biologic Tissue

Absorption of UV–IR radiation in matter arises from the wavelength-dependent resonant absorption of radiation by molecular electrons of optically absorbing molecular species (Grossweiner, 1989). Because of the chemical inhomogeneity of biologic tissues, the degree of absorption of incident radiation strongly depends upon its wavelength. The most prevalent or concentrated UV–IR absorbing molecular species in biologic tissues are listed in Table 13.1 along with associated high-absorbance wavelengths. These species include the peptide bonds; the phenylalanine, tyrosine, and tryptophan residues of proteins, all of which absorb in the UV range; oxy- and deoxyhemoglobin of blood which absorb in the visible to near-IR range; melanin, which absorbs throughout the UV to near-IR range, which decreases absorption occurring with increasing wavelength; and water, which absorbs maximally in the mid-IR range (Hale and Querry, 1973; Miller and Veitch, 1993; White et al., 1968). Biomedical lasers and their emitted radiation wavelength values also are tabulated in Table 13.1. The correlation between the wavelengths of clinically useful lasers and wavelength regions of absorption by constituents of biological tissues is evident. Additionally, exogenous light-absorbing chemical species may be intentionally present in tissues. These include:

1. Photosensitizers, such as porphyrins, which upon excitation with UV–visible light initiate photochemical reactions which are cytotoxic to the cells of the tissue, for example, a cancer which concentrates the photosensitizer relative to surrounding tissues (Spikes, 1989).
2. Dyes such as indocyanine green which, when dispersed in a concentrate fibrin protein gel can be used to localize 810 nm *GaAlAs* diode laser radiation and the associated heating to achieve

TABLE 13.1 UV–IR-Radiation-Absorbing Constituent of Biological Tissues and Biomedical Laser Wavelengths

Constituent	Tissue Type	Optical Absorption			
		Wavelength[a] (nm)	Relative[b] Strength	Laser Type	Wavelength (nm)
Proteins	All				
Peptide bond		<220 (r)	++++++	ArF	193
Amino acid					
Residues					
Tryptophan		220–290 (r)	+		
Tyrosine		220–290 (r)	+		
Phenylalanine		220–2650 (r)	+		
Pigments					
Oxyhemoglobin	Blood	414 (p)	+++	Ar ion	488–514.5
	Vascular tissues	537 (p)	++	Frequency	532
		575 (p)	++	Doubled	
		970 (p)	+	Nd:YAG	
		690–1100 (r)		Diode	810
				Nd:YAG	1064
Deoxyhemoglobin	Blood	431 (p)	+++	Dye	400–700
	Vascular tissues	554 (p)	++	Nd:YAG	1064
Melanin	Skin	220–1000 (r)	++++	Ruby	693
Water	All	2.1 (p)	+++	Ho:YAG	2100
		3.02 (p)	++++++	Er:YAG	2940
		>2.94 (r)	++++	CO_2	10,640

[a] (p): Peak absorption wavelength; (r): wavelength range.
[b] The number of +signs qualitatively ranks the magnitude of the optical absorption.

localized thermal denaturation and bonding of collagen to affect joining or welding of tissue (Bass et al., 1992; Oz et al., 1989).

3. Tattoo pigments including graphite (black) and black, blue, green, and red organic dyes (Fitzpatrick, 1994; McGillis et al., 1994).

13.2 Penetration and Effects of UV–IR Laser Radiation into Biologic Tissue

Both scattering and absorption processes affect the variations of the intensity of radiation with propagation into tissues. In the absence of scattering, absorption results in an exponential decrease of radiation intensity described simply by Beers law (Grossweiner, 1989). With appreciable scattering present, the decrease in incident intensity from the surface is no longer monotonic. A maximum in local internal intensity is found to be present due to efficient back-scattering, which adds to the intensity of the incoming beam as shown, for example, by Miller and Veitch (1993) for visible light penetrating into the skin and by Rastegar et al. (1992) for 1.064 μm *Nd:YAG* laser radiation penetrating into the prostate gland. Thus, the relative contributions of absorption and scattering of incident laser radiation will stipulate the depth in a tissue at which the resulting tissue effects will be present. Since the absorbed energy can be released in a number of different ways including thermal vibrations, fluorescence, and resonant electronic energy transfer according to the identity of the absorber, the effects on tissue are in general different. Energy release from both hemoglobin and melanin pigments and from water is by molecular vibrations resulting in a local temperature rise. Sufficient continued energy absorption and release can result in local temperature increases which, as energy input increases, result in protein denaturation (41–65°C), water evaporation and boiling (up to ≈ 300°C under confining pressure of tissue), thermolysis of proteins, generation of gaseous decomposition products and of carbonaceous residue or char (≥300°C). The generation of residual char is minimized by sufficiently rapid energy input to support rapid gasification reactions. The clinical effect of this chain of thermal events is tissue ablation. Much smaller values of energy input result in coagulation of tissues due to protein denaturation.

Energy release from excited exogenous photosensitizing dyes is via formation of free-radical species or energy exchange with itinerant dissolved molecular oxygen (Spikes, 1989). Subsequent chemical reactions following free-radical formation or formation of an activated or more reactive form of molecular oxygen following energy exchange can be toxic to cells with takeup of the photosensitizer.

Energy release following absorption of *visible (VIS) radiation* by fluorescent molecular species, either endogenous to tissue or exogenous, is predominantly by emission of longer wavelength radiation (Lakowicz, 1983). Endogenous fluorescent species include tryptophan, tyrosine, phenylalanine, flavins, and metal-free porphyrins. Comparison of measured values of the intensity of fluorescence emission from hyperplastic (transformed precancerous) cervical cells to cancerous cervical cells with normal cervical epithelial cells shows a strong potential for diagnostic use in the automated diagnosis and staging of cervical cancer (Mahadevan et al., 1993).

13.3 Effects of Mid-IR Laser Radiation

Because of the very large absorption by water of radiation with wavelength in the IR range ≥2.0 μm, the radiation of *Ho:YAG, Er:YAG*, and CO_2 lasers is absorbed within a very short distance of the tissue surface, and scattering is essentially unimportant. Using published values of the water absorption coefficient (Hale and Querry, 1973) and assuming an 80% water content and that the decrease in intensity is exponential with distance, the depth in the "average" soft tissue at which the intensity has decreased to 10% of the incident value (the optical penetration depth) is estimated to be 619, 13, and 170 μm, respectively, for Ho:YAG, Er:YAG, and CO_2 laser radiation. Thus, the absorption of radiation from these laser sources and thermalization of this energy results essentially in the formation of a surface heat source. With sufficient energy input, tissue ablation through water boiling and tissue thermolysis occur at the surface. Penetration of heat to underlying tissues is by diffusion alone; thus, the depth of coagulation of tissue below the surface region of ablation is limited by competition between thermal diffusion and the rate of descent of the heated surface impacted by laser radiation during ablation of tissue. Because of this competition, coagulation depths obtained in soft biologic tissues with use of mid-IR laser radiation are typically ≤205–500 μm, and the ability to achieve sealing of blood vessels leading to hemostatic ("bloodless") surgery is limited (Judy et al., 1992; Schroder et al., 1987).

13.4 Effects of Near-IR Laser Radiation

The 810-nm and 1064-μm radiation, respectively, of the GaAlAs diode laser and Nd:YAG laser penetrate more deeply into biologic tissues than the radiation of longer-wavelength IR lasers. Thus, the resulting thermal effects arise from absorption at greater depth within tissues, and the depths of coagulation and degree of hemostasis achieved with these lasers tend to be greater than with the longer-wavelength IR lasers. For example, the optical penetration depths (10% incident intensity) for 810-nm and 1.024-μm radiation are estimated to be 4.6 and ≃8.6 mm, respectively, in canine prostate tissue (Rastegar et al., 1992). Energy deposition of 3600 J from each laser onto the urethral surface of the canine prostate results in maximum coagulation depths of 8 and 12 mm, respectively, using diode and Nd:YAG lasers (Motamedi et al., 1993). Depths of optical penetration and coagulation in porcine liver, a more vascular tissue than prostate gland, of 2.8 and ≃9.6 mm, respectively, were obtained with a Nd:YAG laser beam, and of 7 and 12 mm, respectively, with an 810-nm diode laser beam (Rastegar et al., 1992). The smaller penetration depth obtained with 810-nm diode radiation in liver than in prostate gland reflects the effect of greater vascularity (blood content) on near-IR propagation.

13.5 Effects of Visible-Range Laser Radiation

Blood and vascular tissues very efficiently absorb radiation in the visible wavelength range due to the strong absorption of hemoglobin. This absorption underlies, for example, the use of

1. The argon ion laser (488–514.5 nm) in the localized heating and thermal coagulation of the vascular choroid layer and adjacent retina, resulting in the anchoring of the retina in treatment of retinal detachment (Katoh and Peyman, 1988).
2. The argon ion laser (488–514.5 nm), frequency-doubled Nd:YAG laser (532 nm), and dye laser radiation (585 nm) in the coagulative treatment of cutaneous vascular lesions such as port wine stains (Mordon et al., 1993).
3. The argon ion (488–514.5 nm) and frequency-doubled Nd:YAG lasers (532 nm) in the ablation of pelvic endometrial lesions which contain brown iron-containing pigments (Keye et al., 1983).

Because of the large absorption by hemoglobin and iron-containing pigments, the incident laser radiation is essentially absorbed at the surface of the blood vessel or lesion, and the resulting thermal effects are essentially local (Miller and Veitch, 1993).

13.6 Effects of UV Laser Radiation

Whereas exposure of tissue to IR and visible-light-range laser energy result in removal of tissue by thermal ablation, exposure to *argon fluoride* (*ArF*) laser radiation of 193-nm wavelength results predominantly in ablation of tissue initiated by a photochemical process (Garrison and Srinivasan, 1985). This ablation arises from repulsive forces between like-charged regions of ionized protein molecules that result from ejection of molecular electrons following UV photon absorption (Garrison and Srinivasan, 1985). Because the ionization and repulsive processes are extremely efficient, little of the incident laser energy escapes as thermal vibrational energy, and the extent of thermal coagulation damage adjacent to the site of incidence is very limited (Garrison and Srinivasan, 1985). This feature and the ability to tune very finely the fluence emitted by the ArF laser so that micrometer depths of tissue can be removed have led to ongoing clinical trials to investigate the efficiency of the use of the ArF laser to selectively remove tissue from the surface of the human cornea for correction of short-sighted vision to eliminate the need for corrective eyewear (Van Saarloos and Constable, 1993).

13.7 Effects of Continuous and Pulsed IR–Visible Laser Radiation and Associated Temperature Rise

Heating following absorption of IR–visible laser radiation arises from molecular vibration during loss of the excitation energy and initially is manifested locally within the exposed region of tissue. If incidence of the laser energy is maintained for a sufficiently long time, the temperature within adjacent regions of biologic tissue increases due to heat diffusion. The mean squared distance $\langle X^2 \rangle$ over which appreciable heat diffusion and temperature rise occur during exposure time t can be described in terms of the thermal diffusion time τ by the equation:

$$\langle X^2 \rangle = \tau t \qquad (13.1)$$

where τ is defined as the ratio of the thermal conductivity to the product of the heat capacity and density. For soft biologic tissues τ is approximately 1×10^3 cm^2 s^{-1} (Meijering et al., 1993). Thus, with continued energy input, the distance over which thermal diffusion and temperature rise occurs increases. Conversely, with use of pulsed radiation, the distance of heat diffusion can be made very small; for example, with exposure to a 1-µs pulse, the mean thermal diffusion distance is found to be approximately 0.3 µm, or about 3–10% of a biologic cell diameter. If the laser radiation is strongly absorbed and the ablation of tissues is efficient, then little energy diffuses away from the site of incidence, and lateral thermally induced coagulation of tissue can be minimized with pulses of short duration. The effect of limiting lateral thermal damage is desirable in the cutting of cornea (Hibst et al., 1992) and sclera of the eye (Hill et al., 1993), and joint cartilage (Maes and Sherk, 1994), all of which are avascular (or nearly so, with cartilage), and the hemostasis arising from lateral tissue coagulation is not required.

13.8 General Description and Operation of Lasers

Lasers emit a beam of intense electromagnetic radiation that is essentially monochromatic or contains at most a few nearly monochromatic wavelengths and is typically only weakly divergent and easily focused into external optical systems. These attributes of laser radiation depend on the key phenomenon which underlies laser operation, that of light amplification by stimulated emission of radiation, which in turn gives rise to the acronym *LASER*.

In practice, a laser is generally a generator of radiation. The generator is constructed by housing a light-emitting medium within a cavity defined by mirrors which provide feedback of emitted radiation through the medium. With sustained excitation of the ionic or molecular species of the medium to give a large density of excited energy states, the spontaneous and attendant stimulated emission of radiation from these states by photons of identical wavelength (a lossless process), which is amplified by feedback due to photon reflection by the cavity mirrors, leads to the generation of a very large photon density within the cavity. With one cavity mirror being partially transmissive, say 0.1–1%, a fraction of the cavity energy is emitted as an intense beam. With suitable selection of a laser medium, cavity geometry, and peak wavelengths of mirror reflection, the beam is also essentially monochromatic and very nearly collimated.

Identity of the lasing molecular species or laser medium fixes the output wavelength of the laser. Laser media range from gases within a tubular cavity, organic dye molecules dissolved in a flowing inert liquid carrier and heat sink, to impurity-doped transparent crystalline rods (solid state lasers) and semiconducting diode junctions (Lengyel, 1971). The different physical properties of these media in part determine the methods used to excite them into lasing states.

Gas-filled, or gas lasers are typically excited by dc or rf electric current. The current either ionizes and excites the lasing gas, for example, argon, to give the electronically excited and lasing Ar+ ion, or ionizes a gaseous species in a mixture also containing the lasing species, for example, N_2, which by efficient energy transfer excites the lasing molecular vibrational states of the CO_2 molecule.

Dye lasers and so-called solid-state lasers are typically excited by intense light from either another laser or from a flashlamp. The excitation light wavelength range is selected to ensure efficient excitation at the absorption wavelength of the lasing species. Both excitation and output can be continuous, or the use of a pulsed flashlamp or pulsed exciting laser to pump a solid-state or dye laser gives pulsed output with high peak power and short pulse duration of 1 µs to 1 ms. Repeated excitation gives a train of pulses. Additionally, pulses of higher peak power and shorter duration of approximately 10 ns can be obtained from solid lasers by intracavity Q-switching (Lengyel, 1971). In this method, the density of excited states is transiently greatly increased by impeding the path between the totally reflecting and partially transmitting mirror of the cavity interrupting the stimulated emission process. Upon rapid removal of the impeding device (a beam-interrupting or -deflecting device), stimulated emission of the very large population of excited lasing states leads to emission of an intense laser pulse. The process can give single pulses or can be repeated to give a pulse train with repetition frequencies typically ranging from 1 Hz to 1 kHz.

Gallium–aluminum (GaAlAs) lasers are, as are all semiconducting diode lasers, excited by electrical current which creates excited hole-electron pairs in the vicinity of the diode junction. Those carrier pairs are the lasing species which emit spontaneously and with photon stimulation. The beam emerges parallel to the function with the plane of the function forming the cavity and thin-layer surface mirrors providing reflection. Use of continuous or pulsed excitation current results in continuous or pulsed output.

13.9 Biomedical Laser Beam Delivery Systems

Beam delivery systems for biomedical lasers guide the laser beam from the output mirror to the site of action on tissue. Beam powers of up to 100 W are transmitted routinely. All biomedical lasers incorporate a coaxial aiming beam, typically from a HeNe laser (632.8 nm) to illuminate the site of incidence on tissue.

Usually, the systems incorporate two different beam-guiding methods, either (1) a flexible fused silica (SiO$_2$) optical fiber or light guide, generally available currently for laser beam wavelengths between $\simeq$400 nm and $\simeq$2.1 μm, where SiO$_2$ is essentially transparent and (2) an articulated arm having beam-guiding mirrors for wavelengths greater than circa 2.1 μm (e.g., CO$_2$ lasers), for the Er:YAG and for pulsed lasers having peak power outputs capable of causing damage to optical fiber surfaces due to ionization by the intense electric field (e.g., pulsed ruby). The arm comprises straight tubular sections articulated together with high-quality power-handling dielectric mirrors at each articulation junction to guide the beam through each of the sections. Fused silica optical fibers usually are limited to a length of 1–3 m and to wavelengths in the visible-to-low midrange IR (<2.1 μm), because longer wavelengths of IR radiation are absorbed by water impurities (<2.9 μm) and by the SiO$_2$ lattice itself (wavelengths > 5 μm), as described by Levi (1980).

Since the flexibility, small diameter, and small mechanical inertia of optical fibers allow their use in either flexible or rigid endoscopes and offer significantly less inertia to hand movement, fibers for use at longer IR wavelengths are desired by clinicians. Currently, researchers are evaluating optical fiber materials transparent to longer IR wavelengths. Material systems showing promise are fused Al$_2$O$_3$ fibers in short lengths for use with near-3-μm radiation of the Er:YAG laser and *Ag halide* fibers in short lengths for use with the CO$_2$ laser emitting at 10.6 μm (Merberg, 1993). A flexible hollow Teflon waveguide 1.6 mm in diameter having a thin metal film overlain by a dielectric layer has been reported recently to transmit 10.6 μm CO$_2$ radiation with attenuation of 1.3 and 1.65 dB/m for straight and bent (5-mm radius, 90-degree bend) sections, respectively (Gannot et al., 1994).

13.9.1 Optical Fiber Transmission Characteristics

Guiding of the emitted laser beam along the optical fiber, typically of uniform circular cross-section, is due to total internal reflection of the radiation at the interface between the wall of the optical fiber core and the cladding material having refractive index n_1 less than that of the core n_2 (Levi, 1980). Total internal reflection occurs for any angle of incidence θ of the propagating beam with the wall of the fiber core such that θ > θ$_c$ where

$$\sin\theta_c = \left(\frac{n_1}{n_2}\right) \tag{13.2}$$

or in terms of the complementary angle α$_c$

$$\cos\alpha_c = \left(\frac{n_1}{n_2}\right) \tag{13.3}$$

For a focused input beam with apical angle α$_m$ incident upon the flat face of the fiber as shown in Figure 13.1, total internal reflection and beam guidance within the fiber core will occur (Levi, 1980) for

$$NA = \sin(\alpha_m/2) \leq [n_2^2 - n_1^2]^{0.5} \tag{13.4}$$

where NA is the numerical aperture of the fiber.

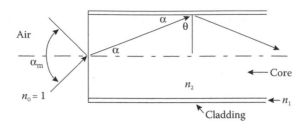

FIGURE 13.1   Critical reflection and propagation within an optical fiber.

This relationship ensures that the critical angle of incidence of the interface is not exceeded and that total internal reflection occurs (Levi, 1980). Typical values of NA for fused SiO_2 fibers with polymer cladding are in the range of 0.36–0.40. The typical values of $\alpha_m = 14°$ used to insert the beam of the biomedical laser into the fiber is much smaller than those values ($\simeq 21$–$23°$) corresponding to typical NA values. The maximum value of the propagation angle α typically used in biomedical laser systems is $\simeq 4.8°$.

Leakage of radiation at the core–cladding interface of the fused SiO_2 fiber is negligible, typically being 0.3 dB/m at 400 nm and 0.01 dB/m at 1.064 µm. Bends along the fiber length always decrease the angle of the incidence at the core–cladding interface. Bends do not give appreciable losses for values of the bending radius sufficiently large that the angle of incidence θ of the propagating beam in the bent core does not become less than θ_c at the core–cladding interface (Levi, 1980). The relationship given by Levi (1980) between the bending radius r_b, the fiber core radius r_o, the ratio (n_2/n_1) of fiber core to cladding refractive indices, and the propagation angle α in Figure 13.1 which ensures that the beam does not escape is

$$\frac{n_1}{n_2} > \frac{1-\rho}{1+\rho}\cos\alpha \tag{13.5}$$

where $\rho = (r_o/r_b)$. The inequality will hold for all $\alpha \le \alpha_c$ provided that

$$\frac{n_1}{n_2} \le \frac{1-\rho}{1+\rho} \tag{13.6}$$

Thus, the critical bending radius r_{bc} is the value of r_b such that Equation 13.6 is an equality. Use of Equation 13.6 predicts that bends with radii ≥12, 18, and 30 mm, respectively, will not result in appreciable beam leakage from fibers having 400–, 600–, and 1000-µm diameter cores, which are typical in biomedical use. Thus, use of fibers in flexible endoscopes usually does not compromise beam guidance.

Because the integrity of the core–cladding interface is critical to beam guiding, the clad fiber is encased typically in a tough but flexible protective fluoropolymer buffer coat.

13.9.2 Mirrored Articulated Arm Characteristics

Typically two or three relatively long tubular sections or arms of 50–80 cm length make up the portion of the articulated arm that extends from the laser output fixturing to the handpiece, endoscope, or operating microscope stage used to position the laser beam onto the tissue proper. Mirrors placed at the articulation of the arms and within the articulated handpiece, laparoscope, or operating microscope stage maintain the centration of the trajectory of the laser beam along the length of the delivery system. Dielectric multilayer mirrors (Levi, 1980) are routinely used in articulated devices. Their low–high reflectivity ≤99.9 + % and power-handling capabilities ensure efficient power transmission down the arm. Mirrors in articulated devices typically are held in kinetically adjustable mounts for rapid stable alignment to maintain beam concentration.

13.9.3 Optics for Beam Shaping on Tissues

Since the rate of heating on tissue, and hence rates of ablation and coagulation, depend directly on energy input per unit volume of tissue, selection of ablation and coagulation rates of various tissues is achieved through control of the energy density (J/cm^2 or $W\ s/cm^2$) of the laser beam. This parameter is readily achieved through use of optical elements such as discrete focusing lenses placed on the hand-piece or rigid endoscope which controls the spot size upon the tissue surface or by affixing a so-called contact tip to the end of an optical fiber. These are conical or spherical in shape with diameters ranging from 300 to 1200 µm and with very short focal lengths. The tip is placed in contact with the tissue and generates a submillimeter-sized focal spot in tissue very near the interface between the tip and tissue. One advantage of using the contact tip over a focused beam is that ablation proceeds with small lateral depth of attendant coagulation (Judy et al., 1993a). This is because the energy of the tightly focused beam causes tissue thermolysis essentially at the tip surface and because the resulting tissue products strongly absorb the beam resulting in energy deposition and ablation essentially at the tip surface. This contrasts with the radiation penetrating deeply into tissue before thermolysis which occurs with a less tightly focused beam from a free lens or fiber. An additional advantage with the use of contact tips in the perception of the surgeon is that the kinesthetics of moving a contact tip along a resisting tissue surface more closely mimics the "touch" encountered in moving a scalpel across the tissue surface.

Recently a class of optical fiber tips has been developed which laterally directs the beam energy from a silica fiber (Judy et al., 1993b). These tips, either a gold reflective micromirror or an angled refractive prism, offer a lateral angle of deviation ranging from 35 to 105° from the optical fiber axis (undeviated beam direction). The beam reflected from a plane micromirror is unfocused and circular in cross-section, whereas the beam from a concave mirror and refractive devices is typically elliptical in shape, fused with distal diverging rays. Fibers with these terminations are currently finding rapidly expanding, large-scale application in coagulation (with 1.064-µm Nd:YAG laser radiation) of excess tissue lining the urethra in treatment of benign prostatic hypertrophy (Costello et al., 1992). The capability for lateral beam direction may offer additional utility of these terminated fibers in other clinical specialties.

13.9.4 Features of Routinely Used Biomedical Lasers

Currently four lasers are in routine large-scale clinical biomedical use to ablate, dissect, and to coagulate soft tissue. Two, the carbon dioxide (CO_2) and argon ion (Ar-ion) lasers, are gas-filled lasers. The other two employ solid-state lasing media. One is the Neodymium–yttrium–aluminum–garnet (Nd:YAG) laser, commonly referred to as a solid-state laser, and the other is the gallium–aluminum arsenide (GaAlAs) semiconductor diode laser. Salient features of the operating characteristics and biomedical applications of those lasers are listed in Tables 13.2 through 13.5. The operational descriptions are

TABLE 13.2 Operating Characteristics of Principal Biomedical Lasers

Characteristics	Ar Ion Laser	CO_2 Laser
Cavity medium	Argon gas, 133 Pa	10% CO_2, 10% Ne, and 80% He; 1330 Pa
Lasing species	Ar + ion	CO_2 molecule
Excitation	Electric discharge, continuous	Electric discharge, continuous, pulsed
Electric input	208 V_{AC}, 60 A	110 V_{AC}, 15 A
Wall plug efficiency	≃0.06%	≃10%
Characteristics	Nd:YAG laser	GaAlAs diode laser
Cavity medium	Nd-doped YAG	n–p junction, GaAlAs diode
Lasing species	Nd3t in YAG lattice	Hole-electron pairs at diode junction
Excitation	Flashlamp, continuous, pulsed	Electric current, continuous pulsed
Electric input	208/240 V_{AC}, 30 A continuous 110 V_{AC}, 10 A pulsed	110 V_{AC}, 15 A
Wall plug efficiency	≃1%	≃23%

TABLE 13.3   Output Beam Characteristics of Ar Ion and CO_2 Biomedical Lasers

Output Characteristics	Argon Laser	CO_2 Laser
Output power	2–8 W, continuous	1–100 W, continuous
Wavelength (s)	Multiple lines (454.6–528.7 nm), 488, 514.5, dominant	10.6 μm
Electromagnetic wave propagation mode	TEM_∞	TEM_∞
Beam guidance, shaping	Fused-silica optical fiber with contact tip or flat ended for beam emission, lensed handpiece. Slit lamp with ocular lens	Flexible articulated arm with mirrors; lensed handpiece or mirrored-microscope platen

TABLE 13.4   Output Beam Characteristics of Nd:YAG and GaAlAs Diode Biomedical Lasers

Output Characteristics	Nd:YAG Lasers	GaAlAs Diode Laser
Output power	1–100 W continuous at 1.064 millimicron 1–36 W continuous at 532 nm (frequency doubled with KTP)	1–25 W continuous
Wavelength (s)	1.064 μm/532 nm	810 nm
Electromagnetic wave propagation modes	Mixed modes	Mixed modes
Beam guidance and shaping	Fused SiO_2 optical fiber with contact tip directing mirrored or refracture tip	Fused SiO_2 optical fiber with contact tip or laterally directing mirrored or refracture tip

TABLE 13.5   Clinical Uses of Principal Biomedical Lasers

Ar Ion Laser	CO_2 Laser
Pigmented (vascular) soft-tissue ablation in gynecology, general and oral surgery, otolaryngology, vascular lesion coagulation in dermatology, and retinal coagulation in ophthalmology	Soft-tissue ablation–dissection and bulk tissue removal in dermatology; gynecology; general, oral, plastic, and neurosurgery; otolaryngology; podiatry; urology
Nd:YAG Laser	**GaAlAs Diode Laser**
Soft tissue, particularly pigmented vascular tissue, ablation–dissection, and bulk tissue removal—in dermatology; gastroenterology; gynecology; general, arthroscopic, neuroplastic, and thoracic surgery; urology; posterior capsulotomy (ophthalmology) with pulsed 1.064 millimicron and ocular lens	Pigmented (vascular) soft-tissue ablation–dissection and bulk removal in gynecology; gastroenterology; general, surgery, and urology; FDA approval for otolaryngology and thoracic surgery pending

typical of the lasers currently available commercially and do not represent the product of any single manufacturer.

13.9.5 Other Biomedical Lasers

Some important biomedical lasers have smaller-scale use or currently are being researched for biomedical application. The following four lasers have more limited scales of surgical use:

The Ho:YAG (Holmium:YAG) laser, emitting pulses of 2.1 μm wavelength and up to 4 J in energy, used in soft tissue ablation in arthroscopic (joint) surgery (FDA approved).

The Q-switched Ruby (*Cr:Al$_2$O$_3$*) laser, emitting pulses of 694-nm wavelength and up to 2 J in energy is used in dermatology to disperse black, blue, and green tattoo pigments and melanin in pigmented lesions (not melanoma) for subsequent removal by phagocytosis by macrophages (FDA approved).

The flashlamp pumped pulsed dye laser emitting 1- to 2-J pulses at either 577- or 585-nm wavelength (near the 537–577 absorption region of blood) is used for treatment of cutaneous vascular lesions and melanin pigmented lesions except melanoma. Use of pulsed radiation helps to localize the thermal damage to within the lesions to obtain low damage of adjacent tissue.

The following lasers are being investigated for clinical uses:

1. The Er:YAG laser, emitting at 2.94 μm near the major water absorption peak (OH stretch), is currently being investigated for ablation of tooth enamel and dentin (Li et al., 1992).
2. Dye lasers emitting at 630–690 nm are being investigated for application as light sources for exciting dihematoporphyrin ether or benzoporphyrin derivatives in investigation of the efficacy of these photosensitives in the treatment of esophageal, bronchial, and bladder carcinomas for the FDA approved process.

Defining Terms

Biomedical Laser Radiation Ranges

Infrared (IR) radiation: The portion of the electromagnetic spectrum within the wavelength range 760 nm–1 mm, with the regions 760 nm–1.400 μm and 1.400–10.00 μm, respectively, called the near- and mid-IR regions.
Ultraviolet (UV) radiation: The portion of the electromagnetic spectrum within the wavelength range 100–400 nm.
Visible (VIS) radiation: The portion of the electromagnetic spectrum within the wavelength range 400–760 nm.

Laser Medium Nomenclature

Argon fluoride (ArF): Argon fluoride eximer laser (an eximer is a diatomic molecule which can exist only in an excited state).
Ar ion: Argon ion.
CO_2: Carbon dioxide.
$Cr:Al_2O_3$: Ruby laser.
Er:YAG: Erbium–yttrium–aluminum–garnet.
GaAlAs: Gallium–aluminum laser.
HeNe: Helium–neon laser.
Ho:YAG: Holmium–yttrium–aluminum–garnet.
Nd:YAG: Neodymium–yttrium–aluminum–garnet.

Optical Fiber Nomenclature

Ag halide: Silver halide, halide ion, typically bromine (Br) and chlorine (Cl).
Fused silica: Fused SiO_2.

References

Bass L.S., Moazami N., Pocsidio J. et al. 1992. Change in type I collagen following laser welding. *Lasers Surg. Med.* 12: 500.
Costello A.J., Johnson D.E., and Bolton D.M. 1992. Nd:YAG laser ablation of the prostate as a treatment for benign prostate hypertrophy. *Lasers Surg. Med.* 12: 121.
Fitzpatrick R.E. 1993. Comparison of the Q-switched Ruby, Nd:YAG, and alexandrite lasers in tattoo removal. *Lasers Surg. Med.* (Suppl.) 6: 52.
Gannot I., Dror J., Calderon S. et al. 1994. Flexible waveguides for IR laser radiation and surgery applications. *Lasers Surg. Med.* 14: 184.

Garrison B.J. and Srinivasan R. 1985. Laser ablation of organic polymers: Microscopic models for photo-chemical and thermal processes. *J. Appl. Physiol.* 58: 2909.

Grossweiner L.I. 1989. Photophysics. In: K.C. Smith (ed.), *The Science of Photobiology*, pp. 1–47. New York, Plenum.

Hale G.M. and Querry M.R. 1973. Optical constants of water in the 200 nm to 200 μm wavelength region. *Appl. Opt.* 12: 555.

Hibst R., Bende T., and Schröder D. 1992. Wet corneal ablation by Er:YAG laser radiation. *Lasers Surg. Med.* (Suppl.) 4: 56.

Hill R.A., Le M.T., Yashiro H. et al. 1993. Ab-interno erbium (Er:YAG) laser sclerostomy with iridotomy in Dutch cross rabbits. *Lasers Surg. Med.* 13: 559.

Judy M.M., Matthews J.L., Aronoff B.L. et al. 1993a. Soft tissue studies with 805 nm diode laser radiation: Thermal effects with contact tips and comparison with effects of 1064 nm. Nd:YAG laser radiation. *Lasers Surg. Med.* 13: 528.

Judy M.M., Matthews J.L., Gardetto W.W. et al. 1993b. Side firing laser–fiber technology for minimally invasive transurethral treatment of benign prostate hyperplasia. *Proc. Soc. Photo-Opt. Instr. Eng. (SPIE)* 1982: 86.

Judy M.M., Matthews J.L., Goodson J.R. et al. 1992. Thermal effects in tissues from simultaneous coaxial CO_2 and Nd:YAG laser beams. *Lasers Surg. Med.* 12: 222.

Katoh N. and Peyman G.A. 1988. Effects of laser wavelengths on experimental retinal detachments and retinal vessels. *Jpn. J. Ophthalmol.* 32: 196.

Keye W.R., Matson G.A., and Dixon J. 1983. The use of the argon laser in treatment of experimental endo-metriosis. *Fertil. Steril.* 39: 26.

Lakowicz J.R. 1983. *Principles of Fluorescence Spectroscopy.* New York, Plenum.

Lengyel B.A. 1971. *Lasers.* New York, John Wiley.

Levi L. 1980. *Applied Optics*, Vol. 2. New York, John Wiley.

Li Z.Z., Code J.E., and Van de Merve W.P. 1992. Er:YAG laser ablation of enamel and dentin of human teeth: Determination of ablation rates at various fluences and pulse repetition rates. *Lasers Surg. Med.* 12: 625.

Maes K.E. and Sherk H.H. 1994. Bone and meniscal ablation using the erbium YAG laser. *Lasers Surg. Med.* (Suppl.) 6: 31.

Mahadevan A., Mitchel M.F., Silva E. et al. 1993. Study of the fluorescence properties of normal and neo-plastic human cervical tissue. *Lasers Surg. Med.* 13: 647.

McGillis S.T., Bailin P.L., Fitzpatrick R.E. et al. 1994. Successful treatments of blue, green, brown and reddish-brown tattoos with the Q-switched alexandrite laser. *Laser Surg. Med.* (Suppl.) 6: 52.

Meijering L.J.T., VanGermert M.J.C., Gijsbers G.H.M. et al. 1993. Limits of radial time constants to approximate thermal response of tissue. *Lasers Surg. Med.* 13: 685.

Merberg G.N. 1993. Current status of infrared fiberoptics for medical laser power delivery. *Lasers Surg. Med.* 13: 572.

Miller I.D. and Veitch A.R. 1993. Optical modeling of light distributions in skin tissue following laser irradiation. *Lasers Surg. Med.* 13: 565.

Mordon S., Beacco C., Rotteleur G. et al. 1993. Relation between skin surface temperature and minimal blanching during argon, Nd:YAG 532, and cw dye 585 laser therapy of port-wine stains. *Lasers Surg. Med.* 13: 124.

Motamedi M., Torres J.H., Cammack T. et al. 1993. Thermodynamics of cw laser interaction with prostatic tissue: Effects of simultaneous cooling on lesion size. *Lasers Surg. Med.* (Suppl.) 5: 64.

Oz M.C., Chuck R.S., Johnson J.P. et al. 1989. Indocyanine green dye-enhanced welding with a diode laser. *Surg. Forum* 40: 316.

Rastegar S., Jacques S.C., Motamedi M. et al. 1992. Theoretical analysis of high-power diode laser (810 nm) and Nd:YAG laser (1064 nm) for coagulation of tissue: Predictions for prostate coagulation. *Proc. Soc. Photo-Opt. Instr. Eng. (SPIE)* 1646: 150.

Schroder T., Brackett K., and Joffe S. 1987. An experimental study of effects of electrocautery and various lasers on gastrointestinal tissue. *Surgery* 101: 691.

Spikes J.D. 1989. Photosensitization. In: K.C. Smith (ed.), *The Science of Photobiology*, 2nd ed., pp. 79–110. New York, Plenum.

Van de Hulst H.C. 1957. *Light Scattering by Small Particles.* New York, John Wiley.

Van Saarloos P.P. and Constable I.J. 1993. Improved eximer laser photorefractive keratectomy system. *Lasers Surg. Med.* 13: 189.

White A., Handler P., and Smith E.L. 1968. *Principles of Biochemistry*, 4th ed. New York, McGraw-Hill.

Further Information

Current research on the optical, thermal, and photochemical interactions of radiation and their effect on biologic tissues, are published routinely in the journals: *Laser in Medicine and Surgery, Lasers in the Life Sciences,* and *Photochemistry Photobiology* and to a lesser extent in *Applied Optics and Optical Engineering.*

Clinical evaluations of biomedical laser applications appear in *Lasers and Medicine and Surgery* and in journals devoted to clinical specialties such as *Journal of General Surgery, Journal of Urology, and Journal of Gastroenterological Surgery.*

The annual symposium proceedings of the biomedical section of the *Society of Photo-Optical Instrumentation Engineers (SPIE)* contain descriptions of new and current research on application of lasers and optics in biomedicine.

The book *Lasers* (a second edition by Bela A. Lengyel), although published in 1971, remains a valuable resource on the fundamental physics of lasers—gas, dye, solid-state, and semiconducting diode. A more recent book, *The Laser Guidebook* by Jeffrey Hecht, published in 1992, emphasizes the technical characteristics of the gas, diode, solid-state, and semiconducting diode lasers.

The Journal of Applied Physics, Physical Review Letters, and *Applied Physics Letters* carry descriptions of the newest advances and experimental phenomena in lasers and optics.

The book *Safety with Lasers and Other Optical Sources* by David Sliney and Myron Wolbarsht, published in 1980, remains a very valuable resource on matters of safety in laser use.

Laser safety standards for the United States are given for all laser uses and types in the American National Standard (ANSI) Z136.1-1993, Safe Use of Lasers.

14

Measuring Cellular Traction Forces at the Micro- and Nanoscale

Nathan J. Sniadecki
University of Washington

Christopher S. Chen
University of Pennsylvania

14.1 Introduction

Individual cells exert forces that are essential to the development and function of tissue in an organism. The tension produced by actin and myosin proteins produce traction forces that allow cells to migrate from one locality to another in an organism. These forces are also used by cells to contract in order to change the shape of a tissue or to provide rigidity to its structure. In this chapter, we will discuss the techniques and assays that have been developed to measure traction forces during migration and contraction. These tools have helped to understand how these forces are regulated and the role they play in the biological function of cells.

Traction forces are important at all stages of life because it provides a mechanism for a cell to move to areas of need and repair the integrity of a tissue. At the early stage of an organism, the process of gastrulation drives the movement of cells from positions on the periphery of an embryo to the inside to create the layers that become the ectoderm, mesoderm, and endoderm. Morphogenesis continues the process of folding, movements, and cellular contractility to reach the final form of an organism. Once a final stage of the architecture is reached, the repair and maintenance of the tissue requires further coordinated cell movement. White blood cells exit from the blood stream and crawl through nearby tissue to patrol for pathogens, mutated cells, and debris from dead cells. Cellular locomotion is important in healing the regions where cells have been scrapped away or damaged. Replacement cells migrate into a wound site from adjacent regions to restore the integrity of a tissue's boundary and rebuild the surrounding extracellular matrix.

The movement of cells can also have pathological effects as in the case of cancer where angiogenesis drives the sprouting of endothelial cells to form new blood vessel in the direction of a tumor. New vessels speed up the growth of the tumor by increasing its nutritional supply. However, a more dire consequence of cell locomotion arises when cancer cells migrate away from a tumor and metastasize into other vital tissue, overwhelming the tissue's ability to function properly and thereby possibly causing the organism to die.

The measurement of cellular forces is a difficult task because cells are living entities and are responsive to physical stimuli through a process known as mechanotransduction, which can be defined as a biological response to forces or mechanical properties of the microenvironment.[1,2] Mechanotransduction has been implicated to play a role in proliferation, differentiation, migration, and morphogenesis. In particular to traction forces, a cell is able to adjust the assembly of actin and myosin at different regions within its cytoplasm to change its direction of migration or contraction in response to a physical cue. Perhaps one of the most fascinating and simultaneously challenging aspects of studying traction forces is that they can change in response to the tool itself. If one puts a force transducer on a cell, the cell will adjust its traction forces in proportion to the mechanical stiffness of the transducer. The adaptability of cells to the tools used makes it difficult to characterize the natural state of cells. Thus, one of the major goals of cell mechanics is not only to measure cellular traction forces, but also to identify the mechanism by which cells sense, interpret, and respond to physical stimuli.

14.2 Contractile Apparatus of Cells

As previously introduced, the behavior and function of a cell's contractile apparatus is dependent on two major proteins—actin and myosin. These proteins serve as the contractile machinery that generates strain within a cell's cytoskeleton to produce traction forces. An actin filament is made up of globular monomers known as G-actin that organize into a double-helical strand known as F-actin (Figure 14.1a). Because all actin monomers are orientated in the same direction along the double helix, there is polarity in the filament. Unique properties are associated with the positive "barbed end" and the negative "pointed end" by the different proteins that bind to actin. Actin grows its length by the polymerization of free monomers at either end, but the growth rate at the positive end is significantly larger. Within a cell, actin filaments can be found as bundles of fibers, interwoven meshes, three-dimensional (3D) gels, or intermediaries of the three. These structures form the cytoskeleton that provides mechanical support to the structure of a cell. Actin is a very strong polymer, having a modulus of elasticity between 1 and 2 GPa, and plays an essential role in locomotion by pushing the membrane of a cell forward. However, the role it plays in conjunction with myosin is of major importance to traction forces.

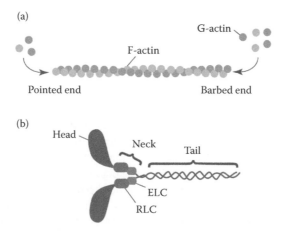

FIGURE 14.1   Actin and myosin proteins. (a) Actin forms a double-helix filament structure known as F-actin. Individual monomers known as G-actin are added at either end of the filament, but the rate of polymerization at the positive barbed end is significantly greater. (b) Myosin has a head region that binds to actin, a neck region that contains essential light chains (ELC) and regulatory light chains (RLC), and the tail region that is a coiled-coil structure.

Myosin converts chemical energy into mechanical work that slides actin filaments past each other to shorten the length of a cell. The structure of myosin has two heads, two necks, and a coiled-coil tail region (Figure 14.1b). Each head of myosin has an actin-binding site and utilizes ATP hydrolysis to move myosin toward the positive end of actin. The conformational change that arise from catalyzing ATP into ADP during ATP hydrolysis causes myosin's head to rotate about a fulcrum point in the neck region (Figure 14.2). The release of energy from ATP hydrolysis causes the head to cock forward to start the power stroke. When the head binds to actin, the phosphate dissociated from ATP is released and elastic energy stored in the cocked head is transferred to actin to complete the power stroke. The neck region plays a role as a stiff rod that increases the fulcrum action of myosin's head with each power stroke. Individual heads of myosin can deliver between 2 and 4 pN of force per power stroke.[3] The tail region of myosin interacts with the tail of another myosin to form a dimer, causing each myosin to be aligned antiparallel to the other. Multiple myosin dimers can self-assemble together into a myosin filament, which has a bipolar structure due to the myosin heads positioned at either end of the filament. The bipolar orientation of myosin filaments allows the heads to move actin filaments in opposite directions, or to create tension in the filaments when actin is restrained from sliding.

In the case of muscle, actin and myosin are arranged as parallel filaments that form a contractile unit called a sarcomere. Actin composes the thin filaments of the sarcomere and myosin forms the thick filaments (Figure 14.3a). Within each sarcomere unit, the positive ends of actin are anchored at the Z-disk by α-actinin, an actin cross-linking protein. Thin filaments are found at either side of the Z-disk and are aligned like the bristles of a hairbrush. Thick filaments are found interdigitated between thin filaments and their bipolar structure allows them to connect opposing thin filaments. Overall, this arrangement forms a structural sequence: Z-disk, thin filaments, thick filaments, thin filaments, Z-disk, and so on. Thin filaments are oriented with their negative ends facing each other and their positive ends at the Z-disk. When activated, myosin heads walk toward the positive ends of actin at both ends of the thick filament. This movement shortens the distance between opposing Z-disks by sliding actin filaments closer together. The structural sequence of the sarcomere is repeated along the length of a muscle cell and determines the overall distance the muscle can shorten.

The contractile apparatus in nonmuscle cells has many of the same proteins found in sarcomeres. Bundles of actin and myosin are known as stress fibers, which provide the cytoskeletal tension required for migration or contraction. Stress fibers are composed of bundles of actin filaments that are held

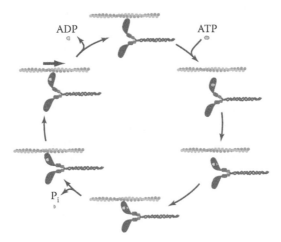

FIGURE 14.2 Actin–myosin power stroke cycle. At the top of the cycle, myosin releases from actin when ATP becomes bound. Myosin ATPase activity causes the dissociation of ATP into ADP and P_i, which changes the conformation of myosin for the power stroke. When myosin binds to actin, P_i is released and the head of myosin pulls on actin to impart a force on actin. The remaining ADP is then released and the power stroke cycle begins anew.

(a)

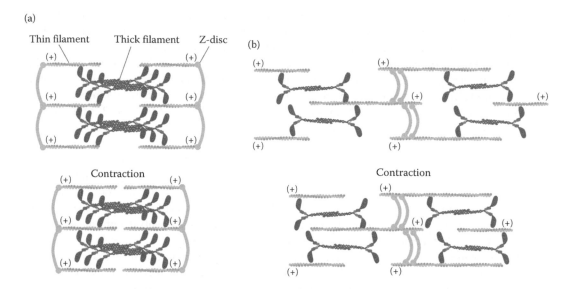

FIGURE 14.3 Contractile apparatus in cells. (a) A sarcomere is a highly organized contractile unit in muscle cells that uses actin thin filaments and myosin thick filaments to shorten the length of a muscle. (b) A stress fiber is a loosely organized contractile structure in nonmuscle cells that is essential for migration and contraction.

together by α-actinin and myosin (Figure 14.3b). The bands of α-actinin and myosin are observed to be periodic along the length of a stress fiber and the bands alternate with each other. In order for stress fibers to be contractile, the positive ends of actin cannot be oriented in the same direction or else myosin would simply walk along the filaments instead of sliding them past one another. Instead, actin filaments in a stress fiber need to have antiparallel alignment for the fiber to contract its length. The ends of a stress fiber are bound to adhesion sites with the extracellular matrix that allow the cell to deliver traction forces from the tension in the fiber.

For a cell to move, it requires the formation of new adhesions at its front end and the release of old adhesions at its back end. A useful conceptualization is that migration is a cycle of front protrusion, new adhesions, contraction, and release at the rear. A cell extends its membrane forward by actin polymerization to find new ligands for its integrin receptors to form a focal complex. Integrins are transmembrane receptors that mediate adhesion by binding to ligands in the extracellular matrix. On the cytoplasmic side, focal adhesion proteins connect integrins to the contractile apparatus of the cytoskeleton. Tension applied at a focal complex produces a traction force that pulls a cell forward. The tension also causes the complex to grow in size by recruiting additional focal adhesion proteins. These larger adhesion structures are referred to as focal adhesions and are found to be more stable than focal complexes, likely because of the abundant focal adhesion proteins that are able to aggregate additional integrins together to reinforce the bond strength to the extracellular matrix. To complete the migration step, a cell moves its body forward by contracting its length so as to create high force at its rear, breaking the bonds of a focal adhesion or contributing to its disassembly.

14.3 Design Consideration for Traction Force Assays

The difficulty in measuring traction forces arise because integrin-mediated adhesions can be as small as 100 nm in diameter and so the sensors must be able to resolve forces at a similar length scale. It is easy to see that this excludes most conventional force transducers, for instance, strain gages and metal springs. However, the same principles of elasticity that govern these tools are used to measure a cell's traction forces. To state simply, the strength of a force on a material is proportional to its deformation. Using this concept, known as Hooke's law, researchers have employed materials and techniques that have the appropriate physics and dimensions for measuring traction forces.

At the length scale of cells, the ratio of forces relative to each other is rather nonintuitive. In scaling down to the nanometer scale, a body force has a smaller effect on an object than a surface force. The former scales with length to the third power (L^3), whereas the latter scales with length to the second power (L^2). It is even more dramatic when one considers forces that scale only with length (L^1). To illustrate, an ant can lift up to a hundred times its own weight (L^3) because the strength of its muscles scale with their cross-sectional area (L^2), due to the number of thick filaments. However, an ant is easily trapped inside a droplet of water because of its surface tension, which scales with the length of the air–water interface (L^1). The implications of scaling laws for assaying traction forces is apparent when one considers that the weight of a cell with a 10 μm diameter is approximately 5 nN, yet the force at one of its focal adhesions can be larger than 100 nN.

The materials used in conventional force transducers and springs are not very feasible at the length scale of a cell. A typical metal has an elastic modulus that is greater than 50 GPa and so the shear strain for an area the size of a focal complex under the load of a traction force would be at most a few tenths of a percent. Given that a focal complex is already a difficult nanoscale structure to resolve with high-powered microscopy, the prospect of detecting a physical distortion that is a very small fraction of its size is nearly impossible. Therefore, softer structures are used instead of those that have low elastic moduli (Section 14.4.2) or slender dimensions (Section 14.4.3) because they can adequately measure a traction force by their larger degree of deformation.

To make slender objects for transducing traction forces, as in the case of cantilever force sensors, it is important to have control over the manufacturing dimensions. For this reason, nanotechnology and microfabrication have been used to construct the measurement devices. For example, cantilever beams have been built so thin and slender that although the elastic modulus of the materials are between 1 MPa and 100 GPa, the spring constant of the structure is in the range of 1–100 nN/μm. The structural flexibility allows the beam to deflect a few micrometers under the load of a traction force, which is an amount that is readily measured under a high-powered microscope.

The use of nanotechnology and microfabrication has also allowed thousands to millions of traction forces sensors to be manufactured at the same time. Large-scale production of the sensors is a major advantage in biological experiments. Cells within a culture or tissue are not identical. They have different degrees of metabolic activities, signaling reactions, cell cycle states, and differentiation cues due to stochastic processes. To overcome the "noise" in biological systems, large data sets are often required to make conclusions that are statistically significant. A supply of traction forces sensors that are plentiful and easy to prepare is a major benefit.

Not only must the mechanics of the new tools be tailored to the range of traction forces to be measured, but how to resolve the deflections must also be considered. Using a microscope to observe the deflection of a tool is a relatively noninvasive technique. Microscopy does require that the substrate be optically transparent, which limits materials available for fabrication. Additionally, one must consider whether to observe the forces exerted by one cell with high spatial and temporal accuracy, but with a limited data population, or whether to interrogate a large number of cells at a low magnification but with less measurement sensitivity. Overall, these considerations should act as a simple warning that one must treat each new system with a degree of guarded optimism on what kind of studies are possible because of the limits in its performance.

14.4 Traction Force Assays for Cells

To investigate traction forces and their role in physiology and pathology, tools have been made from materials that are biocompatible with cells and functionalized with proteins that allow cells to adhere through their integrin receptors. In general, studying traction forces involves culturing them on flexible substrates that physically deform under the applied load. Traction forces assays owe much to the work of Robert Hooke. In 1665, he was the first to use the term "cell" based on his observations with an early microscope and it is his theory of elasticity that is used predominantly to measure their forces.

14.4.1 Silicone Membrane Wrinkling

In the early 1980s, Albert Harris pioneered the first method for measuring traction forces.[4] His technique used a thin membrane of silicone rubber that wrinkled from the traction forces of a cell (Figure 14.4a). To create the silicone membrane, a film of liquid prepolymer was spread on a glass coverslip and briefly exposed to an open flame. The heat treatment created a thin skin of cured silicone rubber on top of the remaining silicone liquid. The skin was approximately 1 μm in thickness and the underlying silicone liquid served as a lubricant layer between the coverslip and the skin. Cells seeded onto the silicone membrane slowly pulled on the skin with a tangential force, producing wrinkles that were observed easily under an optical microscope. This technique was a breakthrough in that traction forces had been hypothesized previously, but had not been confirmed experimentally.

Albert Harris' technique could assess where there were regions of compression and tension beneath a cell by the shape and pattern of the wrinkles, which was useful in understanding the structures cells use to crawl. It was observed that the wrinkles were different between cell types, but there was no means to measure the strength of the traction forces that produced them, except to compare which cells produced more or less wrinkles than others. This tool also made major impact in assessing the enzymes and regulatory proteins that regulate traction forces by comparing the amount of wrinkles between different treatments or inhibitors given to cells.[5–9] Paradoxically, traction forces were found to be weakest among cell types that had the fastest migration speeds.[10] What was more puzzling was that fibroblasts were observed to have traction forces that were far larger than was required for cell migration. From this observation, traction forces were newly considered as factors in morphogenesis because fibroblasts were observed to pull matrix fibers into alignment, which bore a striking resemblance to the fiber arrangements seen in ligaments and tendons.

The silicone membrane wrinkling technique was later improved upon with an additional fabrication step to drastically reduce the stiffness of the substrate and provide a semiquantitative way to measure traction forces (Figure 14.4b). After flame curing, UV irradiation was used to weaken the elasticity of the silicone skin.[11,12] To calibrate the softer membranes, a known force from a glass pipette was applied to the surface and the length of the wrinkles that formed was measured. It was found that the length of a wrinkle increased linearly with the applied tip force. The improved wrinkling assay was used to study the change in contractility during cytokinesis, where daughter cells form by cleavage of the cytoplasm

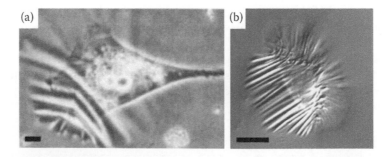

FIGURE 14.4 Silicone wrinkling membrane. (a) Fibroblast exerts traction forces that are strong enough to wrinkle the silicone rubber membrane. (Reproduced from Harris, A. K., Stopak, D. and Wild, P. *Nature* **290**, 249–251, 1981.) (b) Keratocyte produces significantly more wrinkles on silicone membranes made softer by UV irradiation. (Reproduced from Burton, K., Park, J. H. and Taylor, D. L. *Mol Biol Cell* **10**, 3745–3769, 1999.) Scale bars, 10 μm.

and then pull apart from each other. The increased number of wrinkles on the softer membranes allowed for assessing the different subcellular forces that occur during migration. At the lamellipodia of a migrating keratocyte, the wrinkles were radial and remain anchored to spots, possibly focal adhesion, as the cell advanced forward. Once these spots were translocated to the boundary between the lamellipodia and cell body, the wrinkles transitioned to compressive wrinkles. Overall, the improved spatial resolution of traction forces revealed that migration is a coordination of pulling forces at the front and detachment forces at the rear.

14.4.2 Traction Force Microscopy

Traction force microscopy is a technique that employs an elastic substrate, but instead of using wrinkles to indicate how strong a cell is as it distorts a substrate, beads or markers are embedded on the substrate to quantify traction forces by their displacement. The early approach developed in traction force microscopy was similar to Albert Harris' in that a thin silicone membrane on a liquid layer was used to detect traction forces, but micrometer-sized latex beads were stuck on the film and the membrane was kept taut so as to not wrinkle (Figure 14.5a). This approach had improved accuracy because traction forces could be measured quantitatively by the displacement of the beads.[13–15] The rigidity of the silicone membranes was rather high and so the technique was limited to analyzing cell types that were very contractile, like fibroblasts or keratocytes. Polyacrylamide gels were later adopted as the elasticity of the gels could be adjusted by the amount of bis-acrylamide cross-linker, so that a wider range of cell types could be studied.[16] Fluorescent beads were mixed into the polyacrylamide gel during the synthesis to act as markers of displacement and only those near the top surface of the gel were used for measuring traction forces (Figure 14.5b).

To compute traction forces, the positions of the beads are subtracted from their positions once the cell has been removed.[15,16] The subtraction creates a vector field that describes the deformation of the substrate from equilibrium. The displacements can then be used to solve for the traction forces by assuming that the membrane is an elastic material. Specifically, the membrane can be regarded as a semi-infinite half-space of an incompressible, elastic material with tangential forces applied only at the boundary

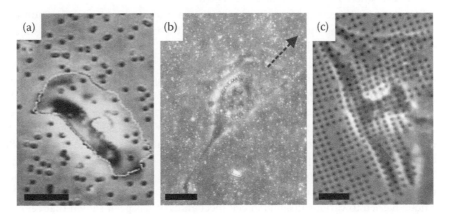

FIGURE 14.5 Traction force microscopy. (a) Keratocyte migrated on silicone membrane airbrushed with latex beads (scale bar, 20 μm). (Reproduced from Oliver, T., Dembo, M. and Jacobson, K. *Cell Motil Cytoskeleton* **31**, 225–240, 1995.) (b) Traction forces from a migrating fibroblast (arrow indicts direction of migration) are measured from the displacement of fluorescent beads embedded in a polyacrylamide gel (scale bar, 20 μm). (Reproduced from Munevar, S., Wang, Y. and Dembo, M. *Biophys J* **80**, 1744–1757, 2001.) (c) Contracting fibroblast distorts the regular array of micropatterned markers used to measure traction forces (scale bar, 20 μm). (Reproduced from Balaban, N. Q. et al. *Nat Cell Biol* **3**, 466–472, 2001.)

plane. Under these assumptions, the displacement vector field of the beads from the traction force vector field T is related by an integral relation:

$$u_i(x, y) = \iint G_{ij}(x - r, y - s)T_j(r, s) \mathrm{d}r \mathrm{d}s \tag{14.1}$$

where (x, y) is the position of bead and (s, r) is the position of the point-force. The problem is confined to the displacement of beads on the top surface of the substrate, so a two-dimensional (2D) solution is expected, where $1 \leq i, j \leq 2$ are the directional indices. Green's function G_{ij} relates the displacements u to the traction forces T beneath a cell. Because traction forces are discrete points, the integral becomes a set of linear equations $u_i = G_{ij}T_j$ which is inverted to solve for T_j. If one makes the assumption that Poisson's ratio is 0.5 because the substrate is incompressible, then Green's function has the form:

$$G_{ij}(\bar{x}) = \frac{3}{4\pi E}\left(\frac{\delta_{ij}}{|\bar{x}|} + \frac{x_i x_j}{|\bar{x}|^3}\right) \tag{14.2}$$

where E is the modulus of elasticity of the substrate and δ_{ij} is the Kronecker delta.

What may not be apparent in Equations 14.1 and 14.2 is that the beads embedded in the substrate do not move as an ideal elastic spring, in which their displacement is linearly proportional to an applied force. Instead, a single traction force displaces a bead proportionally to the stiffness E of the gel but also inversely to the distance $|\bar{x}|$ between them. The system of linear equations indicates that a bead is moved from the combined effect of multiple traction forces acting nearby. What is not certain in the experiments is how many points of force a cell exerts. This implies that the length of T could be greater than u, and so inverting the system of linear equations is not straightforward. To address this problem, regularization schemes are used that apply additional criteria on what range of solutions are feasible. These criteria include incorporating the constraint that the sum of all of the traction forces must balance because of equilibrium, the least complex solution be used, and whenever possible, traction forces are only applied at points where focal adhesions are detected.

If focal adhesions are not assessed for the last criterion, a grid-meshing approximation is superimposed on the area of cell during the calculation to solve for the traction forces at all regions beneath a cell. Because the beads are randomly seeded in the gel, there can be insufficient displacement information within regions of a cell to make an accurate estimation of the traction forces. The placement of mesh grids in these sparser areas leads to an ill-posed problem in solving for the force map because often more traction forces are assumed than there are displacement markers beneath a cell's area. To address this detection limitation, microfabricated regular arrays of fluorescent beads have been imprinted onto the elastomeric substrate for improved force tracking (Figure 14.5c).[17,18] The deformation of the marker pattern on the substrate is readily observed under a microscope. The patterns are formed with 800 nm or smaller spots that were spaced at 2 μm intervals. The calculation for the force mapping is similar to the random seeding but with significant reduction in the number of possible solutions due to the uniform density of displacement markers throughout the cell area.

The technique has led to various insights in cell mechanics. It has been shown that cells are able to adjust the strength of their traction forces in response to physical cues like rigidity or adhesivity of their environment.[19,20] How a cell responds to its physical environment with its traction forces has been implicated as a hallmark of cancer.[21–23] The technique has been used in combination with nanoscale manipulations like magnetic beads, laser nanoscissors, and nanoindentation to examine the mechanics of the cytoskeleton to verify different theories about its solidity or fluidity.[24–26] Overall, traction force microscopy is a relatively popular technique for measuring traction forces because the polyacrylamide gels are able to be fabricated with equipment commonly available in most laboratories.

14.4.3 Microfabricated Cantilever Force Sensors

In the previous methods, the use of a continuous membrane for measuring cell forces has the disadvantage that the traction forces are convoluted by the observed bead displacements. Because the calculation is not direct, constraints or assumptions are required to solve the inverse problem. A technique to transduce individual traction forces comes from the use of microfabricated cantilevers. The first demonstration of these sensors was a horizontal silicon cantilever that was made with microfabrication techniques (Figure 14.6a).[27,28] As a cell migrates across the surface, it bends the cantilever under the load of the traction force. Because the sensor is mechanically decoupled from the substrate, the deflection of the cantilever directly reports only the local force. The simple spring equation relates the deflection of the cantilever beam δ to the cellular traction force:

$$F = K\delta \qquad (14.3)$$

where K is the measured spring constant for the cantilever ($\approx$75 nN/μm). The fabrication steps involved in manufacturing the device were rather labor-intensive and expensive so these devices were reused between experiments. Although this technique could directly calculate a cell's traction force, it could only detect force at one point beneath a migrating cell. The beam could also defect only in its transverse direction and was very stiff in the longitudinal direction. Because of this, deflection was not due to the full strength of the traction force but to a portion of the traction force in the transverse direction. It was assumed that a cells' traction force acted in the same direction as its migration. This led to the calculation of traction forces by dividing by the sine of the angle between the migration direction and longitudinal axis of the beam.

A new approach was developed afterwards that modified the force sensor design by using vertical cantilevers.[29,30] With each cantilever placed perpendicular to the surface of the substrate, the spacing between force sensors could be significantly reduced and made it possible to have a high-density array of force sensors. This arrangement improved both the spatial resolution and the scope of possible experiments. Like Albert Harris' approach, the force sensor arrays were made from silicone rubber, but used a new manufacturing approach known as soft lithography.[31] Master templates for the cantilevers were

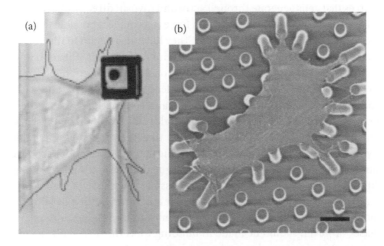

FIGURE 14.6 Microfabricated cantilever force sensors. (a) A silicon cantilever is constructed underneath a substrate. Its deflection is used to measure the traction force of a migrating fibroblast. (Reproduced from Galbraith, C. G. and Sheetz, M. P. *Proc Natl Acad Sci USA* **94**, 9114–9118, 1997.) (b) Local traction forces of a smooth muscle cell a measured with an array of vertical cantilever posts made from silicone elastomer (scale bar, 10 μm). (Reproduced from Tan, J. L. et al. *Proc Natl Acad Sci USA* **100**, 1484–1489, 2003.)

made from silicon or photoresist using microfabrication techniques.[32] Silicone rubber was then poured onto the masters, cured, and then peeled to create a replica of the master. The cost per device is inexpensive once the master has been built and many replicates can be made from the same master.

The deflection of a cantilever post is detectable under an optical microscope. As with the horizontal design, the deflection of a post is related by a simple cantilever beam relationship between force and displacement:

$$F = \left(\frac{3ED^4}{64L^3} \right) \delta \tag{14.4}$$

where E is the modulus of elasticity of the silicone, D the diameter of the cantilever post, and L its length. Unlike the horizontal cantilever devices, the deflection of the post are not limited to one axis, but can bend in all directions and so the deflection observed is a true vector quantity with which to gauge traction forces.

With the close proximity between sensors, the array of vertical cantilevers can examine traction forces at a higher density than previous methods and examine the forces at individual focal adhesions. Because the spring constant of these structure can be tailored by changing the length or diameter of the array (1–200 nN/μm), it has been possible to further examine the changes that a cell's contractile apparatus has with the stiffness of its microenvironment.[33–35] Another advantage is that each cantilever can deflect independently, which means that each array has millions of isolated sensors. This allows for studies that were not readily possible with previous techniques, like assessing the traction forces of large monolayers of cells as well as the tugging force between adjacent cells.[36–38] The array of cantilevers does have a nonphysiological topology, which may provide unique physical stimuli to the cells. However, fabrication technology allows the cantilevers to approach nanoscale dimensions, which makes it possible to have a higher density of force sensors that closely mimic a continuous substrate for a cell.[39]

14.5 Conclusion

The mechanical forces that cells generate through actin and myosin directly affect the function of tissue. The use of deformable substrates to measure traction forces has made it possible to better understand the proteins and structures associated with these forces. They have also begun to illuminate the mechanism that cells use to detect and respond to physical cues in their environment. The tools and techniques continue to improve both accuracy and precision as new approaches are incorporated from engineering and physics. Each new design comes closer to matching the length scale of cells, and with it brings a giant step in understanding the mechanisms of cell migration and contraction.

As the field moves forward, several issues need to be addressed to improve these techniques further. First, the reactions that cells have to the environments that the tools present should be considered. Topology, rigidity, and adhesivity of the tool can cause a mechanotransduction response that is independent of the response tested. On one hand, some would argue that these stimuli are nonphysiological and so little insight into the inner mechanisms of a cell is possible when using the tools. However, it should be noted that a plastic tissue culture dish is a rigid, planar environment that has little resemblance to an *in vivo* environment, yet the insights into cell biology from standard tissue culture have been immense. A stronger emphasis, however, should be made in building tools that can replicate mechanical cues so as to better analyze traction forces and to understand the role of mechanotransduction in cell biology. Second, because the devices used in measuring traction forces are built in-house, it is likely that they were calibrated in the early phase of their development, but subsequent tests and checks on their accuracy are sporadic. There are also major deviations in how the techniques are implemented in other laboratories. It is hard to compare the findings between studies if the methods used were widely different. It would be more advantageous if standard protocols were adopted or tools were made widely available so that a healthy degree of congruency and verification could be made in the field. Lastly, construction of these devices needs to be simple enough so that widespread use is possible. By reducing the barrier to use these tools, a larger effort can be directed at studying the numerous protein interactions that occur during traction force generation. Understanding the interactions between mechanical forces and biological response, how cells migrate, and how cells change the structure–function relations of tissues can provide valuable insight in the treatment of diseased states.

To achieve these goals, there are many future directions that the techniques described can be advanced. Foremost is the integration of traction force assays with other powerful microscopy techniques, such as fluorescent recovery after photobleaching (FRAP), GFP protein-labeling, fluorescent resonant emission transfer (FRET), super-resolution fluorescence microscopy, and 3D microscopy. These optical techniques allow one to detect proteins at the single molecular level, and in combination with traction force assays, provide a correlation between molecular activity and cell mechanics. To some degree, this direction has already been pursued.[17,40] Yet, there are still insights to be gained on the assembly of focal adhesions during migration and the interactions that myosin has with actin. Incorporating nanotechnology materials or devices may provide powerful new sensors that improve both spatial resolution and force measurement.[41] Because the size of an adhesion is hundreds of nanometers and the range of forces for single myosin motor is a few piconewtons, the ability to resolve these structures would provide greater insight into the mechanical behavior of cells. Additionally, the constructions of 3D measurement techniques, such as with gels or more complex sensing devices, would extend the current 2D understanding of traction forces into an environment more pertinent to cellular interactions in living tissue. Early attempts have been made that provide some understanding of 3D forces, but the substrates are still planar and constrain how the cell organizes its cytoskeleton and adhesions along those planes.[42,43] Lastly, strong exploration into the development of devices or techniques that are usable for *in vivo* studies of traction forces would open new areas of treatment for diseases in the cardiovascular and skeletal systems. From the activity and improvements so far, there is good reason to anticipate significant developments to come in understanding traction forces and cell mechanics.

Acknowledgments

NJS acknowledge support in part from grants from the National Science Foundation's CAREER Award and the National Institutes of Health (HL097284). CSC acknowledges support in part by grants from the National Institutes of Health (EB00262, EB08396, HL73305, HL90747, GM74048).

References

1. Sniadecki, N. J., Desai, R. A., Ruiz, S. A. and Chen, C. S. Nanotechnology for cell-substrate interactions. *Ann Biomed Eng* **34**, 59–74, 2006.
2. Chen, C. S. Mechanotransduction—A field pulling together? *J Cell Sci* **121**, 3285–3292, 2008.
3. Finer, J. T., Simmons, R. M. and Spudich, J. A. Single myosin molecule mechanics: Piconewton forces and nanometre steps. *Nature* **368**, 113–119, 1994.
4. Harris, A. K., Wild, P. and Stopak, D. Silicone rubber substrata: A new wrinkle in the study of cell locomotion. *Science* **208**, 177–179, 1980.
5. Chrzanowska-Wodnicka, M. and Burridge, K. Rho-stimulated contractility drives the formation of stress fibers and focal adhesions. *J Cell Biol* **133**, 1403–1415, 1996.
6. Helfman, D. M., Levy, E. T., Berthier, C., Shtutman, M., Riveline, D., Grosheva, I., Lachish-Zalait, A., Elbaum, M. and Bershadsky, A. D. Caldesmon inhibits nonmuscle cell contractility and interferes with the formation of focal adhesions. *Mol Biol Cell* **10**, 3097–3112, 1999.
7. Danowski, B. A., Imanaka-Yoshida, K., Sanger, J. M. and Sanger, J. W. Costameres are sites of force transmission to the substratum in adult rat cardiomyocytes. *J Cell Biol* **118**, 1411–1420, 1992.

8. Hinz, B., Celetta, G., Tomasek, J. J., Gabbiani, G. and Chaponnier, C. Alpha-smooth muscle actin expression upregulates fibroblast contractile activity. *Mol Biol Cell* **12**, 2730–2741, 2001.

9. Bogatcheva, N. V., Verin, A. D., Wang, P., Birukova, A. A., Birukov, K. G., Mirzopoyazova, T., Adyshev, D. M., Chiang, E. T., Crow, M. T. and Garcia, J. G. Phorbol esters increase MLC phosphorylation and actin remodeling in bovine lung endothelium without increased contraction. *Am J Physiol Lung Cell Mol Physiol* **285**, L415–426, 2003.

10. Harris, A. K., Stopak, D. and Wild, P. Fibroblast traction as a mechanism for collagen morphogenesis. *Nature* **290**, 249–251, 1981.

11. Burton, K. and Taylor, D. L. Traction forces of cytokinesis measured with optically modified elastic substrata. *Nature* **385**, 450–454, 1997.

12. Burton, K., Park, J. H. and Taylor, D. L. Keratocytes generate traction forces in two phases. *Mol Biol Cell* **10**, 3745–3769, 1999.

13. Lee, J., Leonard, M., Oliver, T., Ishihara, A. and Jacobson, K. Traction forces generated by locomoting keratocytes. *J Cell Biol* **127**, 1957–1964, 1994.

14. Oliver, T., Dembo, M. and Jacobson, K. Traction forces in locomoting cells. *Cell Motil Cytoskeleton* **31**, 225–240, 1995.

15. Dembo, M., Oliver, T., Ishihara, A. and Jacobson, K. Imaging the traction stresses exerted by locomoting cells with the elastic substratum method. *Biophys J* **70**, 2008–2022, 1996.

16. Dembo, M. and Wang, Y. L. Stresses at the cell-to-substrate interface during locomotion of fibroblasts. *Biophys J* **76**, 2307–2316, 1999.

17. Balaban, N. Q., Schwarz, U. S., Riveline, D., Goichberg, P., Tzur, G., Sabanay, I., Mahalu, D., Safran, S., Bershadsky, A., Addadi, L. and Geiger, B. Force and focal adhesion assembly: A close relationship studied using elastic micropatterned substrates. *Nat Cell Biol* **3**, 466–472, 2001.

18. Schwarz, U. S., Balaban, N. Q., Riveline, D., Bershadsky, A., Geiger, B. and Safran, S. A. Calculation of forces at focal adhesions from elastic substrate data: The effect of localized force and the need for regularization. *Biophys J* **83**, 1380–1394, 2002.

19. Wang, H. B., Dembo, M., Hanks, S. K. and Wang, Y. Focal adhesion kinase is involved in mechanosensing during fibroblast migration. *Proc Natl Acad Sci U S A* **98**, 11295–11300, 2001.

20. Reinhart-King, C. A., Dembo, M. and Hammer, D. A. The dynamics and mechanics of endothelial cell spreading. *Biophys J* **89**, 676–689, 2005.

21. Munevar, S., Wang, Y. and Dembo, M. Traction force microscopy of migrating normal and H-ras transformed 3T3 fibroblasts. *Biophys J* **80**, 1744–1757, 2001.

22. Paszek, M. J., Zahir, N., Johnson, K. R., Lakins, J. N., Rozenberg, G. I., Gefen, A., Reinhart-King, C. A. et al. Tensional homeostasis and the malignant phenotype. *Cancer Cell* **8**, 241–254, 2005.

23. Ghosh, K., Thodeti, C. K., Dudley, A. C., Mammoto, A., Klagsbrun, M. and Ingber, D. E. Tumor-derived endothelial cells exhibit aberrant Rho-mediated mechanosensing and abnormal angiogenesis in vitro. *Proc Natl Acad Sci U S A* **105**, 11305–11310, 2008.

24. Wang, N., Naruse, K., Stamenovic, D., Fredberg, J. J., Mijailovich, S. M., Tolic-Norrelykke, I. M., Polte, T., Mannix, R. and Ingber, D. E. Mechanical behavior in living cells consistent with the tensegrity model. *Proc Natl Acad Sci U S A* **98**, 7765–7770, 2001.

25. Kumar, S., Maxwell, I. Z., Heisterkamp, A., Polte, T. R., Lele, T. P., Salanga, M., Mazur, E. and Ingber, D. E. Viscoelastic retraction of single living stress fibers and its impact on cell shape, cytoskeletal organization, and extracellular matrix mechanics. *Biophys J* **90**, 3762–3773, 2006.

26. Krishnan, R., Park, C. Y., Lin, Y. C., Mead, J., Jaspers, R. T., Trepat, X., Lenormand, G. et al. Reinforcement versus fluidization in cytoskeletal mechanoresponsiveness. *PLoS One* **4**, e5486, 2009.

27. Galbraith, C. G. and Sheetz, M. P. A micromachined device provides a new bend on fibroblast traction forces. *Proc Natl Acad Sci U S A* **94**, 9114–9118, 1997.

28. Galbraith, C. G. and Sheetz, M. P. Keratocytes pull with similar forces on their dorsal and ventral surfaces. *J Cell Biol* **147**, 1313–1324, 1999.

29. Tan, J. L., Tien, J., Pirone, D. M., Gray, D. S., Bhadriraju, K. and Chen, C. S. Cells lying on a bed of microneedles: An approach to isolate mechanical force. *Proc Natl Acad Sci U S A* **100**, 1484–1489, 2003.

30. du Roure, O., Saez, A., Buguin, A., Austin, R. H., Chavrier, P., Siberzan, P. and Ladoux, B. Force mapping in epithelial cell migration. *Proc Natl Acad Sci U S A* **102**, 2390–2395, 2005.

31. Xia, Y. and Whitesides, G. M. Soft Lithography. *Annu Rev Mater Sci* **28**, 153–184, 1998.

32. Sniadecki, N. J. and Chen, C. S. Microfabricated silicone elastomeric post arrays for measuring traction forces of adherent cells. *Methods Cell Biol* **83**, 313–328, 2007.

33. Saez, A., Buguin, A., Silberzan, P. and Ladoux, B. Is the mechanical activity of epithelial cells controlled by deformations or forces? *Biophys J* **89**, L52–54, 2005.

34. Saez, A., Ghibaudo, M., Buguin, A., Silberzan, P. and Ladoux, B. Rigidity-driven growth and migration of epithelial cells on microstructured anisotropic substrates. *Proc Natl Acad Sci U S A* **104**, 8281–8286, 2007.

35. Ghibaudo, M., Saez, A., Trichet, L., Xayaphoummine, A., Browaeys, J., Silberzan, P., Buguin, A. and Ladoux, B. Traction forces and rigidity sensing regulate cell functions. *Soft Matter* **4**, 1836–1843, 2008.

36. Nelson, C. M., Jean, R. P., Tan, J. L., Liu, W. F., Sniadecki, N. J., Spector, A. A. and Chen, C. S. Emergent patterns of growth controlled by multicellular form and mechanics. *Proc Natl Acad Sci U S A* **102**, 11594–11599, 2005.

37. Ruiz, S. A. and Chen, C. S. Emergence of patterned stem cell differentiation within multicellular structures. *Stem Cells* **26**, 2921–2927, 2008.

38. Liu, Z., Tan, J. L., Cohen, D. M., Yang, M. T., Sniadecki, N. J., Ruiz, S. A., Nelson, C. M. and Chen, C. S. Mechanical tugging force regulates the size of cell-cell junctions. *Proc Natl Acad Sci U S A* **107**, 9944–9949, 2010.

39. Yang, M. T., Sniadecki, N. J. and Chen, C. S. Geometric considerations of micro- to nanoscale elastomeric post arrays to study cellular traction forces. *Adv Mater* **19**, 3119–3123, 2007.

40. Kong, H. J., Polte, T. R., Alsberg, E. and Mooney, D. J. FRET measurements of cell-traction forces and nano-scale clustering of adhesion ligands varied by substrate stiffness. *Proc Natl Acad Sci U S A* **102**, 4300–4305, 2005.

41. Sniadecki, N. J., Anguelouch, A., Yang, M. T., Lamb, C. M., Liu, Z., Kirschner, S. B., Liu, Y., Reich, D. H. and Chen, C. S. Magnetic microposts as an approach to apply forces to living cells. *Proc Natl Acad Sci U S A* **104**, 14553–14558, 2007.

42. Beningo, K. A., Dembo, M. and Wang, Y. L. Responses of fibroblasts to anchorage of dorsal extracellular matrix receptors. *Proc Natl Acad Sci U S A* **101**, 18024–18029, 2004.

43. Maskarinec, S. A., Franck, C., Tirrell, D. A. and Ravichandran, G. Quantifying cellular traction forces in three dimensions. *Proc Natl Acad Sci U S A* **106**, 22108–22113, 2009.

15

Blood Glucose Monitoring

David D. Cunningham
Eastern Kentucky University

The availability of blood glucose monitoring devices for home use has significantly impacted the treatment of diabetes with the American Diabetes Association currently recommending that Type 1 insulin-dependent diabetic individuals perform blood glucose testing four times per day. Grave health issues are associated with high and low blood glucose levels. Injection of too much insulin without enough food lowers blood sugar into the hypoglycemic range, glucose below 60 mg/dL, resulting in mild confusion or in more severe cases loss of consciousness, seizure, and coma. On the other hand, long-term high blood sugar levels lead to diabetic complications such as eye, kidney, heart, nerve, or blood vessel disease (Diabetes Control and Complications Trial Research Group 1993). Complications were tracked in a large clinical study showing that an additional 5 years of life, 8 years of sight, 6 years free from kidney disease, and 6 years free of amputations can be expected for a diabetic following tight glucose control versus the standard regimen (Diabetes Control and Complications Trial Research Group 1996).

Glucose monitoring and control in the perioperative setting also has a significant effect on patient outcomes since a large percentage of nondiabetic patients, as well as diabetic patients, become hyperglycemic during induction with anesthesia, throughout surgery, and several hours postsurgery. A study published in 2001 showed critically ill patients intensively controlled to between 80 and 110 mg/dL glucose had fewer complications and a 34% lower in-hospital mortality than conventionally managed patients where treatment was initiated when glucose was >215 mg/dL and maintained between 180 and 200 mg/dL (van den Berghe et al. 2001). Subsequently, in 2006, a standard of care for critically ill patients, recommending glucose be kept as close to 110 mg/dL as possible and generally <140 mg/dL, was widely adopted. Unfortunately, additional studies of intensive control in the ICU generally found an increased incidence of hypoglycemia and failed to confirm the initial found benefit in survival, so the guidelines were withdrawn in 2008 (NICE-SUGAR Study Investigators 2009). The accuracy required of the glucose measurements to allow tight glucose control and avoid hypoglycemia received relatively little attention during the studies discussed above, but the painful experience of resetting treatment guidelines has brought the subject of glucose measurement into sharp focus among clinical researchers (Rice et al. 2010).

TABLE 15.1   Landmarks in Glucose Monitoring

1941—Effervescent tablet test for glucose in urine
1956—Dip and read test strip for glucose in urine
1964—Dry reagent blood glucose test strip requiring timing, wash step, and visual comparison to a color chart
1970—Meter to read reflected light from a test strip, designed for use in the doctor's office
1978—Major medical literature publications on home blood glucose monitoring with portable meters
1981—Finger lancing device automatically lances and retracts tip
1987—Electrochemical test strip and small meter in the form of a pen
1997—Multiple test strip package for easy loading into meter
2001—Alternate-site blood sampling for virtually painless testing

The current Food and Drug Administration (FDA) and ISO guidelines on the accuracy of self-monitoring blood glucose systems have been in place since 1996 and state that 95% of the readings must be within 20% of a reference method value for glucose values ≥75 mg/dL and within 15 mg/dL of reference values for glucose values <75 mg/dL. In June 2009, an initiative was launched by ISO with strong support by the FDA to tighten the requirements so that 95% of the readings are within 15% of a reference method value for glucose values ≥75 mg/dL and within 10 mg/dL of reference values for glucose values <75 mg/dL, with implementation by 2012. While industry will certainly meet any government-mandated standard, the cost of the systems may rise and new features such as faster time to result and lower blood sample requirements may not advance as rapidly. The continued need for simple, accurate glucose measurements has led to continuous improvements in sample test strips, electronic meters, sample acquisition techniques, and more recently, continuous monitoring systems.

Self-monitoring blood glucose systems based on single-use test strips are available from a number of companies through pharmacy and mail order; however, the more recently introduced continuous monitoring systems require a prescription. Some of the landmarks in glucose testing are shown in Table 15.1. The remainder of the chapter comprises a history of technical developments with an explanation of the principles behind optical and electrochemical sensing, including examples of the biochemical reactions used in commercial products.

15.1 Historical Methods of Glucose Monitoring

Diabetes is an ancient disease that was once identified by the attraction of ants to the urine of an affected individual. Later, physicians would often rely on the sweet taste of the urine in diagnosing the disease. Once the chemical-reducing properties of glucose were discovered, solutions of a copper salt and dye, typically *o*-toluidine, were used for laboratory tests, and by the 1940s the reagents had been formulated into tablets for use in test tubes of urine. More specific tests were developed using glucose oxidase, which could be impregnated on a dry paper strip. The reaction of glucose with glucose oxidase produces hydrogen peroxide that can subsequently react with a colorless dye precursor in the presence of hydrogen peroxide to form a visible color (see Equation 15.3). The first enzyme-based test strips required addition of the sample to the strip for 1 min and subsequent washing of the strip. Visual comparison of the color on the test strip to the color on a chart was required to estimate the glucose concentration. However, the measurement of glucose in urine is not adequate since only after the blood glucose level is very high for several hours does glucose "spill-over" into the urine. Other physiological fluids such as sweat and tears are not suitable because the glucose level is much lower than in blood.

Whole blood contains hemoglobin inside the red blood cells that can interfere with the measurement of color on a test strip. To prevent staining of the test strip with red blood cells, an ethyl cellulose layer was applied over the enzyme and dye-impregnated paper on a plastic support (Mast 1967). In another early commercially available test strip, the enzymes and dye were incorporated into a homogeneous water-resistant film that prevented penetration of red blood cells into the test strips and enable their easy rcmoval upon washing (Rey et al. 1971). Through various generations of products, the formulations of the strips were improved to eliminate the washing/wiping steps and electronic meters were developed to measure the color.

15.2 Development of Colorimetric Test Strips and Optical Reflectance Meters

Optically based strips are generally constructed with various layers that provide a support function, a reflective function, an analytical function, and a sample-spreading function as illustrated in Figure 15.1. The support function serves as a foundation for the dry reagent and may also contain the reflective function. Otherwise, insoluble reflective or scattering materials such as TiO_2, $BaSO_4$, MgO, or ZnO are added to the dry reagent formulation. The analytical function contains the active enzyme. The reaction schemes used in several commercial products are described in greater detail later. The spreading function must rapidly disperse the sample laterally after application and quickly form a uniform sample concentration on the analytically active portion of the strip. Swellable films and semipermeable membranes, particularly glass fiber fleece has been used to spread and separate plasma from whole blood. Upon formation of the colored reaction product, the amount of diffuse light reflected from the analytical portion of the strip decreases according to the following equation:

$$\%R = (I_u/I_s)\, R_s \tag{15.1}$$

where I_u is the reflected light from the sample, I_s is the reflected light from a standard, and R_s is the percent reflectivity of the standard. The Kubelka–Munk equation gives the relationship in a more useful form:

$$C \propto K/S = (1 - R)^2/2R \tag{15.2}$$

where C is the concentration, K is the absorption coefficient, S is the scattering coefficient, and R is the percent reflectance divided by 100.

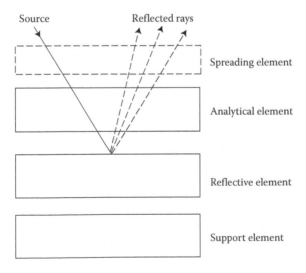

FIGURE 15.1 Basic functions of a reflectance-based test strip. (From Henning TP and Cunningham DD. Biosensors for personal diabetes management. In: *Commercial Biosensors*, pp. 3–46, 1998. Copyright Wiley-VCH Verlag GmbH & Co. KGaA. Reproduced with permission.)

The analytical function of the strip is based on an enzyme reaction with glucose and subsequent color-forming reactions. Although the most stable enzymes are chosen for product development, some loss in activity occurs during manufacturing due to factors such as pH, temperature, physical sheer stress, organic solvents, and various other denaturing actions or agents. Additional inactivation occurs during the storage of the product. In general, sufficient enzyme and other reagents are incorporated into the strip so that the assay reactions near completion in a conveniently short time. Reagent formulations often include thickening agents, builders, emulsifiers, dispersion agents, pigments, plasticizers, pore formers, wetting agents, and the like. These materials provide a uniform reaction layer required for good precision and accuracy. The cost of the materials in the strip must be low since it is used only once.

Many color-forming reactions have been developed into commercial products as indicated in the following examples. Manufacturers often use the same chemistry across multiple brands of strips and meters as indicated by the brief description of the active ingredients given in the test strip package insert. The glucose oxidase/peroxidase reaction scheme used in the Lifescan OneTouch™ (Phillips et al. 1990) and SureStep™ test strips is mentioned later. Glucose oxidase catalyzes the oxidation of glucose forming gluconic acid and hydrogen peroxide. The oxygen concentration in blood (ca. 0.3 mM) is much lower than the glucose concentration (3–35 mM), so oxygen from the atmosphere must diffuse into the test strip to bring the reaction to completion. Peroxidase catalyzes the reaction of the hydrogen peroxide with 3-methyl-2-benzothiazolinone hydrazone (MBTH) and 3-dimethylaminobenzoic acid (DMAB). A naphthalene sulfonic acid salt replaces DMAB in the SureStep strip.

$$\text{Glucose} + \text{oxygen} \xrightarrow{\text{GOx}} \text{gluconic acid} + H_2O_2$$
$$H_2O_2 + \text{MBTH} + \text{DMA} \xrightarrow{\text{peroxidase}} \text{BMBTH-DMAB (blue)}$$

(15.3)

The hexokinase reaction scheme used in the Bayer GLUCOMETER ENCORE™ test strip is shown later. Hexokinase, ATP, and magnesium react with glucose to produce glucose-6-phosphate. The glucose-6-phosphate reacts with glucose-6-phosphate dehydrogenase and NAD^+ to produce NADH. The NADH then reacts with diaphorase and reduces the tetrazolium indicator to produce a brown compound (formazan). The reaction sequence requires three enzymes but is insensitive to oxygen.

$$\text{Glucose} + \text{ATP} \xrightarrow[\text{Mg}^{+2}]{\text{HK}} \text{G-6-P} + \text{ADP}$$
$$\text{G-6-P} + NAD^+ \xrightarrow{\text{G-6-PDH}} \text{6-PG} + \text{NADH} + H^+$$
$$\text{NADH} + \text{tetrazolium} \xrightarrow{\text{diaphorase}} \text{formazan (brown)} + NAD^+$$

(15.4)

The reaction scheme originally used in the Roche Accu-Chek™ Instant™ test strip is shown later (Hoenes et al. 1995). Bis-(2-hydroxy-ethyl)-(4-hydroximinocyclohex-2,5-dienylidene) ammonium chloride (BHEHD) is reduced by glucose to the corresponding hydroxylamine derivative and further to the corresponding diamine under the catalytic action of glucose oxidase. Note that while oxygen is not required in the reaction, oxygen in the sample may compete with the intended reaction creating an oxygen dependency. The diamine reacts with a 2,18 phosphomolybdic acid salt to form molybdenum blue. More recent forms of the Accu-Chek Instant, Compact™, and Integra™ brand test strips were formulated with the oxygen-independent enzyme glucose dehydrogenase containing pyrroloquinoline quinine (GDH-PQQ) and the same reagents used to form molybdenum blue.

$$\text{Glucose} + \text{BHEHD} \xrightarrow{\text{GOx}} \text{diamine}$$
$$P_2Mo_{18}O_{62}^{-6} + \text{diamine} \longrightarrow MoO_{2.0}(OH) \text{ to } MoO_{2.5}(OH)_{0.5} \text{ (molybdenum blue)}$$

(15.5)

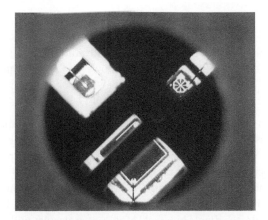

FIGURE 15.2 Photograph of light-emitting diodes and photodetector on the OneTouch meter. Photodetector at bottom, 635 nm light-emitting diode at top left, 700 nm light-emitting diode at top right. Optics viewed through the 4.5 mm hole in the strip after removal of the test strip reagent membrane. (Courtesy of John Grace.)

The reaction scheme used in the Roche Accu-Chek Easy™ test strip is shown later (Freitag 1990). Glucose oxidase reacts with ferricyanide and forms potassium ferric ferrocyanide (Prussian Blue). Again, oxygen is not required but may compete with the intended reaction.

$$\text{Glucose} + \text{GOx (ox)} \rightarrow \text{GOx (red)} \tag{15.6}$$

$$\text{GOx (red)} + [\text{Fe(CN)}_6]^{-3} \rightarrow \text{GOx (ox)} + [\text{Fe(CN)}_6]^{-4}$$

$$3[\text{Fe(CN)}_6]^{-4} + 4\text{FeCl}_3 \rightarrow \text{Fe}_4[\text{Fe(CN)}_6]_3 \text{ Prussian blue}$$

Current optical test strips and reflectance meters typically require 1.5–10 µL of blood and read out an answer in 10–30 s. A significant technical consideration in the development of a product is the measurement of samples spanning the range of red blood cell concentrations (percent hematocrit) typically found in whole blood. Common hematocrit and glucose ranges are 30–55% and 40–500 mg/dL (2.2–28 mM), respectively. The Lifescan OneTouch meter contains two light-emitting diodes (635 and 700 nm), which allows measurement of the color due to red blood cell and the color due to the dye. Reflectance measurements from both LEDs are measured with a single photodetector as shown in Figure 15.2. All glucose meters measure the detector signal at various timepoints and if the curve shape is not within reasonable limits an error message is generated. Some meters measure and correct for ambient temperature. Of course, optical systems are subject to interference from ambient light conditions and may not work in direct sunlight. Optical systems have gradually lost market share to electrochemical systems that were introduced commercially in 1987. Optical test strips generally require a larger blood sample and take longer to produce the result than electrochemical strips. Presently, optical reflectance meters are more costly to manufacture, require larger batteries, and are more difficult to calibrate than electrochemical meters.

15.3 Emergence of Electrochemical Strips

Electrochemical systems are based on the reaction of an electrochemically active mediator with an enzyme. The mediator is oxidized at a solid electrode with an applied positive potential. Electrons will flow between the mediator and electrode surface when a minimum energy is attained. The energy of the electrons in the mediator is fixed based on the chemical structure but the energy of the electrons in the solid electrode can be changed by applying a voltage between the working electrode and a second electrode. The rate of the electron transfer reaction between the mediator and a working electrode surface is given by the Butler–Volmer equation (Bard and Faulkner 1980). When the potential is large enough all the mediator reaching the electrode reacts rapidly and the reaction becomes diffusion controlled. The current from a diffusion-limited reaction follows the Cottrell equation:

$$i = (nFAD^{1/2}C)/(\pi^{1/2}t^{1/2}) \tag{15.7}$$

where i is the current, n is the number of electrons, F is Faraday's constant, A is the electrode area, C is the concentration, D is the diffusion coefficient, and t is the time. The current from a diffusion-controlled electrochemical reaction will decay away as the reciprocal square root of time. This means that the maximum electrochemical signal occurs at short times as opposed to color-forming reactions where the color becomes more intense with time. The electrochemical method relies on measuring the current from the electron transfer between the electrode and the mediator. However, when a potential is first applied to the electrode, the dipole moments of solvent molecules will align with the electric field on the surface of the electrode causing a current to flow. Thus, at very short times, this charging current interferes with the analytical measurement. Electrochemical sensors generally apply a potential to the electrode surface and measure the current after the charging current has decayed sufficiently. With small volumes of sample, coulometric analysis can be used to measure the current required for complete consumption of glucose (Feldman et al. 2000).

The reaction scheme used in the first commercial electrochemical test strip from MediSense (now Abbott Diabetes Care) is shown later. Electron transfer rates between the reduced form of glucose oxidase and ferricinium ion derivatives are very rapid compared with the unwanted side reaction with oxygen (Cass et al. 1984; Forrow et al. 2002). The Abbott Diabetes Care Precision QID™ strip includes the 1,1′-dimethyl-3-(2-amino-1-hydroxyethyl) ferrocene mediator, which has the desirable characteristics of high solubility in water, fast electron-shuttling (bimolecular rate constant of 4.3×10^5 M^{-1} s^{-1}), stability, and pH independence of the redox potential (Heller and Feldman 2008). Electrochemical oxidation of the ferrocene derivative is performed at 0.6 V. Oxidation of interferences, such as ascorbic acid and acetaminophen present in blood, are corrected for by measuring the current at a second electrode on the strip that does not contain glucose oxidase.

$$\text{Glucose + GOx (oxidized)} \rightarrow \text{gluconolactone + GOx (reduced)}$$

$$\text{GOx (reduced) + ferricinium}^+ \rightarrow \text{GOx (oxidized) + ferrocene} \tag{15.8}$$

$$\text{Ferrocene} \rightarrow \text{ferricinium}^+ + \text{electron (reaction at solid electrode surface)}$$

Several electrochemical test strips use ferricyanide rather than ferrocene as the electrochemical mediator although the potential required for oxidation is higher than for ferrocene derivatives. The LifeScan OneTouch FastTake™ and Ultra™ brand test strips include glucose oxidase and either 11 or 22 μg ferricyanide per strip. The strip readout is reduced from 15 to 5 s with the larger amount of ferricyanide mediator. Many Roche Accu-Chek strips, including the Comfort Curve™, Compete™, Advantage™, Aviva™, and Active™, are formulated with the oxygen-independent enzyme GDH-PQQ and ferricyanide as the mediator. An organic mediator, nitrosoanaline is used with GDH-PQQ in the Roche Accu-Chek Performa™ test strip.

The reaction scheme used in the Abbott Diabetes Care Precision-Xtra™ and Sof-Tact™ test strips is shown later. The GDH enzyme does not react with oxygen and the phenanthroline quinine mediator can be oxidized at 0.2 V, which is below the oxidation potential of most interfering substances.

$$\text{Glucose + GDH/NAD}^+ \rightarrow \text{GDH/NADH + gluconolactone}$$

$$\text{GDH/NADH + PQ} \rightarrow \text{GDH/NAD}^+ + \text{PQH}_2 \tag{15.9}$$

$$\text{PQH}_2 \rightarrow \text{PQ + electrons (reaction at solid electrode surface)}$$

The working electrode on most commercially available electrochemical strips is made by screen printing a conductive carbon ink on a plastic substrate; however, more expensive noble metal electrodes are also used. Historically, test strips have been manufactured, tested, and assigned a calibration code. The calibration code provided with each package of strips is sometimes manually entered into the meter by the user but other systems automatically read the calibration code from the strips. Meters designed for use in the hospital often have bar code readers to download calibration, quality control, and patient information. Test strips are supplied in bottles or individual foil wrappers to protect them from moisture over their shelf-life, typically about 1 year. The task of opening and inserting individual test strip into the meter has been minimized by packaging multiple test strips in the form of a disk-shaped cartridge or a drum that is placed into the meter. Disks or drums typically contain 10–17 test strips.

15.4 Enzyme Selectivity and Falsely Elevated Readings

Formulations containing GDH-PQQ became popular due to the lack of oxygen interference and the high catalytic activity of the enzyme relative to glucose oxidase (5000 U/mg vs 300 U/mg). However, GDH-PQQ oxidizes a wide range of sugars with reaction rates generally in the order: glucose (100%), maltose (58%), lactose (58%), galactose (10%), mannose (10%), and xylose (10%). Normally, the concentration of the other sugars is so much lower than the glucose concentration in blood that there is little interference. Until recently, it was not appreciated that patients receiving peritoneal dialysis using the osmotic agent icodextrin absorb and metabolize the icodextrin to shorter polysaccharides, mainly maltose, causing erroneously high glucose measurements. In addition, some injected drug products contain maltose as a part of the formulation, which also leads to high glucose readings. To address this issue, the FDA recently issued a public health notification recommending against the use of GDH-PQQ in glucose test strips (FDA Public Health Notification 2009). Research studies have shown that site-directed mutagenesis of GDH-PQQ can reduce the reactivity to maltose to about 10% that of glucose but cannot achieve the selectivity of either glucose oxidase or NADH-dependent glucose dehydrogenase (Igarashi et al. 2004). Besides adequate activity and selectivity, any new enzyme developed for use in test strips must have good thermal stability. Protein engineering approaches for improving enzyme stability include increasing the hydrophobic interaction in the interior core region of the protein, reducing the water-accessible hydrophobic surface area, and stabilizing the dipoles of the helical structure.

15.5 Improvements in User Interactions with the System and Alternate Site Testing

Both Type 1 and Type 2 diabetic individuals do not currently test as often as recommended by physicians, so systems developed in the last few years have aimed to improve compliance with physician recommendations while maintaining accuracy. Historically, the biggest source of errors in glucose testing involved interaction of the user with the system. Blood is typically collected by lancing the edge of the end of the finger to a depth of about 1.5 mm. Squeezing or milking is required to produce a hanging drop of blood. The target area on test strips is clearly identified by design. A common problem is smearing a drop of blood on top of a strip resulting in a thinner than normal layer of blood over part of the strip and a low reading. Many strips now require that the blood drop be applied to the end or side of the strip where capillary action is used to fill the strip. Partial filling can be detected electrochemically or by observation of the fill window on the strip. The small capillary space in the Abbott Diabetes Care Freestyle™ electrochemical strip requires only 300 nL of blood.

Progressively thinner diameter lancets have come to the market with current sizes typically in the 28–31 gauge range. Most lancets are manufactured with three grinding steps to give a tri-bevel point. After loading the lancet into the lancing device, a spring system automatically lances and retracts the point. The depth of lancing is commonly adjustable through the use of several settings on the device or use of a different end-piece cap. Unfortunately, the high density of nerve endings on the finger makes the process painful and some diabetic individuals do not test as often as they should due to the pain and residual soreness caused by fingersticks. Recently, lancing devices have been designed to lance and apply pressure on the skin of body sites other than the finger, a process termed "alternate site testing." The use of alternate site sampling lead to the realization that capillary blood from alternate sites can have slightly different glucose and hematocrit values than blood from a fingerstick due to the more arterial nature of blood in the fingertips. The pain associated with lancing alternate body sites is typically rated as painless a majority of the time and less painful than a fingerstick over 90% of the time. A low-volume test strip, typically 1 μL or less, is required to measure the small blood samples obtained from alternate sites. Some care and technique is required to obtain an adequate amount of blood and transfer it into the strips when using small blood samples.

Significant insight into blood collection from the skin was uncovered during the development of an alternative site device, the Abbott Diabetes Care Sof-Tact meter, which automatically extracts and transfers blood to the test strip (see Figure 15.3). The device contains a vacuum pump, a lancing device, and a test strip that is automatically indexed over the lancet wound after lancing. The vacuum turns off after sufficient blood enters the strip to make an electrical connection. The key factors and practical limits of blood extraction using vacuum combined with skin stretching were investigated to assure that sufficient blood could be obtained for testing (Cunningham et al. 2002). The amount of blood extracted increases with the application of heat or vacuum prior to lancing, the level of vacuum, the depth of lancing, the time of collection, and the amount of skin stretching (see Figure 15.4). Particularly important is the diameter and height that skin is allowed to stretch into a nosepiece after the application of vacuum as shown in Figure 15.5. Vacuum combined with skin stretching increases blood extraction by increasing the lancet wound opening, increasing the blood available for extraction by vasodilatation, and reducing the venous return of blood through the capillaries. The electrochemical test strip used with the meter can be inserted into a secondary support and used with a fingerstick sample when the battery is low.

The size of a meter is often determined by the size of the display although electrochemical meters can be made smaller than reflectance meters. The size and shape of one electrochemical meter, with a

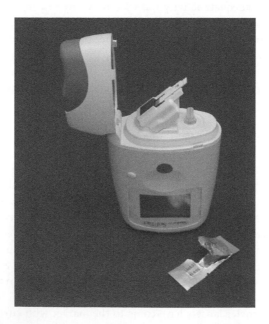

FIGURE 15.3   Sof-Tact meter with cover opened to load test strip and lancet. Test strip is inserted into an electrical connector. The hole in the opposite end of the test strip allows the lancet to pass through. The white cylindrical lancet is loaded into the lancet tip holder in the housing. To perform a test, the cover is closed, the gray area of the cover placed against the skin and the front button depressed.

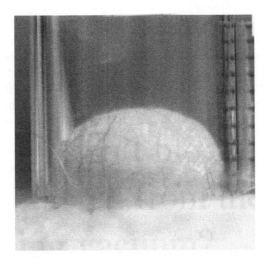

FIGURE 15.4 Photograph of skin on the forearm stretching up into a glass tube upon application of vacuum. Markings on tube at right in 1 mm increments. (Courtesy of Douglas Young.)

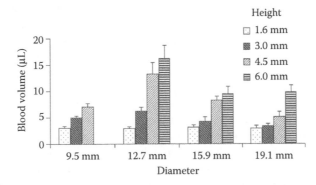

FIGURE 15.5 Effect of skin stretching by vacuum on blood volume extracted from lancet wounds on the forearm. Mean blood volume ± SE in 30 s with −7.5 psig vacuum for nosepieces of different inner diameter and inside step height. (From Cunningham et al., 2002. *J Appl Physiol* 92: 1089–1096. With permission.)

relatively small display, is indistinguishable from a standard ink pen. All meters store recent test results in memory and many allow downloading of the results to a computer. The variety of meters available in the market is mainly driven by the need to satisfy the desires of various customer segments that are driven by different factors, such as cost, ease of use, or incorporation of a specific design or functional feature. Advanced software functions are supplied with some meters to allow entry of exercise, food, and insulin doses, and a personal digital assistant–meter combination was brought to market.

15.6 Continuous Glucose Sensors

All the currently marketed continuous glucose-sensing systems in the United States have similar components. The sensor is contained within a sharp metal housing that is inserted through the skin, then the metal portion is retracted leaving the sensor in the skin. The sensor has a glucose oxidase working electrode portion located under the skin and electrical contacts that are connected to a battery-operated electrochemical potentiostat outside the skin. The electrical components often wirelessly transmit data to a remote display unit where the most recent glucose result and trend data are available. After insertion into the skin, the sensor is calibrated using blood glucose test strips, so a test strip meter is often incorporated into the system for this purpose. Initial calibration and recalibration requirements of the systems has become progressively less demanding over the past several years, but insertion of the sensor into the body changes the sensitivity of present-day sensors enough that some calibration is required. Mechanistic studies of the body's reaction to sensor insertion and testing of more biocompatible coatings is a very active area of investigation both in academia and in industry. However, limited information is available on advances in the area of biocompatible coatings, due to the proprietary nature of the work. Sensors are currently approved for use for up to 7 days, with the risk of infection at the insertion site becoming a concern at longer times.

The sensors marketed by Medtronic and Dexcom are based on a first-generation scheme where the working electrode oxidizes hydrogen peroxide generated by the reaction of glucose and oxygen as catalyzed by glucose oxidase. The working electrode must be covered with a material that is more permeable to oxygen than to glucose since the typical 0.1–0.3 mM concentration of oxygen in the body is much lower than the 2–30 mM concentration of glucose. The Medtronic sensor is a three-electrode system with a working, counter, and reference electrode, so the reference electrode area can be fairly small since no current passes through the reference electrode. The electrodes are fabricated on a thin flexible piece of plastic apparently using thin-film deposition techniques with a membrane polymer coating composed of a diisocyanate, a diamino silane, and a diol, which forms a polyurethane polyurea polymer (VanAntwerp 1999; Henning 2010). The Dexcom sensor is a two-electrode system consisting of a thin platinum wire and a larger silver wire with a silver chloride coating on the outside. During the oxidation of the hydrogen peroxide at about 0.6 V, the silver chloride is reduced. The glucose-limiting membrane is apparently a hydrophilic block copolymer of polyethylene glycol and a polyurethane mixed with a hydrophobic polyurethane polymer (Tapsak et al. 2007). Both the Medtronic and Dexcom sensors are inserted about 12 mm into the skin at a 45° angle but the form of the inserter and the method of electrical contact are of different design (Henning 2010).

The Abbott Diabetes Care sensor is based on a second-generation scheme where an exogenous mediator, in this case an osmium redox polymer, rather than oxygen reacts with the glucose oxidase (Feldman et al. 2003). The mediator can be added at higher effective concentrations than oxygen, eliminating the problem of low oxygen concentration. The sensor is a three-electrode design screen printed on a plastic substrate as shown in Figure 15.6. The reduced mediator is oxidized at a low potential, 0.04 V, so common electrochemical interferences in blood such as acetaminophen and ascorbic acid will not react at the working electrode. The current density of second-generation sensors can be much higher than in the first-generation system since the diffusion of glucose does not have to be reduced to below that of oxygen. The Abbott Diabetes Care sensor is inserted about 5 mm into the skin at a 90° angle.

The GlucoDay™ system based on microdialysis sampling of interstitial fluid was developed in Europe and introduced commercially by Menarini Diagnostics (Poscia et al. 2003). A microdialysis fiber 5 mm

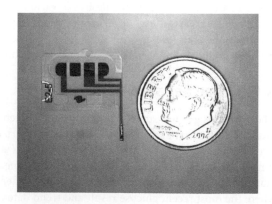

FIGURE 15.6 Abbott Diabetes Care sensor showing size relative to a U.S. dime. (Courtesy of Abbott Diabetes Care.)

long is inserted through the skin by a medical professional, perfused with a buffer solution at a flow rate of ~10 μL/min using a micropump, and the glucose content of the solution measured with a first-generation glucose sensor. The system is calibrated with a blood glucose test strip and the monitoring conducted for up to 48 h, after which the fiber is removed. At present, the high level of professional medical personnel involvement is a significant commercial limitation of the technology.

One 12-h device, the Cygnus GlucoWatch™ based on transdermal reverse iontophoresis (Kurnik et al. 1998) gained FDA approval but the acceptance of the device in the market was poor due to the need to calibrate the device with multiple fingersticks and poor precision and accuracy. The device is no longer commercially available.

15.7 Future Directions

Advances in self-monitoring glucose test strips and meters are difficult to predict given the already highly refined nature of the products in terms of cost of manufacture, size, reliability, ease of use, and time-to-result. Accuracy may be improved through the use of more advanced electrochemical measurements with improved signal-processing strategies or the use of redundant arrays of electrodes on a single strip. Emerging fabrication technologies such as nanoimprint lithography and electrochemical or electrode-less deposition of metals are capable of producing very fine detail without the use of expensive masks. The significant international investment in nanotechnology is producing a wide variety of advanced materials that prove useful in new products. Newly engineered enzymes and electron transfer chemistries may emerge to address selectivity, activity, stability, and other crucial factors. In this regard, several methods have already been reported to electrically connect the glucose oxidase catalytic center to an electrode, gold nanoparticle, or carbon nanotube (Cunningham and Stenken 2010).

The performance of continuous glucose monitoring systems has been rapidly improving and should soon reach the state where the signal is reliable enough to provide input into an insulin infusion pump to produce a "closed-loop" system. However, development of an appropriate algorithm to translate the glucose value into the correct insulin infusion pump setting is quite challenging. A strictly hardware-based system is ignorant of many important factors affecting future blood glucose levels, such as the size of the meal the patient will eat, the amount of exercise planned, or the level of daily stress encountered. So, systems allowing user input of information or "open-loop" control systems may prove more successful. Long-term sensing may involve surgical implantation of a battery-operated unit although many issues remain with the long-term stability of the sensor, miniaturization of the sensing electronics, and data transmitter and biocompatibility of the various materials of construction.

Many fluorescence-based sensing approaches have been investigated by academic and industrial groups. Perhaps the most interesting system involves the injection of glucose-sensitive fluorescent microspheres into the skin to create a "tattoo." The glucose measurement is then made by placing an appropriately designed intensity or time-based fluorometer over the skin area. Many reversible glucose-binding fluorescent systems have been reported with boronic acid derivatives, lectins, or glucose-binding proteins serving as the glucose-selective agent and fluorescent dyes, preferably with absorbance wavelengths above that of hemoglobin, serving as the reporter (McShane and Stein 2010). The *in vivo* stability of the glucose-selective agent and fluorescent dye will likely become more apparent as results from ongoing animal trials are published. Additional work may be needed to overcome the host response to the microspheres and to decrease the immunogenicity of the protein component, if used.

A number of noninvasive spectroscopic approaches have been investigated; however, the amount of clinical data reported to date is very limited. Near-infrared spectroscopy has received the most focused attention with careful analysis of instrumental capabilities and calculation of the net analytical signal indicating currently available hardware can generate glucose-specific information from physiological levels of glucose in body tissue. Additional work is needed to show how this information can be obtained in a reliable and practical manner. Raman spectroscopy and surface-enhanced Raman spectroscopic approaches have advanced through initial animal studies demonstrating partial proof-of-principle.

Likewise, the optical rotation of polarized light by glucose has been utilized to measure glucose particularly in the accessible portion of the aqueous humor of the eye.

Glucose changes also affect the osmotic strength of interstitial fluid, and sensors based on chemical swelling or shrinking of polymers, optical changes in the refractive index, and osmotic effects on electrochemical capacitance have been refined through *in vitro* studies. Prospective clinical trials are needed to more clearly identify the potential of these approaches.

Glucose monitoring of alternative body fluids such as sweat, saliva, gingival crevicular, or tear fluid has been investigated but these fluids generally have a lower glucose concentration than blood and the glucose content of these samples, obtained using traditional methods, does not change in a fixed proportion to the blood glucose concentration. Future studies may explore the possibility that acquisition of smaller physiological samples may show better correlation with blood glucose levels due to the lower anatomical and physiological stress required to obtain smaller volumes of fluid. Further miniaturization and refinement in the design of devices for the collection of small blood or interstitial fluid samples as well as insertion of sensing components into or through the skin is anticipated. Overall, the future of blood glucose monitoring looks very challenging and exciting.

Defining Terms

Alternate site testing: Lancing sites other than the finger to obtain blood in a less painful manner. The small volume of blood obtained from alternate sites requires use of a test strip requiring 1 µL or less of blood.

Type 1 Diabetes: The immune system destroys insulin-producing islet cells in the pancreas, usually in children and young adult, so regular injections of insulin are required (also referred to as juvenile diabetes).

Type 2 Diabetes: A complex disease based on gradual resistance to insulin and diminished production of insulin. Treatment often progresses from oral medications to insulin injections as disease progresses. Also referred to as adult onset diabetes and non-insulin-dependent diabetes mellitus (NIDDM).

References

Bard AJ and Faulkner LR. 1980. *Electrochemical Methods*. New York: John Wiley & Sons. pp. 103, 143.

Cass A, Davis G, Francis G, Hill H, Aston W, Higgins I, Plotkin E, Scott L, and Turner A. 1984. Ferrocene-mediated enzyme electrode for amperometric determination of glucose. *Anal Chem* 56:667–671.

Cunningham DD, Henning T, Shain E, Hannig J, Barua E, and Lee R. 2002. Blood extraction from lancet wounds using vacuum combined with skin stretching. *J Appl Phys* 92:1089–1096.

Cunningham DD and Stenken JA (eds), 2010. *In Vivo Glucose Sensing*. New York: John Wiley & Sons.

Diabetes Control and Complications Trial Research Group. 1993. The effect of intensive treatment of diabetes on the development and progression of long-term complications in insulin-dependent diabetes mellitus. *N Eng J Med* 329:977–986.

Diabetes Control and Complications Trial Research Group. 1996. Lifetime benefits and costs of Intensive therapy as practiced in the diabetes control and complications Trial. *JAMA* 276:1409–1415.

FDA Public Health Notification issued August 13, 2009: Potentially Fatal Errors with GDH-PQQ* Glucose Monitoring Technology. http://www.fda.gov/MedicalDevices/Safety/AlertsandNotices/PublicHealthNotifications/ucm176992.htm, accessed April 15, 2010.

Feldman B, Brazg R, Schwartz S, and Weinstein R. 2003. A continuous glucose sensor based on wired enzyme technology—Results from a 3-day trial in patients with type 1 diabetes. *Diabetes Technol Ther* 5:769–779.

Feldman B, McGarraugh G, Heller A, Bohannon N, Skyler J, DeLeeuw E, and Clarke D. 2000. FreeStyle: A small-volume electrochemical glucose sensor for home blood glucose testing. *Diabetes Technol Ther* 2:221–229.

Forrow NJ, Sanghera GS, and Walters SJ. 2002. The influence of structure in the reaction of electrochemically generated ferrocenium derivatives with reduced glucose oxidase. *J Chem Soc Dalton Trans* 3187.

Freitag H. 1990. Method and reagent for determination of an analyte via enzymatic means using a ferricyanide/ferric compound system. *United States Patent* 4,929,545.

Heller A and Feldman B. 2008. Electrochemical glucose sensors and their applications in diabetes management. *Chem Rev* 108:2482–2505.

Henning TP. 2010. Commercially available continuous glucose monitoring systems. In: *In Vivo Glucose Sensing*, eds D Cunningham and J Stenken, pp. 113–156. New York: John Wiley & Sons.

Henning TP and Cunningham DD 1998. Biosensors for personal diabetes management. In: *Commercial Biosensors*, ed. G. Ramsey, pp. 3–46. New York: John Wiley & Sons.

Hoenes J, Wielinger H, and Unkrig V. 1995. Use of a soluble salt of a heteropoly acid for the determination of an analyte, a corresponding method of determination as well as a suitable agent thereof. *United States Patent* 5,382,523.

Igarashi S, Hirokawa T, and Sode K. 2004. Engineering PQQ glucose dehydrogenase with improved substrate specificity: Site-directed mutagenesis studies on the active center of PQQ glucose dehydrogenase. *Biomol Eng* 21:81–89

Kurnik RT, Berner B, Tamada J, and Potts RO, 1998. Design and simulation of a reverse iontophoretic glucose monitoring device. *J Electrochem Soc* 145:4119–4125.

Mast RL. 1967. Test article for the detection of glucose. *United States Patent* 3,298,789.

McShane M and Stein E. 2010. Fluorescence-based glucose sensors. In: *In Vivo Glucose Sensing*, eds D Cunningham and J Stenken, pp. 113–156. New York: John Wiley & Sons.

NICE-SUGAR Study Investigators. 2009. Intensive versus conventional glucose control in critically ill patients. *N Engl J Med* 360:1283–1297.

Phillips R, McGarraugh G, Jurik F, and Underwood R. 1990. Minimum procedure system for the determination of analytes. *United States Patent* 4,935,346.

Poscia A, Mascini M, Moscone D et al. 2003. A microdialysis technique for continuous subcutaneous glucose monitoring in diabetic patients. *Biosens Bioelectron* 18:891–898.

Rey H, Rieckman P, Wiellager H, and Rittersdorf W. 1971. Diagnostic agent. *United States Patent* 3,630,957.

Rice MJ, Pitkin AD, and Coursin DB. 2010. Glucose measurement in the operating room: More complicated than it seems. *Anesth Analg* 110:1056–65.

Tapsak MA, Rhodes RK, Rathbun K, Shults MC, and McClure JD. 2007. Techniques to improve polyurethane membranes for implantable glucose sensors. *United States Patent* 7,226,978.

VanAntwerp WP. 1999. Polyurethane/polyurea compositions containing silicon for biosensor membranes. *United States Patent* 5,882,494.

Van den Berghe G, Wouters P, Weekers F et al. 2001. Intensive insulin therapy in the critically ill patients. *N Engl J Med* 345:1359–67.

Further Information

Test results of glucose meters are often compared with results from a reference method and presented in the form of a Clarke error grid that defines zones with different clinical implications. Clarke, WL, Cox, DC, Gonder-Frederick, LA, Carter, W, and Pohl, SL. 1987. Evaluating clinical accuracy of systems for self-monitoring of blood glucose. *Diabetes Care* 10: 622–628.

Error grid analysis has recently been extended for the evaluation of continuous glucose monitoring sensors. Kovatchev BP, Gonder-Frederick LA, Cox DJ, and Clarke WL. 2004. Evaluating the accuracy of continuous glucose-monitoring sensors. *Diabetes Care* 27:1922–1928.

Reviews and descriptions of many marketed products are available online at: www.childrenwithdiabetes.com.

Interviews of several people involved with the initial development of blood glucose meters are available online at: www.mendosa.com/history.htm.

16

Atomic Force Microscopy: Opportunities and Challenges for Probing Biomolecular Interactions

Gary C.H. Mo
University of Toronto

Christopher M. Yip
University of Toronto

16.1 Introduction

Discerning and understanding structure–function relationships is often predicated on our ability to measure these properties over a range of relevant length scales. A key concept in the fields of nanoscience and nanotechnology is that directly manipulating atomic and molecular interactions in matter can ultimately control a material's macroscopic physical, chemical, and electronic properties. This is often a consequence of understanding how complex molecular architectures, be they organic, inorganic, or biological, are derived from their constituent building blocks. To study phenomena at such a basic level, tools capable of performing functional measurements, in real time, over critical length scales are required. Such tools would enable researchers to visualize complex biomolecular structures, ideally in their native context, while simultaneously mapping their functional properties.

Powerful functional imaging tools such as single molecule fluorescence and nonlinear optical microscopies, such as coherent anti-Raman Stokes (CARS) and second-harmonic generation (SHG), through to the various electron microscopies (SEM/TEM/STEM) provide a suite of tools for characterizing phenomena under a vast range of conditions and situations. Indeed recent advances in these established techniques provide ample evidence of their continued evolution, including the exciting new development of super-resolution optical imaging [1–6] and live cell electron microscopies [7]. An exceptionally powerful complement to these conventional imaging techniques has been atomic force microscopy (AFM), or scanning probe microscopy (SPM), which, since its inception in the mid-1980s, has developed into one of the most useful tools for characterizing molecular-scale phenomena and interactions, and directly mapping their contribution to macroscopic mechanical properties, structures, and ultimately function.

This chapter explores some of the recent advances in SPM where it has been applied to the study of biomolecular structures and functions—from single molecules to large aggregates and complexes to live cells—and introduce some new innovations in the field of correlated imaging tools designed to address many of the key limitations of this family of techniques.

16.2 Background

SPM is founded on a simple fundamental principle: Direct mapping of the interactions between a nominally atomically sharp raster-scanning tip and a surface can be used to generate real-space images of surfaces. One can reasonably describe these images as isosurfaces of a parameter as a function of (x,y,z) space. Notably, these isosurfaces can be interpreted as maps of a diverse set of interactions, ranging from repulsive or attractive forces to local variations in temperature, adhesion, viscoelasticity, and even charge. SPM has become a well-accepted and established technique for characterizing surfaces and interfacial processes with atomic or molecular-scale resolution [8–11]. It has made a tremendous impact in the biological sciences and the fields of cellular and molecular biophysics [12], due in large part to its unique ability to resolve molecular structures and interaction forces in real time and often *in situ* [13–20]. This growth has been fostered by a continually evolving suite of SPM-based imaging modes, including intermittent contact or tapping mode [21], force volume mapping [22–28], and even spatially resolved nanomechanical property measurements [29]. These attributes are particularly compelling for the study of protein–protein and protein–substrate interactions, including both model and live cell membranes [30], and investigations of cellular dynamics and structures.

16.3 SPM Basics

The family of scanning probe microscopes arguably emerged from early efforts by Young on the "Topographiner" [31]; however, the scanning tunneling microscope (STM), which operates on the principle of measuring the tunneling current between two conducting surfaces separated by a very small distance [32], is often viewed as the forefather of the field. For biology, a more useful variant is AFM, which maps local variations in the inter-molecular and inter-atomic forces between a tip and a surface [33]. By moving the tip relative to the sample surface in the x–y plane, a surface contour map that reflects relative differences in interaction intensity as a function of surface position can be generated. The high spatial and force resolution afforded the atomic force or scanning probe microscope (SPM) is a consequence of the precise control maintained over the tip–sample separation distance through the use of piezoelectric scanners and sophisticated feedback control schemes. In a conventional SPM, the surface is scanned with a nominally atomically sharp tip mounted on the underside of an extremely sensitive cantilever. The spatial resolution of the SPM is a consequence of the sample itself, with near-atomic scale resolution often achievable on atomically flat surfaces, such as a crystal. On softer, more compliant surfaces, such as cells or surfaces with significant variations in surface structure, the resolution can be somewhat reduced. Similarly, although the theoretical force sensitivity of these tips is on the order of 10^{-14} Newtons (N), practical limitations reduce this value to ~10^{-10} N.

The relative motion of the tip and sample is controlled through the use of piezoelectric crystal scanners. The user sets the desired applied force or amplitude dampening in the case of the intermittent contact imaging. Deviations from these set point values are detected as *error* signals on a four-quadrant position-sensitive photodetector (PSPD), and then fed into the main computer (Figure 16.1). The error signal provided to the instrument is then used to generate a feedback signal that is used as the input to the feedback control software. The tip–sample separation distance is then dynamically changed in real

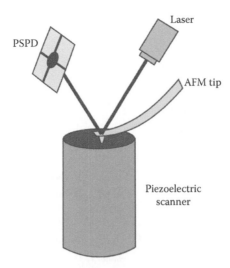

FIGURE 16.1 Schematic representation of the atomic force microscope. In this configuration, the sample would be mounted on the scanner and scanned under a fixed AFM tip. The laser is focused on the AFM tip and the position of the reflected laser spot is monitored on a position-sensitive photodetector (PSPD).

time and adjusted to return to the desired set point force. It is the amount of motion required to return to the desired set point value that is then converted into the observed isosurface. Although tip deflection is the simplest feedback signal, there are a host of other signals that could be used to control the tip–sample mapping, including tip oscillation (amplitude/phase), friction, surface charge, and even temperature.

16.4 Imaging Mechanisms

16.4.1 Contact

During imaging, the AFM tracks gradients in interaction force(s), either attractive or repulsive, between the tip and the surface (Figure 16.2). Similar to how the STM mapped out local variations in tip–sample tunneling current, the AFM uses this force gradient to generate an iso-force surface image. In contact mode imaging, the tip–sample interaction is maintained at a specific, user-defined load. This operating mode arguably provides the best resolution for imaging of surfaces and structures. It also provides direct access to the so-called friction force imaging where transient twisting of the cantilever during scanning can be used to develop maps of relative surface friction [34,35]. The ability to quantify such data is limited because of challenges in determining the torsional stiffness of the cantilevers, a problem exacerbated by the geometry of the cantilever. In contact mode the image represents a constant attractive (or repulsive) tip–sample force that is chosen by the user. Incorrect selection of this load results in sample damage (excessive force) or poor tracking (insufficient force). Subtle manipulation of these imaging forces affords the user the unique ability to both probe local structure and determine the response of the structure to the applied force.

16.4.2 Noncontact

In noncontact mode imaging, the AFM tip is actively oscillated near its resonance frequency at a distance of tens to hundreds of Angströms away from sample surface. The resulting image represents an isosurface corresponding to regions of constant amplitude dampening. As the forces between the tip and the surface are very small, noncontact mode AFM is ideally suited for imaging softer samples, such as proteins, surfactants, or membranes. In this mode, one often uses cantilevers with a higher spring

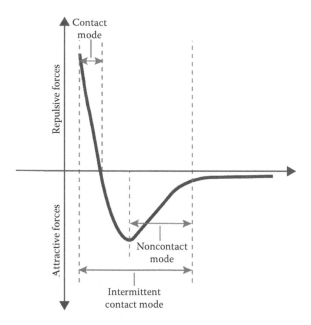

FIGURE 16.2 Schematic representation of the interaction forces between the AFM tip and an arbitrary surface as a function of separation distance. The schematic illustrates the regions of attractive and repulsive forces and the domains of AFM operation (contact/intermittent contact/noncontact).

constant than those employed during normal contact mode imaging. The net result is a very small feedback signal, which can make instrument control difficult and imaging challenging [36,37].

16.4.3 Intermittent Contact

This method, in which the tip alternates from the repulsive to the attractive regions of the tip–sample interaction curve, has become the method of choice currently for most AFM imaging. In early contact mode work, it was quickly realized that poorly adhering molecules could be rapidly displaced by the sweeping motion of the AFM cantilever. This "snow-plow" effect has been largely ameliorated by vertically oscillating the tip during imaging, which removes the lateral forces present during contact mode imaging. As the vertical oscillations occur at a drive frequency that is several orders of magnitude higher than the raster-scanning frequency, it is possible to obtain comparable lateral and vertical resolution as the continuous contact techniques. Because one detects the relative damping of the tip's free vertical oscillation during imaging, an intermittent contact mode AFM image can be viewed as an iso-energy dissipation landscape. Intermittent contact imaging provides access to other imaging modes, including phase imaging, which measures the phase shift between the applied and detected tip oscillations. This derivative signal is particularly useful for tracking spatial distributions of the relative modulus, viscoelasticity, and adhesive characteristics of surfaces, and has proven to be very powerful for studying polymeric materials [26,34,35,38–50]. Phase imaging is particularly useful for studying biological and biomimetic systems, including adsorbed proteins and supported lipid bilayers, even in the absence of topographic contrast [45,51–54].

In intermittent contact imaging, the cantilever can be oscillated either acoustically or magnetically. In the former, the cantilever is vertically oscillated by a piezoelectric crystal typically mounted under the cantilever at a characteristic resonant frequency. In air, this is typically a single value, determined largely by the stiffness of the cantilever. In fluid, mechanical coupling of the cantilever motion with the fluid, and the fluid cell, can result in a complex power spectrum with multiple apparent resonant peaks. In this case, choosing the appropriate peak to operate with can be difficult and experience is often the best guide. Selection of the appropriate cantilever for intermittent contact imaging will depend on the physical imaging environment (air/fluid). In air, one typically uses the so-called "diving board" tips, which have a relatively high resonance peak of approximately 250 kHz (depending on the manufacturer). In fluid, viscous coupling between the tip and the surrounding fluid results in an increase in the apparent resonant frequency of the tip. This allows the use of the conventional V-shaped contact-mode cantilevers. In magnetic mode, a magnetic AFM tip/cantilever assembly is placed in an oscillating magnetic field [55–57]. It is the interaction of the magnetic tip with the field that induces the tip oscillations. This is a fundamentally simpler approach with arguably finer control over the drive amplitude; however, this approach can be complicated by issues such as the quality of the coating and the nature of the sample.

16.4.3.1 Applications

The breadth of possible applications for SPM seems almost endless. As has been described earlier, the concepts underlying the instrument are simple and the technology itself has effectively become turnkey. This does not mean that SPM is a very transparent tool—it is critical that the user has a good grasp of the physical principles that underpin the generation of an SPM image. Similarly, the user must have a good understanding of the nature of their samples, and how they might behave during imaging—an aspect that is of particular interest to those investigating cellular phenomena. Recent reviews by Bottomley et al., and others provide an excellent perspective on the diverse range of topics that are being studied by this and related techniques [9–11,13,58]. In the following sections, we will explore how *in situ* SPM/AFM-based investigations have provided novel insights into the structure and function of biomolecular assemblies. SPM has made in-roads in several different arenas, which can be separated into several key areas: [1] imaging; [2] force spectroscopy; and [3] nanomechanical property measurement. We will focus in a few specific areas, rather than attempting to cover the whole scope of the field.

16.5 Imaging

The real-space imaging capabilities, coupled with the ability to simultaneously display derivative images, such as phase (viscoelasticity), friction, and temperature, are perhaps the most attractive attributes of the SPM. In the case of biomolecules, it is the ability to perform such imaging but in buffer media, under a variety of solution conditions and temperatures, in real time that has really powered the acceptance of this technique by the biomedical community [59–63]. Such capabilities are allowing researchers to gain a glimpse of the mechanics and dynamics of protein assembly and function, and the role of extrinsic factors, such as pH, temperature, or other ligands on these processes [64]. For example, *in situ* SPM has been used successfully to visualize and characterize voltage and pH-dependent conformational changes in two-dimensional arrays of OmpF [21], whereas several groups have used *in situ* SPM to characterize transcription and DNA-complex formation and individual proteins [65–73].

The raster-scanning action of the tip does, however, complicate *in situ* imaging. Processes occurring faster than the raster-scanning acquisition time of the SPM can be missed, or worse, create an artifact associated with the motion of the object. The magnitude of this problem obviously depends on the kinetics of the processes under study. This is particularly important when one is viewing live cell data in which conventional raster-scanning rates are necessarily slow (~1 Hz) [74–76]. Advances in tip and controller technology help to improve the stability of the SPM under fast-scan conditions. Strategies may include tips with active piezoelectric elements [77] smaller cantilevers with high-quality factors, or faster data acquisition and control hardware [78]. A particularly useful and low-cost option for improving time resolution is to simply *disable* one of the scanning directions so that the AFM image is a compilation of line scans taken at the same location as a function of time [79]. This would, therefore, generate an isosurface wherein one image axis reflects time and not position. This approach has been used quite successfully to examine single molecule dynamics in a study of the chaperonin GroES–GroEL complex [80].

Although recent efforts have resulted in particularly compelling new hardware and software implementations for faster biological AFM imaging, including live cells and protein dynamics [76,78,81–85], they continue to rely on a single cantilever probe to perform the imaging. A particularly compelling albeit challenging from the fabrication and control perspectives approach may be to consider the use of multiple imaging tips. Such a strategy would effectively parallelize the imaging process. The potential of such an approach remains largely unproven to date although SPM tip arrays have been developed for data storage applications and sensor applications [86–89].

16.6 Crystallography

In situ SPM has been used with great success to study the mechanisms associated with crystal growth [90], from amino acids [91], to zeolite crystallization [92], and biomineralization [93–95]. For protein crystals, studies have ranged from early investigations of lysozyme [96], to insulin [97], antibodies [98,99], and recently the mechanisms of protein crystal repair [99]. The advantages of SPM for characterizing protein crystallization have been very well discussed in reviews by McPherson and Vekilov [100,101]. Ordered crystalline materials formed through chemical cross-linking are also amenable to high-resolution imaging [102]. It is worth mentioning that the high spatial and temporal resolution capabilities of the SPM are ideal for examining and measuring the thermodynamic parameters for these processes. These range from local variations in free energy and their correlation with conventional models of crystal growth to relating step advancement rates to the product of the density of surface kink sites and the frequency of attachment [103]. Recently, Guo et al. [104] probed the nanomechanical properties of insulin crystals by AFM, providing intriguing insights into inter-planar strength and the local compressibility of the protein within its crystalline lattice in direct comparison with data obtained on insulin fibrils.

A particular challenge for SPM studies of crystal growth is that interpreting the data paradoxically often requires that one already has a known crystal structure or a related isoform for comparison of packing motifs and molecular orientation. *De novo* determination of two-dimensional crystal packing motifs can be readily achieved; however, extrapolations to possible space group symmetries are much more difficult [105–107]. Recently, the focus has shifted toward understanding the growth process. The ability to perform extended duration *in situ* imaging presents the crystallographer with the unique opportunity of directly determining the mechanisms and kinetics of crystal nucleation and growth [99,100,103,106,108–118]. Unlike x-ray approaches, the SPM cannot readily report on atomic-level details of the crystal and the molecular units. Rather, it provides details on crystal and molecular packing motifs with the individual molecules appearing as amorphous blob to the AFM, even when packed into a lattice, making it difficult to assign a specific secondary structure to the protein. Despite these challenges, *in situ* AFM studies of molecular and protein crystals have proven to be quite enlightening. Recent work by Danesh et al., resolved the difference between various crystal polymorphs including face-specific dissolution rates for drug candidates [119–121] while Guo et al. examined the effect of specific proteins on the crystallization of calcium oxalate monohydrate [122]. In a particularly interesting study, Frincu et al., investigated cholesterol crystallization from bile solutions using calcite as a model substrate [123]. In this work, the authors were able to use *in situ* SPM to characterize the role of specific substrate interactions in driving the initial nucleation events associated with cholesterol crystallization. Extended-duration imaging allowed the researchers to characterize the growth rates and the onset of Ostwald ripening under physiological conditions. They were able to confirm their observations and models by calculating the interfacial energies associated with the attachment of the cholesterol crystal to the calcite substrate. In their comprehensive review of the thermodynamics and kinetics of calcium phosphate biomineralization, Wang and Nancollas explored how AFM can be used to directly extract novel insights into the initial nucleation steps associated with crystal growth and phase formation [124]. Biomineralization and its health implications have stimulated numerous studies of calcium oxalate crystallization as it relates to kidney stones and strategies of their remediation [125–127]. These include studies of strategies for modifying the kinetics and habit of calcium oxalate crystals with small peptides, as reported by Wang et al. [128]. Milhiet et al. used detergent-disrupted bilayers to form two-dimensional crystals of several membrane proteins, enabling them to directly probe the structure of the exposed extracellular domains [129]. In our own work, we demonstrated that the self-assembly of small molecule dye aggregates into crystalline arrays with unique, structure-dependent spectroscopic properties on phospholipid bilayers was dependent on both electrostatic effects as well as substrate packing [130]. This work was particularly interesting as it revealed the role of the nucleating interface in controlling the structure, orientation, and packing of the dye aggregate nuclei, portending the design of other structured interfaces for controlling aggregate orientation, size, and properties. It is this powerful combination of *in situ* real-time characterization with theoretical modeling that has made *in situ* SPM particularly compelling for studying molecular self-assembly at interfaces.

16.6.1 Protein Aggregation and Fibril Formation

In a related context, the self-assembly of proteins into fibrillar motifs has been an area of active research for many years, owing in large part to the putative links to diseases such as Alzheimer's, Huntington's, and even diabetes in the context of *in vitro* insulin fibril formation [131,132]. A particular challenge for the field of protein aggregation lies in the complex map of association pathways and structures. Determining what are on- and off-pathway aggregates and their relationship to the disease pathology has proven to be quite difficult, owing in large part to the numerous intermolecular interactions that drive these self-assembly mechanisms. Directly identifying these pathways, tracking biomolecular self-association, and finding a causal link to a particular disease would be a tremendous asset for the design of drug inhibitors. Because *in situ* SPM can easily acquire real-space information on dynamic molecular-scale processes and structures that are difficult to assay clinically, it is ideal for *in situ* studies of protein aggregation and fibrillogenesis. These have included investigations of collagen [133–137], human stefin B [138], spider silk [139–142], insulin amyloid polypeptide (IAPP), amylin, β-amyloid, and synuclein [143–152]. *In situ* observation of Aβ assemblies has enabled direct observation of low molecular weight oligomers [153], whereas high-resolution imaging of islet amyloid polypeptide has been performed using frequency-modulation techniques [154]. In an intriguing study, Friedrichs et al. captured the reorientation of collagen fibrils in cells *in vitro* using AFM [155].

Perhaps, driven more by an applied technology perspective, *in situ* SPM has provided unique chemical insights not only into the process of fibrillization [156,157], but also the role of the nucleating substrate on directing the kinetics, orientation, and structure of the emerging fibril [158,159]. As noted by Kowalewski in their investigation of β-amyloid formation on different surfaces chemically and/or structural dissimilar substrate may in fact facilitate growth biasing the apparent kinetics and orientation of the aggregate [160]. Because SPM imaging requires a supporting substrate, there is often a tacit assumption that this surface is passive and would not adversely influence the aggregation or growth process. However, what has become immediately obvious from a number of studies is that these surfaces can, and do, alter the nucleation and growth patterns [161,162]. Characterization, either theoretical or experimental using the *in situ* capabilities of the SPM, will, in principle, identify how the local physical/electronic/chemical nature of the surface drives fibril formation.[163]. One must ensure that appropriate controls were in place, or performed, so that the aggregate as seen by the SPM is clearly the responsible agent for nucleation. All of this certainly brings up the questions of [1] is the aggregate observed by these *in situ* tools truly the causative agent; [2] what role is the substrate playing in the aggregation or assembly pathway. The first point is a particularly compelling one when it concerns the studies of protein adsorption and assembly. Although the SPM can certainly resolve nanometer-sized objects on the substrate, the adsorption of the smallest species cannot be guaranteed. Correlating solution with surface self-assembly mechanisms and structures, especially in the context of biomolecular complexes and phenomena, can be challenging and often one must resort to complementary, corroborative tools such as light scattering.

16.6.2 Membrane Protein Structure and Assemblies

One area in which SPM has made a significant impact has been in the structural characterization of membrane dynamics and protein–membrane interactions and assembly. Supported planar lipid bilayers (SPB) are particularly attractive as model cell membranes [164] and recent work has provided very detailed insights of their local dynamics and structure [165–171], as well as the dynamics of domain formation [172–175]. Exploiting the *in situ* high-resolution imaging capabilities of the SPM and the conformal nature of supported bilayers, workers have been able to follow thermal phase transitions (gel-fluid) in supported bilayers [174,176,177] and Langmuir–Blodgett films [178]. Thermal transitions in mixed composition supported bilayers have been studied by *in situ* SPM [174,179], where the so-called ripple phase domains were seen to form as the system entered the gel–fluid coexistence regime [180]. These structural studies not only enrich our understanding on bilayers themselves, but also of their interactions with other biological systems.

In situ SPM has been particularly useful for investigating the dynamics of the so-called lipid rafts, which are small lipid heterogeneities thought to facilitate membrane protein function. With nanometer-scale topographical resolution, AFM observations showed that many membrane lipids and mixtures contain such lipid domains [181]. For example, Rinia et al., investigated the role of cholesterol in the formation of rafts using a complex mixture of dioleoylphosphatidylcholine (DOPC), sphingomyelin (SpM), and cholesterol as the model membrane [182]. In the absence of cholesterol, the mixture phase separates into gel-state SpM and fluid-state DOPC domains. As the cholesterol content increased, the authors reported the formation of SpM/cholesterol-rich domains or "lipid rafts" within the (DOPC) fluid domains. In related work, Van Duyl et al. (2003) observed similar domain formation for (1:1) SpM/DOPC SPBs containing 30 mol% cholesterol [183]. With cholesterol, the formation of these domains is not restricted to liquid–liquid coexistence phases [179]. The effect of dynamically changing the cholesterol levels on raft formation and structure was reported by Lawrence et al. [184]. By adding either water-soluble cholesterol or methyl-β-cyclodextrin (Mβ-CD), a cholesterol-sequestering agent, the authors were able to directly resolve the effect of adding or removing cholesterol on domain structure and dynamics, including a biphasic response to cholesterol level that was seen as a transient formation of raft domains as the cholesterol level was reduced. The *in situ* imaging capabilities of the SPM have provided direct evidence of domain formation for cardiolipin, a lipid enriched in the mitochondria that form domains only in the presence of phosphatidylethanolamine and not phosphatidylcholine [185]. *In situ* AFM was used to confirm that clustering of galactosylceramides on the extracellular membrane leaflet, a mechanism thought to facilitate virus adhesion, was a cholesterol-dependent process [186]. Our AFM-based studies of the late endosomal lipid bis-(monoacylglycero)-phosphoate (BMP), thought to cause multivesicular morphology through domain formation [187–189] confirmed this mechanism through coupled AFM phase and fluorescence imaging methods.

Using supported planar bilayers as a model substrate has been particularly useful for the study of membrane-associated molecules by AFM. Polycationic dendrimers were found to induce large, 15–40 nm diameter holes in the zwitterionic bilayers and remove fluid-phase lipids from the alveoli-mimicking Survanta bilayers [190,191]. Anesthetics, such as dibucaine and halothane, were found to compromise membrane structure and elasticity [168,184,192–206]. Several studies explored the interactions between membrane-active and membrane-associated proteins and membrane surfaces. For example, *in situ* SPM has revealed that the association of peptides with membranes can lead to dramatic changes in membrane morphology and membrane disruption. This was seen to be the case for the amphipathic peptides: filipin, amphotericin B, mellitin, and amylin [207–210]. In related work, the N-terminal domain of the capsid protein cleavage product of the flock house virus (FHV), has found to cause the formation of interdigitated lipid membrane domains [211]. We have seen similar effects in our studies of peptide-membrane interactions, including antimicrobial peptides and toxins [212–216]. Tilted peptides were found to cause hole formation while leaving the membrane morphology largely intact [217]. In contrast, the protein synaptotagmin can leave indentations but does not produce defects in anionic lipid bilayers

[218]. In related work, AFM studies revealed how membranes of Gram-negative bacteria disintegrate through to the action of antibacterial Sushi peptides [219]. The relative ease with which SPBs can be formed prompted studies of reconstituted membrane proteins, including ion channels and transmembrane receptors [194–203,220] and enzymes, such as ATP synthase and phosphatases [221,222]. The ease of forming complex model membranes from an SPB suspension helped drive investigations of reconstituted membrane protein functionality [16]. For example, *in situ* AFM has been used to examine the role of divalent ions, such as calcium in facilitating membrane protein insertion while inhibiting detergent interdigitation [223]. However, it is worth noting that because model membrane formation is typically performed by simple vesicle fusion, it is difficult to know *a priori* the orientation of a transmembrane protein in the final supported bilayer as protein reconstitution into the vesicle occurs via freeze-thaw or sonication [168,204–206]. The lipid-to-protein ratios can be manipulated to yield the ideal density or to investigate the structural differences caused by steric factors [224]. Ideally, there is a distinct difference in the size and/or shape of the extra- and intra-cellular domains, and statistical analysis of local surface topographies can be employed to at least infer a molecular orientation.

Peptide-membrane interactions are also thought to be critical to the mechanism of neurodegenerative diseases, such as Alzheimer's (AD) and Parkinson's (PD). For example, studies of α-synuclein with supported lipid bilayers revealed the gradual formation and growth of defects within the SPB [225]. Interestingly, the use of a mutant form of α-synuclein revealed a qualitatively slower rate of bilayer disruption. We conducted an analogous experiment to investigate the interaction between the β-amyloid (Aβ) peptide with SPBs prepared from a total brain lipid mixture [226]. *In situ* SPM revealed that the association of monomeric Aβ1-40 peptide with the SPBs resulted in rapid formation of fibrils followed by membrane disruption. Control experiments performed with pure component DMPC bilayers revealed similar membrane disruption; however, the mechanism was qualitatively different with the formation of amorphous aggregates rather than well-formed fibrils. Others have examined similar membrane-induced aggregation and self-assembly phenomena using a diverse range of model membrane compositions and peptides [190,227–229]. What is particularly compelling about these studies, aside from the ability to provide direct visualization of the effect of the interactions in real-time using the SPM, is the ease with which one can reliably fabricate model membranes of quite complex mixtures, ranging from simple homogeneous gel- or fluid-state bilayers through to complex heterogeneous mimics of bacterial and fungal membranes.

16.7 Force Spectroscopy

16.7.1 Fundamentals

By disabling the x- and y-scan directions and monitoring the tip deflection in the z-direction, the AFM is capable of measuring protein–protein and ligand-receptor binding forces, often with sub-picoNewton resolution. The ability to detect such low forces is because of the low spring constant of the AFM cantilever (0.60–0.06 N/m). In these AFM force curve measurements, the tip is modeled as a Hookian spring whereby the amount of tip deflection (Δz) is directly related to the attractive/repulsive forces (F) acting on the tip through the tip spring constant (k). At the start of the force curve, the AFM tip is held at a null position of zero deflection out of contact with the sample surface. The tip–sample separation distance is gradually reduced and then enlarged using a triangular voltage cycle applied to the piezoelectric scanner. This will bring the tip into and out of contact with the sample surface. As the piezo extends, the sample surface contacts the AFM tip causing the tip to deflect upward until a maximum applied force is reached and the scanner then begins to retract. We should note that when the gradient of the attractive force between the tip and sample exceeds the spring constant of the tip, the tip will "jump" into contact with the sample surface. As the scanner retracts, the upward tip deflection is reduced until it reaches the null position. As the sample continues to move away from the tip, attractive forces between the tip and the surface hold the tip in contact with the surface and the tip begins to deflect in the opposite direction. The tip continues to deflect downwards until the restoring force of the tip cantilever overcomes the attractive forces and the tip jumps out of contact with the sample surface (E), thereby providing us with an estimate of the tip–sample unbinding force, given as:

$$F = -k\Delta z$$

This force spectroscopy approach has found application ranging from mapping effect of varying ionic strength on the interactions between charged surfaces [230–245], to studying electrostatic forces at crystal surfaces [246,247].

16.7.1.1 Single Molecule Force Spectroscopy

Specific intermolecular interactions can be measured in single molecule force spectroscopy using ligand-modified SPM tips [248]. In principle, if we can measure the forces associated with the binding of a ligand to its complementary receptor, we may be able to correlate these forces with association energies [249]. By tethering a ligand of interest, in the correct orientation, to the force microscope tip and bringing the now-modified tip into contact with an appropriately functionalized surface, one can now conceivably directly measure the attractive and repulsive intermolecular forces between single molecules as a function of the tip–sample separation distance. The vertical tip jump during pull-off can be used to estimate the interaction force, which can be related to the number of binding sites, adhesive contact area, and the molecular packing density of the bound molecules. In the case of biomolecular systems, multiple intermolecular interactions exist and both dissociation and (re)association events may occur on the time scale of the experiment resulting in broad retraction curve with discrete, possibly quantized, pull-off events. This approach has been used to investigate biomolecular [22,56,250–252] and DNA-nucleotide interactions, along with the local mechanical properties of biomolecules [20,253–261]. Although estimates of the adhesive interaction forces may be obtained from the vertical tip excursions during the retraction phase of the force curve, during pull-off, the width and shape of the retraction curve reflects entropically unfavourable molecular unfolding and elongation processes.

Although simple in principle, it was soon recognized that the force spectroscopy experiment was highly sensitive to sampling conditions. For example, it is currently well recognized that the dynamics of the measurement will significantly influence the shape of the unbinding curve. It is well known that the rate of ligand-receptor dissociation increases with force resulting in a logarithmic dependence of the unbinding force with rate [262], and studies have shown that single molecule techniques, such as AFM, clearly sample an interaction energy landscape [263]. It is, therefore, evident that forces measured by the AFM cannot be trivially related to binding affinities [264]. Beyond these simple sampling rate dependence relationships, we must also be aware of the dynamics of the tip motion during the acquisition phase of the measurement. In particular, when these interactions are mapped in fluid media, one must consider the hydrodynamic drag associated with the (rapid) motion of the tip through the fluid [265]. This drag effect can be considerable when factored into the interaction force determination.

Another key consideration is that, in single molecule force spectroscopy, the ligands of interest are necessarily immobilized at force microscope tips and sample surfaces. In principle, this approach will allow one to directly measure or evaluate the spatial relationship between the ligand and its corresponding receptor site. For correct binding to occur, the ligands of interest must be correctly oriented, have the appropriate secondary and tertiary structure, and be sufficiently flexible (or have sufficiently high unrestricted mobility) that they can bind correctly. An appropriate immobilization strategy would, therefore, require *a priori* information about the ligand's sequence, conformation, and the location of the binding site(s) [266,267]. Strategies that have worked in the past include *N*-nitrilo-triacetic acid linkages [268], His-tags to preferentially orient ligands at surface [269,270], and, most recently, a rather interesting series of tripodal ligands [271–273]. Thiolated peptides can similarly be immobilized on gold-coated tips [274]. The critical consideration in all of these designs is the ability to robustly orient the ligand of interest appropriately. A particularly robust and reliable approach has been to rely on polyethylene glycol tethers to help extend the ligands away from the tip [252,275–281]. Force spectroscopy is not limited to patterned and model surfaces but can be performed on live cell surfaces. Alsteens et al. performed unfolding experiments directly on live cells [282]. Microbial surface ultrastructure and nanomechanical properties can be visualized [283]. Protein binding and AFM force spectroscopy on live cell membranes can be coupled to downstream processes, potentially revealing the mechanical role that the protein has in eliciting a response [284]. This type of *in situ*, pathway-specific biochemistry is often impossible to approach using more conventional techniques. Perhaps more compelling is the ability to perform such experiments under a range of conditions thus allowing the researcher to consider different, suboptimal conditions to examine induced stresses [285].

Recently, efforts have been underway to measure aggregate forces at intact biological interfaces, including bacterial biofilms on metal [286]. Microbeads were used to measure the adhesion and viscoelasticity of bacterial biofilms [287]. In addition to imaging or single molecular pulling/unfolding experiments, AFM has been used as a microscopic manipulator to dissect or deform bacteria cells [288,289]. As with single molecule force spectroscopy, the immobilization of cells becomes important in these studies. One approach is to engineer patterns and grow patches of single cells [290,291].

16.7.1.2 Force Volume

Acquiring force curves at each point on an image plane provides a means of acquiring the so-called force volume maps, a data-intensive imaging approach capable of providing a map of relative adhesion forces and charge densities across surfaces [23,292–294]. This approach has been used successfully to examine polymer surfaces and surfaces under fluid [295,296], as well as live cells [26,292,297]. Increasingly, force volume methodologies have been applied to live cell surfaces to spatially map interaction forces. These include efforts to investigate adhesin [298], polysaccharides [299,300], thiol-monolayers [301] interactions with bacterial or fungal surfaces to better understand the polarity and localization of specific processes. Not unexpectedly, these efforts have shown that specific antigen–antibody interactions are spatially concentrated in domains within the membrane [302].

16.7.1.3 Pulsed Force Mode

As indicated previously, force volume measurements are very time-consuming and this has led to the development of pulsed force mode imaging [303]. Capable of rapidly acquiring topographic, elasticity, and adhesion data, pulsed force mode operates by sampling selected regions of the force–distance curve during contact-mode imaging. During image scanning, an additional sinusoidal oscillation imparted to the tip brings the tip in and out of contact with the surface at each point of the image. Careful analysis of the pulsed force spectrum can yield details about surface elasticity and adhesion [304–309]. Compared with the ~ Hz sample rates present in conventional force volume imaging, in pulsed force mode, spectra are acquired on kHz sampling rates. Although this helps to resolve the issue related to the speed of data acquisition, one must clearly consider the possibilities associated (possible) with rate dependence of the adhesion forces, and as indicated in the previous section, the hydrodynamic forces would play a larger role.

16.7.2 Binding Forces

As discussed earlier, force spectroscopy samples regions of an energy landscape wherein the strength of a bond (and its lifetime) is highly dependent on the rate with which the spectra are collected [263,310]. At low loading rates, intermolecular bonds have long lifetimes but exhibit small unbinding forces, whereas at high loading rates, the same bonds have shorter lifetimes and larger unbinding forces. In the case of biomolecular complexes because multiple interactions are involved in stabilizing the binding interface, the dissociation pathway of a ligand-receptor complex will exhibit several unbinding energy barriers. This would suggest that one could in fact sample any number of dissociation pathways, each with its own set of transitional bonding interactions. Intriguingly, it was recently argued that the free-energy surface of a protein is significantly distorted during a force spectroscopy experiment and that such a distortion can result in certain complexities when one is considering a single molecule event [311]. The influence of experimental instrument parameters, such as loading rate, and their contribution to accurate modeling and interpretation of the rupture forces obtained from the force spectroscopy experiments has been well documented and described in a series of reports by the Akhremitchev group [312,313].

For the majority of single molecule force microscopy studies, individual ligands have been either randomly adsorbed or directly attached to the AFM tip through covalent bond formation. Covalent binding of a molecule to the tip offers a more stable "anchor" during force measurements as a covalent bond is ~10 times stronger than a typical ligand-receptor bond [314]. Covalent binding also facilitates oriented attachment of the ligand as compared to random adsorption where the orientation of the ligand on the tip surface must be statistically inferred. These advantages are tempered with the challenges present in immobilizing molecules to surfaces such as the AFM tip. As mentioned earlier, oriented ligands have been tethered covalently to AFM tips through use of flexible poly(ethylene-glycol) (PEG)-linkers [252]. In this manner, the peptide or ligand is extended away from the tip surface, which provides it with sufficient flexibility and conformational freedom for it to reorient and sample conformational space. Heterobifunctional PEG derivatives have provided the necessary synthetic flexibility for coupling a host of different ligands to the AFM tips [252,276,277,279,280,315–317]. Indeed, this approach remains a complex technical challenge as it requires due consideration of not only these factors but even seemingly mundane aspects such as the tip geometry and tilt, as was discussed in a recent publication by Rivera et al. [318].

Force spectroscopy pertains to mapping or measuring forces between discrete molecules. For example, several groups have investigated antibody–antigen interactions [319,320] and have shown that these unbinding forces may correlate with thermal dissociation rates [321]. Force spectroscopy has been used to study the energetics of protein adsorption [322]. Although the high force sensitivity of this approach is exceptionally attractive, it is equally important to recognize key experimental considerations, including the use of appropriate controls. Recently, various computational approaches, including steered molecular dynamics [323–328], Monte Carlo simulations [329,330], and graphical energy function analyses [331] have been used to simulate these dissociation and unfolding experiments. It has been particularly impressive to see the strong correlation between the structural changes resolved by these computational approaches and the experimentally determined unbinding events although much work remains to be done in terms of determining appropriate computational schemes for extending the simulation times to best match the experimental time frames and instrument parameters.

Force spectroscopy is also being applied to study protein unfolding pathways. It was recognized in early work that during the retraction phase of the AFM force curve, the molecule is subjected to a high tensile stress, and can undergo reversible elongation and unfolding. Careful control over the applied load (and the degree of extension) will allow one to probe molecular elasticity and the energetics involved in the unfolding/folding process [60,142,265,332–347]. Past studies have included investigations of titin [348], IgG phenotypes [349], various polysaccharides [350], and spider silk proteins [351]. The forces associated with protein fibril formation have been studied using force spectroscopy, including studies of the proteins involved in Parkinson's [352], Alzheimer's, and diabetes [353–355]. The Ikai group has done pioneering work with force spectroscopy of cell surface proteins, both using proteins adsorbed to a surface as well as natively presented on the membrane [356,357].

By bringing the AFM tip into contact with the surface-adsorbed molecules, and carefully controlling the rate and extent of withdrawal from the surface, it is now possible to resolve transitions that may be ascribed to unfolding of individual protein domains. Others have employed this "forced unfolding" approach to look at spectrin [358,359], lysozyme [360], and DNA [361]. Caution needs to be exercised during such experiments. Often the protein of interest is allowed to simply absorb to the substrate to form a film. Force curves performed on these films are then conducted in random locations and the retraction phase of the curve analyzed for elongation and unbinding events. This is a highly statistical approach and somewhat problematic. The general premise is that the tip will bind to the protein somewhere and that if sufficient samples are acquired, there will be a statistically relevant number of curves that will exhibit the anticipated number of unbinding and/or unfolding events. What is fundamentally challenging here is that there is no *a priori* means of knowing where the tip will bind to the protein, which would obviously affect its ability to under extension, and it is difficult to assess the interactions between the protein and the supporting substrate, or possibly other entangled proteins. To simplify the optimization and improve the statistical nature of the force spectroscopy experiment, efforts have been made by several groups to develop automated force spectroscopy systems [362].

Where single molecule imaging comes to the forefront is in the combination of imaging and single-molecule force spectroscopy. In the past, force spectroscopy has relied heavily on random sampling of the immobilized proteins, often without direct imaging of the selected protein. Recently, Raab et al. combined dynamic force microscopy, wherein a magnetically coated AFM tip is oscillated in close proximity to a surface by an alternating magnetic field. This enabled the researchers to apply what they termed "recognition imaging" to facilitate mapping of individual molecular recognition sites on a surface [279]. In recognition imaging, specific binding events are detected through dampening of the amplitude of oscillation of the ligand-modifed tip due to specific binding of the antibody on the tip to an antigen on the surface. The resulting AFM antibody-antigen recognition image will display regions of enhanced contrast that can be identified as possible binding sites or domains. In an excellent demonstration of the coupled imaging and force spectroscopy, Oesterhelt et al., studied the unfolding of bacteriorhodopsin by directly adsorbing native purple membrane to a surface, imaging the trimeric structure of the BR, and then carefully pulling on a selected molecule [60]. This allowed them to resolve the force required to destabilize the BR helices from the membrane and by reimaging the same area, show that extraction occurred two helices at a time. Computationally, these phenomena are most often modeled as freely jointed or worm-like chain systems [363]. To assess what exactly "forced unfolding" involves, Paci and Karplus examined the role of topology and energetics on protein unfolding via externally applied forces and compared it against the more traditional thermal unfolding pathways [364].

16.7.2.1 Mechanical properties

The use of the AFM/SPM as a nanomechanical tester has certainly blossomed. During the past 10 years, AFM-based nanoindentation has been used to determine the elastic modulus of polymers [365], biomolecules [366–371], cellular and tissue surfaces [372–380], pharmaceutical solids [381], and even teeth [382]. What is particularly challenging in these applications is the need for careful consideration when extrapolating bulk moduli against the nanoindentation data. Often the classical models need to be adjusted to compensate for the small (nanometer) contact areas involved in the indentation [383]. A particularly important consideration with AFM-based nanoindentation is the sampling geometry. Although traditional indentation instrumentation applies a purely vertical load on the sample, by virtue of the cantilever arrangement of the AFM system, there is also a lateral component to the indentation load. This leads to an asymmetry in the indentation profile. This asymmetry can make it difficult to compare AFM-based nanoindentation with traditional approaches using a center-loaded system. Often this effect is nullified by the use of a spherical tip with a well-defined geometry; however, this entails a further compromise in the ability to perform imaging before the indentation process. This effect has been extensively covered in the literature, especially in the context of polymer blends and composite materials [384–389]. Other considerations include the relative stiffness of the AFM cantilever, the magnitude of the applied load, tip shape which plays a significant role in the indentation process, and possibly the dwell-time. In many cases, the relatively soft cantilever will allow one to perform more precise modulus measurements including the ability to image before, and immediately after, an indentation measurement. At an even more pragmatic level, determining the stiffness both in-plane and torsional, of the cantilever can be challenging, with approaches ranging from the traditional end mass to new techniques based on thermal noise and resonant frequency shifts [390–392]. Accurate determination of these values is essential in order for the correct assessment of the local stiffness to be made.

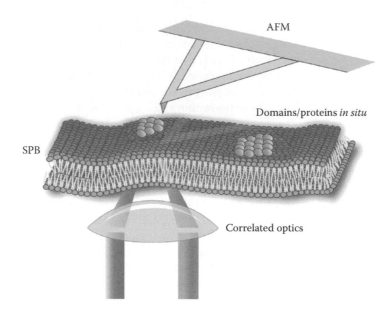

FIGURE 16.3   Schematic representation of a combinatorial AFM-fluorescence microscopy experiment, depicting AFM imaging of a supported planar lipid bilayer (SPB) containing membrane domains and/or proteins.

16.7.2.2 Coupled Imaging

Although AFM/SPM is certainly a powerful tool for following structure and dynamics at surfaces under a wide variety of conditions, it can only provide relative information within a given imaging frame. It similarly cannot confirm (easily) that the structure being imaged is in fact the protein of interest. A confirmation step can involve some *in situ* control, which might be a change in pH or T, or introduction of another ligand or reagent that would cause a change in the same that could be resolved by the SPM. Absent an *in situ* control, or in fact as an adjunct, careful shape/volume analysis is often conducted to characterize specific features in a sample. Image analysis and correlation tools and techniques are often exploited for postacquisition analysis. There has always been an obvious need for techniques or tools that can provide this complementary information, ideally in a form that could be readily integrated into the SPM.

Optical imaging represents perhaps the best tool for integration with SPM. This is motivated by the realization that there are a host of very powerful single molecule optical imaging techniques capable of addressing many of the key limitations of SPM, such as the ability to resolve dynamic events on millisecond time scales. Recent advances in confocal laser scanning (CLSM) and total internal reflection fluorescence (TIRFM) techniques have enabled single molecule detection with subdiffraction limited images [393–402] (Figure 16.3).

16.7.3 Near-Field: SNOM/NSOM

In the family of scanning probe microscopes, perhaps the best example of an integrated optical-SPM system are the scanning near-field (or near-field scanning) optical microscopes (NSOMs) which use near-field excitation of the sample to obtain subdiffraction limited images with spatial resolution comparable to conventional scanning probe microscopes [403–407]. NSOM has been used successfully in single molecule studies of dyes [408], proteins [409–411], and the structure of lignin and ion channels [412,413]. NSOM imaging has also provided insights into ligand-induced clustering of the ErbB2 receptor, a member of the epidermal growth factor (EGF) receptor tyrosine kinase family, in the membrane of live cells [414–416]. Fluorescence lifetime imaging by NSOM has been used to examine the energy and electron-transfer processes of the light harvesting complex (LHC II) [415,416] in intact photosynthetic membranes [417]. NSOM has also been used to monitor the fluorescence resonance energy transfer (FRET) between single pairs of donor and acceptor fluorophores on dsDNA molecules [418]. Challenges that face the NSOM community arguably lie in the robust design of the imaging tips [419,420]. However, NSOM as a tool is enjoying a resurgance of interest of late with recent efforts in polarized NSOM providing detailed insights into protein fibril structure [412,421] and lipid bilayer domains [422–424].

16.7.4 Evanescent Wave: TIRF

Time-resolved single-molecule imaging can be difficult and in the case of the AFM, one may question whether the local phenomena imaged by the AFM are specific to that particular imaging location. This is especially true for studies of dynamic phenomena because the scanning action of the AFM tip effectively acts to increase mass transfer into the imaging volume. Recently, combined AFM/TIRF techniques have been used to study force transmission [373] and single-particle manipulation [425] in cells. These studies helped to address a particularly challenging aspect of SPM, which was that SPM/AFM can only (realistically) infer data about the upper surface of structures and that data on the underside of a structure, for instance the focal adhesions of a cell, are largely invisible to the SPM tip. In the case of cell adhesion, one might be interested in how a cell responds to a local stress applied to its apical surface by monitoring changes in focal adhesion density and size. Using a combined AFM–TIRF system, it then becomes possible to directly interrogate the basal surface of the cell (by TIRF) while applying a load or examining the surface topography of the cell by *in situ* AFM. We recently reported on the design and use of an AFM-objective-based TIRF-based instrument for the study of supported bilayer systems [216,426,427]. By coupling these two instruments together, we were able to identify unequivocally the gel and fluid domains in a mixed dPOPC/dPPC system. What was particularly compelling was the observation of approximately 10–20% difference in the lateral dimension of the features as resolved by TIRF and AFM. Although this likely reflects the inherent diffraction limited nature of TIRFM, we can in fact use the AFM data to confirm the real-space size of the structures that are responsible for the fluorescence image contrast. This combined system also provided another interesting insight. The nonuniform fluorescence intensity across the domains resolved by TIRF may reflect a nonuniform distribution of NBD-PC within dPOPC. It may also be linked to the time required to capture a TIRF image relative to the AFM imaging. At a typical scan rate of 2 Hz, it would require approximately 4 min to capture a conventional 512×512 pixel AFM image, compared with the approximately 30 frame/s video imaging rate of the TIRF camera system. As such the TIRFM system represents an excellent means of visualizing, and capturing, data that occur on time scales faster than what can be readily resolved by the AFM. This further suggests that the differences in fluorescence intensity may reflect real-time fluctuations in the structure of the lipid bilayer that are not detected (or detectable) by AFM imaging. In a particularly intriguing experiment that used TIRF as an excitation source rather than in an imaging mode, Hugel and others were able to measure the effect of a conformational change on the relative stiffness of a photosensitive polymer [428]. By irradiating the sample *in situ*, they were able to initiate a *cis–trans* conformational change that resulted in a change in the backbone conformation of the polymer. Actin/titin in live cells can be followed by a combined TIRF and AFM strategy, simultaneously allowing one to dynamically stimulate the cytoskeleton while recording its fluorescence and mechanical response [429].

16.7.5 Confocal Fluorescence

The functional integration of confocal fluorescence with AFM microscopy is a particularly powerful approach. A complement to TIRF-AFM imging, the confocal approach provides the added advantage of being able to section through the sample along the optical axis. Fluorescently labeled DNA and polystyrene beads have been correlated using fluorescence and AFM to both locate the features and analyze the laser excitation profile of the microscope [430]. Shaw and Yip have investigated dye partitioning and mechanisms of antimicrobial peptide action in model membranes using this correlated confocal-AFM approach [214,431,432]. What was particularly intriguing was the realization, perhaps not unexpectedly but now with direct spatial confirmation, that the addition of an extrinsic fluorophore to a molecule can dramatically affect its chemical properties. In the context of membrane-associated molecules, the addition of a large hydrophobic chromophore can alter the parent molecule's partitioning behavior in the member, possibly affecting its domain specificity and interactions. Our use of the coupled confocal-AFM platform provided direct evidence of this altered domain specificity and also a cautionary note for those who rely solely on fluorescence as a mechanism for identifying membrane structures.

Correlated functional assays also hold great promise for live cell imaging and force microscopy [433]. Confocal fluorescence has been employed to locate regions of focal adhesion before AFM ultrastructural imaging [434]. Two-photon confocal fluorescence was used to confirm the functionality and location of chloroplast grana, and AFM subsequently provided nanometer-scale structural details [435]. Yu et al. [436] performed force spectroscopy of transforming growth factor beta 1 and its receptor on live cell surfaces by locating these receptors through fluorescence, whereas others have taken advantage of sophisticated optical techniques such as Förster resonance energy transfer (FRET) in combined spectroscopic confocal-SPM imaging of biological systems [437,438]. In a particularly compelling approach, Trache et al. have integrated spinning disc confocal, TIRF, and AFM to provide a uniquely powerful platform for studying real-time cellular dynamics, mechanotransduction and signaling using the AFM platform as a nano-stimulator [439–441].

16.8 Summary

As can be readily seen in the brief survey of the SPM field, it is clearly expanding both in terms of techniques and range of applications. The systems are becoming more ubiquitous and certainly more approachable by the general user; however, what is clearly important is that care must be taken in data interpretation, instrument control, and sample preparation. For example, early studies of intermolecular forces often did not exercise the same level of control over their sampling conditions as is commonplace today and this clearly impacts critical analysis of the resulting force spectra. Recognizing the limitations of the tools and hopefully developing strategies that help to overcome these limitations represent a key goal for many SPM users.

As we have seen, fluorescence imaging, either as NSOM/TIRF/CSLM, when coupled with SPM provides an excellent *in situ* tool for characterizing biomolecular interactions and phenomena. Unfortunately, such a scheme requires specific labeling strategies, and it would be preferable to effect such measurements in the absence of a label. Indeed, as we have already presented, the use of extrinsic fluorophores can affect the behavior (folding, partitioning, distribution) of the parent molecule. Recent work has focused on near-field vibrational microscopy to acquire both IR and Raman spectra on nanometer length scales [442–444], whereas a combined Raman–SPM system was used to characterize the surface of an insect compound eye [443]. Indeed, the integration of vibrational spectroscopy with AFM has had a long history, starting with the pioneering work of Knoll and Keilman in 1999 with their tip-based scattering system and now its application to the study of polymer blends [445,446], efforts that have been adopted by various other groups with good results [447,448]. Other approaches to the functional integration of IR with AFM include the innovative exploitation of the photothermal effect with the AFM tip acting as an acousto-optic sensor [449,450]. This intriguing design has enabled submicron scale mapping of both topography and vibrational spectra of polymer domains and viruses and bacteria, portending its broader application in biophysical research. The integration of AFM with ATR-IR has also shown particular promise for tracking crystal growth, electrochemical phenomena as well as phase transitions and protein insertion in lipid bilayers [451–454]. It is critical to note that there is a clear difference in these coupled approaches. The tip-based scattering approaches and, to a lesser extent the photothermal technique, while providing spatial resolution that is on the order of the size of the tip, are inherently linked to the tip–sample interaction, the raster-scanning motion of the tip and the tunability of the IR excitation beam. This latter represents a particular challenge in that obtaining spectral information over a range of wavelengths would require either multiple tip scans, each at a different excitation wavelength, or modulation of the excitation wavelength while the tip is positioned at a specific location. Both of these are time-consuming strategies. These approaches may also not be particularly well suited for examining samples in solution where scattering effects may be difficult to reconcile. The integration of AFM with conventional ATR-IR provides for a completely decoupled approach with the AFM providing topographical insights while the ATR-IR system runs independently. Although this affords full access to all the spectral scanning capabilities of the IR system, it does sacrifice direct correlation of spectral details to a specific topographic feature. This is largely a consequence of the large, micron-sized, sampling region afforded the ATR configuration, especially in a multi-bounce configuration.

It is evident that the creative approaches to both the application of SPM for biology and to address its key challenges as a tool and technique will continue to provide biologists and biophysicist with unique new perspectives on long-standing research questions. This chapter has hopefully provided the reader with some interesting new perspectives on where this technique has been, and where it is headed. We see these new innovations in integrated single molecule correlated functional imaging as enabling tools and clear evidence of the continued evolution of the SPM field and its application to the study of biomolecular interactions.

References

1. Hsu, T. H., Liao, W. Y., Yang, P. C., Wang, C. C., Xiao, J. L., and Lee, C. H. 2007. Dynamics of cancer cell filopodia characterized by super-resolution bright-field optical microscopy, *Opt Express 15*, 76–82.
2. Huang, B., Wang, W., Bates, M., and Zhuang, X. 2008. Three-dimensional super-resolution imaging by stochastic optical reconstruction microscopy, *Science 319*, 810–813.
3. Egner, A., Jakobs, S., and Hell, S. W. 2002. Fast 100-nm resolution three-dimensional microscope reveals structural plasticity of mitochondria in live yeast, *Proc Natl Acad Sci USA 99*, 3370–3375.
4. Shroff, H., White, H., and Betzig, E. 2008. Photoactivated localization microscopy (palm) of adhesion complexes, *Curr Protoc Cell Biol Chapter 4*, Unit 4 21.
5. Shroff, H., Galbraith, C. G., Galbraith, J. A., and Betzig, E. 2008. Live-cell photoactivated localization microscopy of nanoscale adhesion dynamics, *Nat Methods 5*, 417–423.
6. Manley, S., Gillette, J. M., Patterson, G. H., Shroff, H., Hess, H. F., Betzig, E., and Lippincott-Schwartz, J. 2008. High-density mapping of single-molecule trajectories with photoactivated localization microscopy, *Nat Methods 5*, 155–157.
7. de Jonge, N., Peckys, D. B., Kremers, G. J., and Piston, D. W. 2009. Electron microscopy of whole cells in liquid with nanometer resolution, *Proc Natl Acad Sci USA 106*, 2159–2164.
8. Hansma, P. K., Elings, V., Marti, O., and Bracker, C. E. 1988. Scanning tunneling microscopy and atomic force microscopy: Application to biology and technology, *Science 242*, 209–216.
9. Lillehei, P. T., and Bottomley, L. A. 2000. Scanning probe microscopy, *Anal Chem 72*, 189R–196R.
10. Poggi, M. A., Bottomley, L. A., and Lillehei, P. T. 2002. Scanning probe microscopy, *Anal Chem 74*, 2851–2862.
11. Poggi, M. A., Gadsby, E. D., Bottomley, L. A., King, W. P., Oroudjev, E., and Hansma, H. 2004. Scanning probe microscopy, *Anal Chem 76*, 3429–3444.
12. Engel, A., and Muller, D. J. 2000. Observing single biomolecules at work with the atomic force microscope, *Nat Struct Biol 7*, 715–718.
13. Francis, L. W., Lewis, P. D., Wright, C. J., and Conlan, R. S. 2010. Atomic force microscopy comes of age, *Biol Cell 102*, 133–143.
14. Ikai, A. 2010. A review on: Atomic force microscopy applied to nano-mechanics of the cell, *Adv Biochem Eng Biotechnol 119*, 47–61.
15. Goksu, E. I., Vanegas, J. M., Blanchette, C. D., Lin, W. C., and Longo, M. L. 2009. AFM for structure and dynamics of biomembranes, *Biochim Biophys Acta 1788*, 254–266.

16. Frederix, P. L., Bosshart, P. D., and Engel, A. 2009. Atomic force microscopy of biological membranes, *Biophys J 96*, 329–338.
17. Muller, D. J. 2008. AFM: A nanotool in membrane biology, *Biochemistry 47*, 7986–7998.
18. Lamontagne, C. A., Cuerrier, C. M., and Grandbois, M. 2008. AFM as a tool to probe and manipulate cellular processes, *Pflugers Arch 456*, 61–70.
19. Dufrene, Y. F. 2008. Towards nanomicrobiology using atomic force microscopy, *Nat Rev Microbiol 6*, 674–680.
20. Hinterdorfer, P., and Dufrene, Y. F. 2006. Detection and localization of single molecular recognition events using atomic force microscopy, *Nat Methods 3*, 347–355.
21. Moller, C., Allen, M., Elings, V., Engel, A., and Muller, D. J. 1999. Tapping-mode atomic force microscopy produces faithful high-resolution images of protein surfaces, *Biophys J 77*, 1150–1158.
22. Florin, E. L., Moy, V. T., and Gaub, H. E. 1994. Adhesion forces between individual ligand–receptor pairs, *Science 264*, 415–417.
23. Heinz, W. F., and Hoh, J. H. 1999. Spatially resolved force spectroscopy of biological surfaces using the atomic force microscope, *Trends Biotechnol 17*, 143–150.
24. Rief, M., Oesterhelt, F., Heymann, B., and Gaub, H. E. 1997. Single molecule force spectroscopy on polysaccharides by atomic force microscopy, *Science 275*, 1295–1297.
25. Oesterfelt, F., Rief, M., and Gaub, H. E. 1999. Single molecule force spectroscopy by AFM indicates hleical structure of poly(ethylene-glycol) in water, *New J Phys 1*, 6.1–6.11.
26. Walch, M., Ziegler, U., and Groscurth, P. 2000. Effect of streptolysin o on the microelasticity of human platelets analyzed by atomic force microscopy, *Ultramicroscopy 82*, 259–267.
27. A-Hassan, E., Heinz, W. F., Antonik, M., D'Costa, N. P., Nageswaran, S., Schoenenberger, C.-A., and Hoh, J. H. 1998. Relative microelastic mapping of living cells by atomic force microscopy, *Biophys J 74*, 1564–1578.
28. Brown, H. G., and Hoh, J. H. 1997. Entropic exclusion by neurofilament sidearms: A mechanism for maintaining interfilament spacing, *Biochemistry 36*, 15035–15040.
29. Sahin, O., Magonov, S., Su, C., Quate, C. F., and Solgaard, O. 2007. An atomic force microscope tip designed to measure time-varying nanomechanical forces, *Nat Nanotechnol 2*, 507–514.
30. Pelling, A. E., Sehati, S., Gralla, E. B., Valentine, J. S., and Gimzewski, J. K. 2004. Local nanomechanical motion of the cell wall of saccharomyces cerevisiae, *Science 305*, 1147–1150.
31. Young, R., Ward, J., and Scire, F. 1971. The topografiner: An instrument for measuring surface microtopography, *Rev Sci Instr 43*, 999.
32. Binnig, G., Rohrer, H., Gerber, C., and Weibel, E. 1982. Tunneling through a controllable vacuum gap, *Rev Mod Phys 59*, 178–180.
33. Binnig, G., Quate, C. F., and Gerber, C. 1986. Atomic force microscope, *Phys Rev Lett 56*, 930–933.
34. Magonov, S. N., and Reneker, D. H. 1997. Characterization of polymer surfaces with atomic force microscopy, *Ann Rev Mater Sci 27*, 175–222.
35. Paige, M. F. 2003. A comparison of atomic force microscope friction and phase imaging for the characterization of an immiscible polystyrene/poly(methyl methacrylate) blend film, *Polymer 44*, 6345–6352.
36. Dinte, B. P., Watson, G. S., Dobson, J. F., and Myhra, S. 1996. Artefacts in non-contact mode force microscopy: The role of adsorbed moisture, *Ultramicroscopy 63*, 115–124.
37. Lvov, Y., Onda, M., Ariga, K., and Kunitake, T. 1998. Ultrathin films of charged polysaccharides assembled alternately with linear polyions, *J Biomater Sci Polym Ed 9*, 345–355.
38. Magonov, S. N., Elings, V., and Whangbo, M.-H. 1997. Phase imaging and stiffness in tapping mode AFM, *Surface Sci 375*, L385–L391.
39. Magonov, S. and Heaton, M. G. 1998. Atomic force microscopy, part 6: Recent developments in AFM of polymers, *Am Lab 30*(10), 9.
40. Magonov, S. and Godovsky, Y. 1999. Atomic force microscopy, part 8: Visualization of granular nanostructure in crystalline polymers, *Am Lab April 1999*, 52–58.

41. Hansma, H. G., Kim, K. J., Laney, D. E., Garcia, R. A., Argaman, M., Allen, M. J., and Parsons, S. M. 1997. Properties of biomolecules measured from atomic force microscope images: A review, *J Struct Biol 119*, 99–108.

42. Fritzsche, W. and Henderson, E. 1997. Mapping elasticity of rehydrated metaphase chromosomes by scanning force microscopy, *Ultramicroscopy 69*, 191–200.

43. Noy, A., Sanders, C. H., Vezenov, D. V., Wong, S. S., and Lieber, C. M. 1998. Chemically-sensitive imaging in tapping mode by chemical force microscopy: Relationship between phase lag and adhesion, *Langmuir 14*, 1508–1511.

44. Nagao, E. and Dvorak, J. A. 1999. Phase imaging by atomic force microscopy: Analysis of living homoiothermic vertebrate cells, *Biophys J 76*, 3289–3297.

45. Holland, N. B. and Marchant, R. E. 2000. Individual plasma proteins detected on rough biomaterials by phase imaging AFM, *J Biomed Mater Res 51*, 307–315.

46. Czajkowsky, D. M., Allen, M. J., Elings, V., and Shao, Z. 1998. Direct visualization of surface charge in aqueous solution, *Ultramicroscopy 74*, 1–5.

47. Brandsch, R., Bar, G., and Whangbo, M.-H. 1997. On the factors affecting the contrast of height and phase images in tapping mode atomic force microscopy, *Langmuir 13*, 6349–6353.

48. Winkler, R. G., Spatz, J. P., Sheiko, S., Moller, M., Reineker, P., and Marti, O. 1996. Imaging material properties by resonant tapping-force microscopy: A model investigation, *Phys Rev B 54*, 8908–8912.

49. Opdahl, A., Hoffer, S., Mailhot, B., and Somorjai, G. A. 2001. Polymer surface science, *Chem Rec 1*, 101–122.

50. Scott, W. W. and Bhushan, B. 2003. Use of phase imaging in atomic force microscopy for measurement of viscoelastic contrast in polymer nanocomposites and molecularly thick lubricant films, *Ultramicroscopy 97*, 151–169.

51. Krol, S., Ross, M., Sieber, M., Kunneke, S., Galla, H. J., and Janshoff, A. 2000. Formation of three-dimensional protein-lipid aggregates in monolayer films induced by surfactant protein b, *Biophys J 79*, 904–918.

52. Deleu, M., Nott, K., Brasseur, R., Jacques, P., Thonart, P., and Dufrene, Y. F. 2001. Imaging mixed lipid monolayers by dynamic atomic force microscopy, *Biochim Biophys Acta 1513*, 55–62.

53. Argaman, M., Golan, R., Thomson, N. H., and Hansma, H. G. 1997. Phase imaging of moving DNA molecules and DNA molecules replicated in the atomic force microscope, *Nucleic Acids Res 25*, 4379–4384.

54. Sitterberg, J., Ozcetin, A., Ehrhardt, C., and Bakowsky, U. 2010. Utilising atomic force microscopy for the characterisation of nanoscale drug delivery systems, *Eur J Pharm Biopharm 74*, 2–13.

55. Han, W., Lindsay, S. M., and Jing, T. 1996. A magnetically driven oscillating probe microscope for operation in liquids, *Appl Phys Lett 69*, 4111–4113.

56. Florin, E.-L., Radmacher, M., Fleck, B., and Gaub, H. E. 1994. Atomic force microscope with magnetic force modulation, *Rev Sci Instrum 65*, 639–643.

57. Lindsay, S. M., Lyubchenko Yu, L., Tao, N. J., Li, Y. Q., Oden, P. I., Derose, J. A., and Pan, J. 1993. Scanning tunneling microscopy and atomic force microscopy studies of biomaterials at a liquid-solid interface, *J Vac Sci Technol A 11*, 808–815.

58. Lillehei, P. T. and Bottomley, L. A. 2001. Scanning force microscopy of nucleic acid complexes, *Methods Enzymol 340*, 234–251.

59. Conway, K. A., Harper, J. D., and Lansbury, P. T., Jr. 2000. Fibrils formed *in vitro* from alpha-synuclein and two mutant forms linked to Parkinson's disease are typical amyloid, *Biochemistry 39*, 2552–2563.

60. Oesterhelt, F., Oesterhelt, D., Pfeiffer, M., Engel, A., Gaub, H. E., and Muller, D. J. 2000. Unfolding pathways of individual bacteriorhodopsins, *Science 288*, 143–146.

61. Rochet, J. C., Conway, K. A., and Lansbury, P. T., Jr. 2000. Inhibition of fibrillization and accumulation of prefibrillar oligomers in mixtures of human and mouse alpha-synuclein, *Biochemistry 39*, 10619–10626.

62. Moradian-Oldak, J., Paine, M. L., Lei, Y. P., Fincham, A. G., and Snead, M. L. 2000. Self-assembly properties of recombinant engineered amelogenin proteins analyzed by dynamic light scattering and atomic force microscopy, *J Struct Biol 131*, 27–37.

63. Trottier, M., Mat-Arip, Y., Zhang, C., Chen, C., Sheng, S., Shao, Z., and Guo, P. 2000. Probing the structure of monomers and dimers of the bacterial virus phi29 hexamer RNA complex by chemical modification, *RNA 6*, 1257–1266.

64. Thompson, J. B., Paloczi, G. T., Kindt, J. H., Michenfelder, M., Smith, B. L., Stucky, G., Morse, D. E., and Hansma, P. K. 2000. Direct observation of the transition from calcite to aragonite growth as induced by abalone shell proteins, *Biophys J 79*, 3307–3312.

65. Rivetti, C., Vannini, N., and Cellai, S. 2003. Imaging transcription complexes with the atomic force microscope, *Ital J Biochem 52*, 98–103.

66. Seong, G. H., Yanagida, Y., Aizawa, M., and Kobatake, E. 2002. Atomic force microscopy identification of transcription factor NFkappab bound to streptavidin-pin-holding DNA probe, *Anal Biochem 309*, 241–247.

67. Mukherjee, S., Brieba, L. G., and Sousa, R. 2002. Structural transitions mediating transcription initiation by T7 RNA polymerase, *Cell 110*, 81–91.

68. Hun Seong, G., Kobatake, E., Miura, K., Nakazawa, A., and Aizawa, M. 2002. Direct atomic force microscopy visualization of integration host factor- induced DNA bending structure of the promoter regulatory region on the Pseudomonas tol plasmid, *Biochem. Biophys. Res. Commun. 291*, 361–366.

69. Tahirov, T. H., Sato, K., Ichikawa-Iwata, E., Sasaki, M., Inoue-Bungo, T., Shiina, M., Kimura, K. et al. 2002. Mechanism of c-myb-c/ebp beta cooperation from separated sites on a promoter, *Cell 108*, 57–70.

70. Neaves, K. J., Huppert, J. L., Henderson, R. M., and Edwardson, J. M. 2009. Direct visualization of g-quadruplexes in DNA using atomic force microscopy, *Nucleic Acids Res 37*, 6269–6275.

71. Limanskaya, O. Y., and Limanskii, A. P. 2008. Imaging compaction of single supercoiled DNA molecules by atomic force microscopy, *Gen Physiol Biophys 27*, 322–337.

72. Lohr, D., Bash, R., Wang, H., Yodh, J., and Lindsay, S. 2007. Using atomic force microscopy to study chromatin structure and nucleosome remodeling, *Methods 41*, 333–341.

73. Sorel, I., Pietrement, O., Hamon, L., Baconnais, S., Cam, E. L., and Pastre, D. 2006. The Ecori-DNA complex as a model for investigating protein-DNA interactions by atomic force microscopy, *Biochemistry 45*, 14675–14682.

74. Jena, B. P. 2002. Fusion pore in live cells, *News Physiol Sci 17*, 219–222.

75. Cho, S. J., Quinn, A. S., Stromer, M. H., Dash, S., Cho, J., Taatjes, D. J., and Jena, B. P. 2002. Structure and dynamics of the fusion pore in live cells, *Cell Biol Int 26*, 35–42.

76. Ma, H., Snook, L. A., Tian, C., Kaminskyj, S. G. W., and Dahms, T. E. S. 2006. Fungal surface remodelling visualized by atomic force microscopy, *Mycol Res 110*, 879–886.

77. Rogers, B., Manning, L., Sulchek, T., and Adams, J. D. 2004. Improving tapping mode atomic force microscopy with piezoelectric cantilevers, *Ultramicroscopy 100*, 267–276.

78. Fantner, G. E., Schitter, G., Kindt, J. H., Ivanov, T., Ivanova, K., Patel, R., Holten-Andersen, N. et al. 2006. Components for high speed atomic force microscopy, *Ultramicroscopy 106*, 881–887.

79. Petsev, D. N., Thomas, B. R., Yau, S., and Vekilov, P. G. 2000. Interactions and aggregation of apoferritin molecules in solution: Effects of added electrolytes, *Biophys J 78*, 2060–2069.

80. Viani, M. B., Pietrasanta, L. I., Thompson, J. B., Chand, A., Gebeshuber, I. C., Kindt, J. H., Richter, M., Hansma, H. G., and Hansma, P. K. 2000. Probing protein–protein interactions in real time, *Nat Struct Biol 7*, 644–647.

81. Casuso, I., Kodera, N., Le Grimellec, C., Ando, T., and Scheuring, S. 2009. Contact-mode high-resolution high-speed atomic force microscopy movies of the purple membrane, *Biophys J 97*, 1354–1361.

82. Miyagi, A., Tsunaka, Y., Uchihashi, T., Mayanagi, K., Hirose, S., Morikawa, K., and Ando, T. 2008. Visualization of intrinsically disordered regions of proteins by high-speed atomic force microscopy, *ChemPhysChem 9*, 1859–1866.

83. Ando, T., Uchihashi, T., Kodera, N., Yamamoto, D., Miyagi, A., Taniguchi, M., and Yamashita, H. 2008. High-speed AFM and nano-visualization of biomolecular processes, *Pflugers Arch 456*, 211–225.

84. Ando, T., Kodera, N., Naito, Y., Kinoshita, T., Furuta, K., and Toyoshima, Y. Y. 2003. A high-speed atomic force microscope for studying biological macromolecules in action, *ChemPhysChem 4*, 1196–1202.

85. Fantner, G. E., Barbero, R. J., Gray, D. S., and Belcher, A. M. 2010. Kinetics of antimicrobial peptide activity measured on individual bacterial cells using high-speed atomic force microscopy, *Nat Nanotechnol 5*, 280–285.

86. Archibald, R., Datskos, P., Devault, G., Lamberti, V., Lavrik, N., Noid, D., Sepaniak, M., and Dutta, P. 2007. Independent component analysis of nanomechanical responses of cantilever arrays, *Anal Chim Acta 584*, 101–105.

87. Loui, A., Ratto, T. V., Wilson, T. S., McCall, S. K., Mukerjee, E. V., Love, A. H., and Hart, B. R. 2008. Chemical vapor discrimination using a compact and low-power array of piezoresistive microcantilevers, *Analyst 133*, 608–615.

88. Kim, S., Rahman, T., Senesac, L. R., Davison, B. H., and Thundat, T. 2009. Piezoresistive cantilever array sensor for consolidated bioprocess monitoring, *Scanning 31*, 204–210.

89. Kelling, S., Paoloni, F., Huang, J., Ostanin, V. P., and Elliott, S. R. 2009. Simultaneous readout of multiple microcantilever arrays with phase-shifting interferometric microscopy, *Rev Sci Instrum 80*, 093101.

90. Ward, M. D. 2001. Bulk crystals to surfaces: Combining x-ray diffraction and atomic force microscopy to probe the structure and formation of crystal interfaces, *Chem Rev 2001*, 1697–1725.

91. Manne, S., Cleveland, J. P., Stucky, G. D., and Hansma, P. K. 1993. Lattice resolution and solution kinetics on surfaces of amino acid crystals: An atomic force microscope study, *J. Crystal Growth 130*, 333–340.

92. Agger, J. R., Hanif, N., Cundy, C. S., Wade, A. P., Dennison, S., Rawlinson, P. A., and Anderson, M. W. 2003. Silicalite crystal growth investigated by atomic force microscopy, *J Am Chem Soc 125*, 830–839.

93. Teng, H. H., Dove, P. M., Orme, C. A., and De Yoreo, J. J. 1998. Thermodynamics of calcite growth: Baseline for understanding biomineral formation, *Science 282*, 724–727.

94. Costa, N. and Maquis, P. M. 1998. Biomimetic processing of calcium phosphate coating, *Med Eng Phys 20*, 602–606.

95. Wen, H. B., Moradian-Oldak, J., Zhong, J. P., Greenspan, D. C., and Fincham, A. G. 2000. Effects of amelogenin on the transforming surface microstructures of bioglass in a calcifying solution, *J Biomed Mater Res 52*, 762–773.

96. Durbin, S. D. and Feher, G. 1996. Protein crystallization, *Annu Rev Phys Chem 47*, 171–204.

97. Yip, C. M., Brader, M. L., Frank, B. H., DeFelippis, M. R., and Ward, M. D. 2000. Structural studies of a crystalline insulin analog complex with protamine by atomic force microscopy, *Biophys J 78*, 466–473.

98. Kuznetsov, Y. G., Malkin, A. J., Lucas, R. W., and McPherson, A. 2000. Atomic force microscopy studies of icosahedral virus crystal growth, *Colloids Surf B Biointerfaces 19*, 333–346.

99. Plomp, M., McPherson, A., and Malkin, A. J. 2003. Repair of impurity-poisoned protein crystal surfaces, *Proteins 50*, 486–495.

100. McPherson, A., Malkin, A. J., and Kuznetsov Yu, G. 2000. Atomic force microscopy in the study of macromolecular crystal growth, *Annu Rev Biophys Biomol Struct 29*, 361–410.

101. Vekilov, P. G. 2005. Kinetics and mechanisms of protein crystallization at the molecular level, *Methods Mol Biol 300*, 15–52.

102. Barrera, N. P., Ormond, S. J., Henderson, R. M., Murrell-Lagnado, R. D., and Edwardson, J. M. 2005. Atomic force microscopy imaging demonstrates that p2x[2] receptors are trimers but that p2x[6] receptor subunits do not oligomerize, *J Biol Chem 280*, 10759–10765.

103. Yau, S., Thomas, B. R., and Vekilov, P. G. 2000. Molecular mechanisms of crystallization and defect formation, *Phys Rev Lett 85*, 353–356.

104. Guo, S. and Akhremitchev, B. B. 2008. Investigation of mechanical properties of insulin crystals by atomic force microscopy, *Langmuir 24*, 880–887.

105. Larson, S. B., Kuznetsov, Y. G., Day, J., Zhou, J., Glaser, S., Braslawsky, G., and McPherson, A. 2005. Combined use of AFM and x-ray diffraction to analyze crystals of an engineered, domain-deleted antibody, *Acta Crystallogr D Biol Crystallogr 61*, 416–422.

106. Ko, T. P., Kuznetsov, Y. G., Malkin, A. J., Day, J., and McPherson, A. 2001. X-ray diffraction and atomic force microscopy analysis of twinned crystals: Rhombohedral canavalin, *Acta Crystallogr D Biol Crystallogr 57*, 829–839.

107. Yip, C. M., DeFelippis, M. R., Frank, B. H., Brader, M. L., and Ward, M. D. 1998. Structural and morphological characterization of ultralente insulin crystals by atomic force microscopy: Evidence of hydrophobically driven assembly, *Biophys J 75*, 1172–1179.

108. Malkin, A. J., Plomp, M., and McPherson, A. 2002. Application of atomic force microscopy to studies of surface processes in virus crystallization and structural biology, *Acta Crystallogr D Biol Crystallogr 58*, 1617–1621.

109. Plomp, M., Rice, M. K., Wagner, E. K., McPherson, A., and Malkin, A. J. 2002. Rapid visualization at high resolution of pathogens by atomic force microscopy: Structural studies of Herpes Simplex Virus-1, *Am J Pathol 160*, 1959–1966.

110. McPherson, A., Malkin, A. J., Kuznetsov, Y. G., and Plomp, M. 2001. Atomic force microscopy applications in macromolecular crystallography, *Acta Crystallogr D Biol Crystallogr 57*, 1053–1060.

111. Kuznetsov, Y. G., Larson, S. B., Day, J., Greenwood, A., and McPherson, A. 2001. Structural transitions of satellite tobacco mosaic virus particles, *Virology 284*, 223–234.

112. Kuznetsov, Y. G., Malkin, A. J., Lucas, R. W., Plomp, M., and McPherson, A. 2001. Imaging of viruses by atomic force microscopy, *J Gen Virol 82*, 2025–2034.

113. Lucas, R. W., Kuznetsov, Y. G., Larson, S. B., and McPherson, A. 2001. Crystallization of brome mosaic virus and t = 1 brome mosaic virus particles following a structural transition, *Virology 286*, 290–303.

114. Day, J., Kuznetsov, Y. G., Larson, S. B., Greenwood, A., and McPherson, A. 2001. Biophysical studies on the RNA cores of satellite tobacco mosaic virus, *Biophys J 80*, 2364–2371.

115. Kuznetsov, Y. G., Malkin, A. J., and McPherson, A. 2001. Self-repair of biological fibers catalyzed by the surface of a virus crystal, *Proteins 44*, 392–396.

116. Yau, S. T., Thomas, B. R., Galkin, O., Gliko, O., and Vekilov, P. G. 2001. Molecular mechanisms of microheterogeneity-induced defect formation in ferritin crystallization, *Proteins 43*, 343–352.

117. Yau, S. T. and Vekilov, P. G. 2000. Quasi-planar nucleus structure in apoferritin crystallization, *Nature 406*, 494–497.

118. Chen, K. and Vekilov, P. G. 2002. Evidence for the surface-diffusion mechanism of solution crystallization from molecular-level observations with ferritin, *Phys Rev E Stat Nonlin Soft Matter Phys 66*, 021606.

119. Danesh, A., Connell, S. D., Davies, M. C., Roberts, C. J., Tendler, S. J., Williams, P. M., and Wilkins, M. J. 2001. An *in situ* dissolution study of aspirin crystal planes [100] and [001] by atomic force microscopy, *Pharm Res 18*, 299–303.

120. Danesh, A., Chen, X., Davies, M. C., Roberts, C. J., Sanders, G. H., Tendler, S. J., Williams, P. M., and Wilkins, M. J. 2000. The discrimination of drug polymorphic forms from single crystals using atomic force microscopy, *Pharm Res 17*, 887–890.

121. Danesh, A., Chen, X., Davies, M. C., Roberts, C. J., Sanders, G. H. W., Tendler, S. J. B., and Williams, P. M. 2000. Polymorphic discrimination using atomic force microscopy: Distinguishing between two polymorphs of the drug cimetidine, *Langmuir 16*, 866–870.

122. Guo, S., Ward, M. D., and Wesson, J. A. 2002. Direct visualization of calcium oxalate monohydrate crystallization and dissolution with atomic force microscopy and the role of polymeric additives, *Langmuir 18*, 4282–4291.

123. Frincu, M. C., Fleming, S. D., Rohl, A. L., and Swift, J. A. 2004. The epitaxial growth of cholesterol crystals from bile solutions on calcite substrates, *J Am Chem Soc 126*, 7915–7924.

124. Wang, L. and Nancollas, G. H. 2009. Pathways to biomineralization and biodemineralization of calcium phosphates: The thermodynamic and kinetic controls, *Dalton Trans*, 2665–2672.

125. Wesson, J. A. and Ward, M. D. 2006. Role of crystal surface adhesion in kidney stone disease, *Curr Opin Nephrol Hypertens 15*, 386–393.

126. Sheng, X., Jung, T., Wesson, J. A., and Ward, M. D. 2005. Adhesion at calcium oxalate crystal surfaces and the effect of urinary constituents, *Proc Natl Acad Sci USA 102*, 267–272.

127. Sheng, X., Ward, M. D., and Wesson, J. A. 2005. Crystal surface adhesion explains the pathological activity of calcium oxalate hydrates in kidney stone formation, *J Am Soc Nephrol 16*, 1904–1908.

128. Wang, L., Qiu, S. R., Zachowicz, W., Guan, X., Deyoreo, J. J., Nancollas, G. H., and Hoyer, J. R. 2006. Modulation of calcium oxalate crystallization by linear aspartic acid-rich peptides, *Langmuir 22*, 7279–7285.

129. Milhiet, P. E., Gubellini, F., Berquand, A., Dosset, P., Rigaud, J. L., Le Grimellec, C., and Levy, D. 2006. High-resolution AFM of membrane proteins directly incorporated at high density in planar lipid bilayer, *Biophys J 91*, 3268–3275.

130. Mo, G. C. H. and Yip, C. M. 2009. Supported lipid bilayer templated J-aggregate growth: Role of stabilizing cation-pi interactions and headgroup packing, *Langmuir 25*, 10719–10729.

131. Waugh, D. F., Thompson, R. E., and Weimer, R. J. 1950. Assay of insulin *in vitro* by fibril elongation and precipitation, *J Biol Chem 185*, 85–95.

132. Foster, G. E., Macdonald, J., and Smart, J. V. 1951. The assay of insulin *in vitro* by fibril formation and precipitation, *J Pharm Pharmacol 3*, 897–904.

133. Baselt, D. R., Revel, J. P., and Baldeschwieler, J. D. 1993. Subfibrillar structure of Type I collagen observed by atomic force microscopy, *Biophys J 65*, 2644–2655.

134. Cotterill, G. F., Fergusson, J. A., Gani, J. S., and Burns, G. F. 1993. Scanning tunnelling microscopy of collagen I reveals filament bundles to be arranged in a left-handed helix, *Biochem Biophys Res Commun 194*, 973–977.

135. Gale, M., Pollanen, M. S., Markiewicz, P., and Goh, M. C. 1995. Sequential assembly of collagen revealed by atomic force microscopy, *Biophys J 68*, 2124–2128.

136. Watanabe, M., Kobayashi, M., Fujita, Y., Senga, K., Mizutani, H., Ueda, M., and Hoshino, T. 1997. Association of Type VI collagen with d-periodic collagen fibrils in developing tail tendons of mice, *Arch Histol Cytol 60*, 427–434.

137. Taatjes, D. J., Quinn, A. S., and Bovill, E. G. 1999. Imaging of collagen type III in fluid by atomic force microscopy, *Microsc Res Tech 44*, 347–352.

138. Zerovnik, E., Skarabot, M., Skerget, K., Giannini, S., Stoka, V., Jenko-Kokalj, S., and Staniforth, R. A. 2007. Amyloid fibril formation by human stefin b: Influence of pH and TFE on fibril growth and morphology, *Amyloid-J Protein Folding Disord 14*, 237–247.

139. Miller, L. D., Putthanarat, S., Eby, R. K., and Adams, W. W. 1999. Investigation of the nanofibrillar morphology in silk fibers by small angle x-ray scattering and atomic force microscopy, *Int J Biol Macromol 24*, 159–165.

140. Li, S. F., McGhie, A. J., and Tang, S. L. 1994. New internal structure of spider dragline silk revealed by atomic force microscopy, *Biophys J 66*, 1209–1212.

141. Gould, S. A., Tran, K. T., Spagna, J. C., Moore, A. M., and Shulman, J. B. 1999. Short and long range order of the morphology of silk from *Latrodectus hesperus* (black widow. as characterized by atomic force microscopy, *Int J Biol Macromol 24*, 151–157.

142. Oroudjev, E., Soares, J., Arcdiacono, S., Thompson, J. B., Fossey, S. A., and Hansma, H. G. 2002. Segmented nanofibers of spider dragline silk: Atomic force microscopy and single-molecule force spectroscopy, *Proc Natl Acad Sci USA 99 Suppl 2*, 6460–6465.

143. Harper, J. D., Lieber, C. M., and Lansbury, P. T., Jr. 1997. Atomic force microscopic imaging of seeded fibril formation and fibril branching by the Alzheimer's disease amyloid-beta protein, *Chem Biol 4*, 951–959.

144. Harper, J. D., Wong, S. S., Lieber, C. M., and Lansbury, P. T. 1997. Observation of metastable Ab amyloid protofibrils by atomic force microscopy, *Chem Biol 4*, 119–125.

145. Yang, D. S., Yip, C. M., Huang, T. H., Chakrabartty, A., and Fraser, P. E. 1999. Manipulating the amyloid-beta aggregation pathway with chemical chaperones, *J Biol Chem 274*, 32970–32974.

146. Huang, T. H., Yang, D. S., Plaskos, N. P., Go, S., Yip, C. M., Fraser, P. E., and Chakrabartty, A. 2000. Structural studies of soluble oligomers of the alzheimer beta-amyloid peptide, *J Mol Biol 297*, 73–87.

147. Roher, A. E., Baudry, J., Chaney, M. O., Kuo, Y. M., Stine, W. B., and Emmerling, M. R. 2000. Oligomerizaiton and fibril asssembly of the amyloid-beta protein, *Biochim Biophys Acta 1502*, 31–43.

148. Parbhu, A., Lin, H., Thimm, J., and Lal, R. 2002. Imaging real-time aggregation of amyloid beta protein [1–42] by atomic force microscopy, *Peptides 23*, 1265–1270.

149. Yip, C. M., Darabie, A. A., and McLaurin, J. 2002. Abeta42-peptide assembly on lipid bilayers, *J Mol Biol 318*, 97–107.

150. Gorman, P. M., Yip, C. M., Fraser, P. E., and Chakrabartty, A. 2003. Alternate aggregation pathways of the Alzheimer beta-amyloid peptide: Abeta association kinetics at endosomal pH, *J Mol Biol 325*, 743–757.

151. McLaurin, J., Darabie, A. A., and Morrison, M. R. 2002. Cholesterol, a modulator of membrane-associated abeta-fibrillogenesis, *Ann N Y Acad Sci 977*, 376–383.

152. Jansen, R., Dzwolak, W., and Winter, R. 2005. Amyloidogenic self-assembly of insulin aggregates probed by high resolution atomic force microscopy, *Biophys J 88*, 1344–1353.

153. Mastrangelo, I. A., Ahmed, M., Sato, T., Liu, W., Wang, C. P., Hough, P., and Smith, S. O. 2006. High-resolution atomic force microscopy of soluble Ab 42 oligomers, *J Mol Biol 358*, 106–119.

154. Fukuma, T., Mostaert, A. S., Serpell, L. C., and Jarvis, S. P. 2008. Revealing molecular-level surface structure of amyloid fibrils in liquid by means of frequency modulation atomic force microscopy, *Nanotechnology 19*(38), 384010.

155. Friedrichs, J., Taubenberger, A., Franz, C. M., and Muller, D. J. 2007. Cellular remodelling of individual collagen fibrils visualized by time-lapse AFM, *J Mol Biol 372*, 594–607.

156. Zheng, J., Jang, H., Ma, B., and Nussinov, R. 2008. Annular structures as intermediates in fibril formation of Alzheimer Ab[17–42], *J Phys Chem B 112*, 6856–6865.

157. Marek, P., Abedini, A., Song, B. B., Kanungo, M., Johnson, M. E., Gupta, R., Zaman, W., Wong, S. S., and Raleigh, D. P. 2007. Aromatic interactions are not required for amyloid fibril formation by islet amyloid polypeptide but do influence the rate of fibril formation and fibril morphology, *Biochemistry 46*, 3255–3261.

158. Ha, C., Ryu, J., and Park, C. B. 2007. Metal ions differentially influence the aggregation and deposition of Alzheimer's beta-amyloid on a solid template, *Biochemistry 46*, 6118–6125.

159. Elliott, J. T., Woodward, J. T., Umarji, A., Mei, Y., and Tona, A. 2007. The effect of surface chemistry on the formation of thin films of native fibrillar collagen, *Biomaterials 28*, 576–585.

160. Kowalewski, T. and Holtzman, D. M. 1999. *In situ* atomic force microscopy study of Alzheimer's beta-amyloid peptide on different substrates: New insights into mechanism of beta-sheet formation, *Proc Natl Acad Sci USA 96*, 3688–3693.

161. Wang, Z., Zhou, C., Wang, C., Wan, L., Fang, X., and Bai, C. 2003. AFM and STM study of beta-amyloid aggregation on graphite, *Ultramicroscopy 97*, 73–79.

162. Yang, G., Woodhouse, K. A., and Yip, C. M. 2002. Substrate-facilitated assembly of elastin-like peptides: Studies by variable-temperature *in situ* atomic force microscopy, *J Am Chem Soc 124*, 10648–10649.

163. Sherrat, M. J., Holmes, D. F., Shuttleworth, C. A., and Kielty, C. M. 2004. Substrate-dependent morphology of supramolecular assemblies: Fibrillin and type-IV collagen microfibrils, *Biophys J 86*, 3211–3222.

164. Sackmann, E. 1996. Supported membranes: Scientific and practical applications, *Science 271*, 43–48.

165. Richter, R., Mukhopadhyay, A., and Brisson, A. 2003. Pathways of lipid vesicle deposition on solid surfaces: A combined QCM-D and AFM study, *Biophys J 85*, 3035–3047.

166. Leonenko, Z. V., Carnini, A., and Cramb, D. T. 2000. Supported planar bilayer formation by vesicle fusion: The interaction of phospholipid vesicles with surfaces and the effect of gramicidin on bilayer properties using atomic force microscopy, *Biochim Biophys Acta 1509*, 131–147.

167. Dufrene, Y. F. and Lee, G. U. 2000. Advances in the characterization of supported lipid films with the atomic force microscope, *Biochim Biophys Acta 1509*, 14–41.

168. Jass, J., Tjarnhage, T., and Puu, G. 2000. From liposomes to supported, planar bilayer structures on hydrophilic and hydrophobic surfaces: An atomic force microscopy study, *Biophys J 79*, 3153–3163.

169. Blanchette, C. D., Orme, C. A., Ratto, T. V., and Longo, M. L. 2008. Quantifying growth of symmetric and asymmetric lipid bilayer domains, *Langmuir 24*, 1219–1224.

170. Fukuma, T., Higgins, M. J., and Jarvis, S. P. 2007. Direct imaging of individual intrinsic hydration layers on lipid bilayers at Angstrom resolution, *Biophys J 92*, 3603–3609.

171. Richter, R. P. and Brisson, A. R. 2005. Following the formation of supported lipid bilayers on mica: A study combining AFM, QCM-D, and ellipsometry, *Biophys J 88*, 3422–3433.

172. McKiernan, A. E., Ratto, T. V., and Longo, M. L. 2000. Domain growth, shapes, and topology in cationic lipid bilayers on mica by fluorescence and atomic force microscopy, *Biophys J 79*, 2605–2615.

173. Rinia, H. A., Demel, R. A., van der Eerden, J. P., and de Kruijff, B. 1999. Blistering of Langmuir–Blodgett bilayers containing anionic phospholipids as observed by atomic force microscopy, *Biophys J 77*, 1683–1693.

174. Giocondi, M.-C., Vie, V., Lesniewska, E., Milhiet, P.-E., Zinke-Allmang, M., and Le Grimellec, C. 2001. Phase topology and growth of single domains in lipid bilayers, *Langmuir 17*, 1653–1659.

175. Yuan, C., Chen, A., Kolb, P., and Moy, V. T. 2000. Energy landscape of streptavidin–biotin complexes measured by atomic force microscopy, *Biochemistry 39*, 10219–10223.

176. Tokumasu, F., Jin, A. J., and Dvorak, J. A. 2002. Lipid membrane phase behaviour elucidated in real time by controlled environment atomic force microscopy, *J Electron Microsc (Tokyo) 51*, 1–9.

177. Muresan, A. S., Diamant, H., and Lee, K. Y. 2001. Effect of temperature and composition on the formation of nanoscale compartments in phospholipid membranes, *J Am Chem Soc 123*, 6951–6952.

178. Nielsen, L. K., Bjornholm, T., and Mouritsen, O. G. 2000. Fluctuations caught in the act, *Nature 404*, 352.

179. Giocondi, M. C. and Le Grimellec, C. 2004. Temperature dependence of the surface topography in dimyristoylphosphatidylcholine/distearoylphosphatidylcholine multibilayers, *Biophys J 86*, 2218–2230.

180. Leidy, C., Kaasgaard, T., Crowe, J. H., Mouritsen, O. G., and Jorgensen, K. 2002. Ripples and the formation of anisotropic lipid domains: Imaging two-component supported double bilayers by atomic force microscopy, *Biophys J 83*, 2625–2633.

181. Jensen, M. H., Morris, E. J., and Simonsen, A. C. 2007. Domain shapes, coarsening, and random patterns in ternary membranes, *Langmuir 23*, 8135–8141.

182. Rinia, H. A. and de Kruijff, B. 2001. Imaging domains in model membranes with atomic force microscopy, *FEBS Lett 504*, 194–199.

183. van Duyl, B. Y., Ganchev, D., Chupin, V., de Kruijff, B., and Killian, J. A. 2003. Sphingomyelin is much more effective than saturated phosphatidylcholine in excluding unsaturated phosphatidylcholine from domains formed with cholesterol, *FEBS Lett 547*, 101–106.

184. Lawrence, J. C., Saslowsky, D. E., Edwardson, J. M., and Henderson, R. M. 2003. Real-time analysis of the effects of cholesterol on lipid raft behavior using atomic force microscopy, *Biophys J 84*, 1827–1832.

185. Domenech, O., Sanz, F., Montero, M. T., and Hernandez-Borrell, J. 2006. Thermodynamic and structural study of the main phospholipid components comprising the mitochondrial inner membrane, *Biochim Biophys Acta-Biomembranes 1758*, 213–221.

186. Blanchette, C. D., Lin, W. C., Ratto, T. V., and Longo, M. L. 2006. Galactosylceramide domain microstructure: Impact of cholesterol and nucleation/growth conditions, *Biophys J 90*, 4466–4478.

187. Kobayashi, T., Startchev, K., Whitney, A. J., and Gruenberg, J. 2001. Localization of lysobisphosphatidic acid-rich membrane domains in late endosomes, *Biol Chem 382*, 483–485.

188. Hayakawa, T., Makino, A., Murate, M., Sugimoto, I., Hashimoto, Y., Takahashi, H., Ito, K., Fujisawa, T., Matsuo, H., and Kobayashi, T. 2007. pH-dependent formation of membranous cytoplasmic body-like structure of ganglioside G(m1)/bis(monoacylglycero)phosphate mixed membranes, *Biophys J 92*, L13–L15.

189. Frederick, T. E., Chebukati, J. N., Mair, C. E., Goff, P. C., and Fanucci, G. E. 2009. Bis(monoacylglycero) phosphate forms stable small lamellar vesicle structures: Insights into vesicular body formation in endosomes, *Biophys J 96*, 1847–1855.

190. Mecke, A., Lee, D. K., Ramamoorthy, A., Orr, B. G., and Banaszak Holl, M. M. 2005. Membrane thinning due to antimicrobial peptide binding: An atomic force microscopy study of MSI-78 in lipid bilayers, *Biophys J 89*, 4043–4050.

191. Erickson, B., DiMaggio, S. C., Mullen, D. G., Kelly, C. V., Leroueil, P. R., Berry, S. A., Baker, J. R., Orr, B. G., and Holl, M. M. B. 2008. Interactions of poly(amidoamine) dendrimers with Survanta lung surfactant: The importance of lipid domains, *Langmuir 24*, 11003–11008.

192. Lorite, G. S., Nobre, T. M., Zaniquelli, M. E. D., de Paula, E., and Cotta, M. A. 2009. Dibucaine effects on structural and elastic properties of lipid bilayers, *Biophys Chem 139*, 75–83.

193. Leonenko, Z., Finot, E., and Cramb, D. 2006. AFM study of interaction forces in supported planar DPPC bilayers in the presence of general anesthetic halothane, *Biochim Biophys Acta-Biomembranes 1758*, 487–492.

194. Yuan, C. and Johnston, L. J. 2001. Atomic force microscopy studies of ganglioside GM1 domains in phosphatidylcholine and phosphatidylcholine/cholesterol bilayers, *Biophys J 81*, 1059–1069.

195. Fotiadis, D., Jeno, P., Mini, T., Wirtz, S., Muller, S. A., Fraysse, L., Kjellbom, P., and Engel, A. 2001. Structural characterization of two aquaporins isolated from native spinach leaf plasma membranes, *J Biol Chem 276*, 1707–1714.

196. Puu, G., Artursson, E., Gustafson, I., Lundstrom, M., and Jass, J. 2000. Distribution and stability of membrane proteins in lipid membranes on solid supports, *Biosens Bioelectron 15*, 31–41.

197. Puu, G., Gustafson, I., Artursson, E., and Ohlsson, P. A. 1995. Retained activities of some membrane proteins in stable lipid bilayers on a solid support, *Biosens Bioelectron 10*, 463–476.

198. Rinia, H. A., Kik, R. A., Demel, R. A., Snel, M. M. E., Killian, J. A., van Der Eerden, J. P. J. M., and de Kruijff, B. 2000. Visualization of highly ordered striated domains induced by transmembrane peptides in supported phosphatidylcholine bilayers, *Biochemistry 39*, 5852–5858.

199. Bayburt, T. H., Carlson, J. W., and Sligar, S. G. 1998. Reconstitution and imaging of a membrane protein in a nanometer-size phospholipid bilayer, *J Struct Biol 123*, 37–44.

200. Neff, D., Tripathi, S., Middendorf, K., Stahlberg, H., Butt, H. J., Bamberg, E., and Dencher, N. A. 1997. Chloroplast f0f1 atp synthase imaged by atomic force microscopy, *J Struct Biol 119*, 139–148.

201. Takeyasu, K., Omote, H., Nettikadan, S., Tokumasu, F., Iwamoto-Kihara, A., and Futai, M. 1996. Molecular imaging of *Escherichia coli* F0F1-ATPase in reconstituted membranes using atomic force microscopy, *FEBS Lett 392*, 110–113.

202. Lal, R., Kim, H., Garavito, R. M., and Arnsdorf, M. F. 1993. Imaging of reconstituted biological channels at molecular resolution by atomic force microscopy, *Am J Physiol 265*, C851–856.

203. Slade, A., Luh, J., Ho, S., and Yip, C. M. 2002. Single molecule imaging of supported planar lipid bilayer—Reconstituted human insulin receptors by *in situ* scanning probe microscopy, *J Struct Biol 137*, 283–291.

204. Puu, G. and Gustafson, I. 1997. Planar lipid bilayers on solid supports from liposomes—Factors of importance for kinetics and stability, *Biochim Biophys Acta 1327*, 149–161.

205. Reviakine, I. and Brisson, A. 2000. Formation of supported phospholipid bilayers from unilamellar vesicles investigated by atomic force microscopy, *Langmuir 16*, 1806–1815.

206. Radler, J., Strey, H., and Sackmann, E. 1995. Phenomenology and kinetics of lipid bilayer spreading on hydrophilic surfaces, *Langmuir 11*, 4539–4548.

207. Santos, N. C., Ter-Ovanesyan, E., Zasadzinski, J. A., Prieto, M., and Castanho, M. A. 1998. Filipin-induced lesions in planar phospholipid bilayers imaged by atomic force microscopy, *Biophys J 75*, 1869–1873.

208. Milhaud, J., Ponsinet, V., Takashi, M., and Michels, B. 2002. Interactions of the drug amphotericin b with phospholipid membranes containing or not ergosterol: New insight into the role of ergosterol, *Biochim Biophys Acta 1558*, 95–108.

209. Steinem, C., Galla, H.-J., and Janshoff, A. 2000. Interaction of melittin with solid supported membranes, *Phys Chem Chem Phys 2*, 4580–4585.

210. Green, J. D., Kreplak, L., Goldsbury, C., Blatter, X. L., Stolz, M., Cooper, G. S., Seelig, A., Kist-Ler, J., and Aebi, U. 2004. Atomic force microscopy reveals defects within mica supported lipid bilayers induced by the amyloidogenic human amylin peptide, *J Mol Biol 342*, 877–887.

211. Janshoff, A., Bong, D. T., Steinem, C., Johnson, J. E., and Ghadiri, M. R. 1999. An animal virus-derived peptide switches membrane morphology: Possible relevance to nodaviral transfection processes, *Biochemistry 38*, 5328–5336.

212. Shaw, J. E., Epand, R. F., Hsu, J. C., Mo, G. C., Epand, R. M., and Yip, C. M. 2008. Cationic peptide-induced remodelling of model membranes: Direct visualization by *in situ* atomic force microscopy, *J Struct Biol 162*, 121–138.

213. Oreopoulos, J., Epand, R. F., Epand, R. M., and Yip, C. M. 2010. Peptide-induced domain formation in supported lipid bilayers: Direct evidence by combined atomic force and polarized total internal reflection fluorescence microscopy, *Biophys J 98*, 815–823.

214. Shaw, J. E., Epand, R. F., Sinnathamby, K., Li, Z., Bittman, R., Epand, R. M., and Yip, C. M. 2006. Tracking peptide–membrane interactions: Insights from *in situ* coupled confocal-atomic force microscopy imaging of NAP-22 peptide insertion and assembly, *J Struct Biol 155*, 458–469.

215. Alattia, J. R., Shaw, J. E., Yip, C. M., and Prive, G. G. 2006. Direct visualization of saposin remodelling of lipid bilayers, *J Mol Biol 362*, 943–953.

216. Slade, A. L., Schoeniger, J. S., Sasaki, D. Y., and Yip, C. M. 2006. *in situ* scanning probe microscopy studies of tetanus toxin-membrane interactions, *Biophys J 91*, 4565–4574.

217. El Kirat, K., Burton, I., Dupres, V., and Dufrene, Y. F. 2005. Sample preparation procedures for biological atomic force microscopy, *J Microsc 218*, 199–207.

218. Shahin, V. and Barrera, N. P. 2008. Providing unique insight into cell biology via atomic force microscopy, *Int Rev Cytol 265*, 227–252.

219. Li, A., Lee, P. Y., Ho, B., Ding, J. L., and Lim, C. T. 2007. Atomic force microscopy study of the antimicrobial action of sushi peptides on Gram negative bacteria, *Biochimica Biophysica Acta-Biomembranes 1768*, 411–418.

220. Jang, K. E. and Ye, J. C. 2007. Single channel blind image deconvolution from radially symmetric blur kernels, *Opt Express 15*, 3791–3803.

221. Arechaga, I. and Fotiadis, D. 2007. Reconstitution of mitochondrial ATP synthase into lipid bilayers for structural analysis, *J Struct Biol 160*, 287–294.

222. Giocondi, M. C., Seantier, B., Dosset, P., Milhiet, P. E., and Le Grimellec, C. 2008. Characterizing the interactions between GPI-anchored alkaline phosphatases and membrane domains by AFM, *Pflugers Arch 456*, 179–188.

223. Berquand, A., Levy, D., Gubellini, F., Le Grimellec, C., and Milhiet, P. E. 2007. Influence of calcium on direct incorporation of membrane proteins into in-plane lipid bilayer, *Ultramicroscopy 107*, 928–933.

224. Goncalves, R. P., Busselez, J., Levy, D., Seguin, J., and Scheuring, S. 2005. Membrane insertion of rhodopseudomonas acidophila light harvesting complex 2 investigated by high resolution AFM, *J Struct Biol 149*, 79–86.

225. Jo, E., McLaurin, J., Yip, C. M., St George-Hyslop, P., and Fraser, P. E. 2000. α-synuclein membrane interactions and lipid specificity, *J Biol Chem 275*, 34328–34334.

226. Yip, C. M. and McLaurin, J. 2001. Amyloid-beta peptide assembly: A critical step in fibrillogenesis and membrane disruption, *Biophys J 80*, 1359–1371.

227. Hane, F., Drolle, E., and Leonenko, Z. 2010. Effect of cholesterol and amyloid-beta peptide on structure and function of mixed-lipid films and pulmonary surfactant BLES. An atomic force microscopy study, *Nanomedicine. 6*(6), 808–814.

228. Choucair, A., Chakrapani, M., Chakravarthy, B., Katsaras, J., and Johnston, L. J. 2007. Preferential accumulation of Ab[1–42] on gel phase domains of lipid bilayers: An AFM and fluorescence study, *Biochim Biophys Acta 1768*, 146–154.

229. Lam, K. L., Ishitsuka, Y., Cheng, Y., Chien, K., Waring, A. J., Lehrer, R. I., and Lee, K. Y. 2006. Mechanism of supported membrane disruption by antimicrobial peptide protegrin-1, *J Phys Chem B 110*, 21282–21286.

230. Butt, H. 1991. Measureing electrostatic, Van der Waals, and hydration forces in electrolyte solutions with an atomic force microscope, *Biophys J 60*, 1438–1444.

231. Ducker, W. A., Senden, T. J., and Pashley, R. M. 1991. Direct measurement of colloidal forces using an atomic force microscope, *Nature 353*, 239–241.

232. Senden, T. J., and Drummond, C. J. 1995. Surface chemistry and tip–sample interactions in atomic force microscopy, *Colloids and Surfaces 94*(1), 29–51.

233. Bowen, W. R., Hilal, N., Lovitt, R. W., and Wright, C. J. 1998. Direct measurement of interactions between adsorbed protein layers using an atomic force microscope, *J Colloid Interface Sci 197*, 348–352.

234. Lokar, W. J. and Ducker, W. A. 2004. Proximal adsorption at glass surfaces: Ionic strength, pH, chain length effects, *Langmuir 20*, 378–388.

235. Mosley, L. M., Hunter, K. A., and Ducker, W. A. 2003. Forces between colloid particles in natural waters, *Environ Sci Technol 37*, 3303–3308.

236. Lokar, W. J. and Ducker, W. A. 2002. Proximal adsorption of dodecyltrimethylammonium bromide to the silica-electrolyte solution interface, *Langmuir 18*, 3167–3175.

237. Liu, J.-F., Min, G., and Ducker, W. A. 2001. AFM study of cationic surfactants and cationic polyelectrolytes at the silica–water interface, *Langmuir 17*, 4895–4903.

238. Tulpar, A., Subramaniam, V., and Ducker, W. A. 2001. Decay lengths in double-layer forces in solutions of partly associated ions, *Langmuir 17*, 8451–8454.

239. Butt, H.-J., Jaschke, M., and Ducker, W. 1995. Measuring surface forces in aqueous electrolyte solution with the atomic force microscopy, *Bioelectrochem. Bioenergetics 38*, 191–201.

240. Ducker, W. A. Xu, Z., and Israelachvili, J. N. 1994. Measurements of hydrophobic and DLVO forces in bubble-surface interactions in aqueous solutions, *Langmuir 10*, 3279–3289.

241. Ducker, W. A., and Cook, R. F. 1990. Rapid measurement of static and dynamic surface forces, *Appl Phys Lett 56*, 2408–2410.

242. Manne, S. and Gaub, H. E. 1997. Force microscopy: Measurement of local interfacial forces and surface stresses, *Curr Opin Colloid Interface Sci 2*, 145–152.

243. Toikka, G. and Hayes, R. A. 1997. Direct measurement of colloidal forces between mica and silica in aqueous electrolyte, *J Colloid Interface Sci 191*, 102–109.

244. Zhang, J., Uchida, E., Yuama, Y., and Ikada, Y. 1997. Electrostatic interaction between ionic polymer grafted surfaces studied by atomic force microscopy, *J Colloid Interf Sci 188*, 431–438.

245. Hodges, C. S. 2002. Measuring forces with the AFM: Polymeric surfaces in liquids, *Adv Colloid Interface Sci 99*, 13–75.

246. Muster, T. H. and Prestidge, C. A. 2002. Face specific surface properties of pharmaceutical crystals, *J Pharm Sci 91*, 1432–1444.

247. Danesh, A., Davies, M. C., Hinder, S. J., Roberts, C. J., Tendler, S. J., Williams, P. M., and Wilkins, M. J. 2000. Surface characterization of aspirin crystal planes by dynamic chemical force microscopy, *Anal Chem 72*, 3419–3422.

248. Noy, A., Frisbie, C. D., Rozsnyai, L. F., Wrighton, M. S., and Leiber, C. M. 1995. Chemical force microscopy: Exploiting chemically-modified tips to quantify adhesion, friction, and functional group distributions in molecular assemblies., *J Am Chem Soc 117*, 7943–7951.

249. Leckband, D. 2000. Measuring the forces that control protein interactions, *Annu Rev Biophys Biomol Struct 29*, 1–26.

250. Rief, M., Gautel, M., Oesterhelt, F., Fernandez, J. M., and Gaub, H. E. 1997. Reversible unfolding of individual titin immunoglobulin domains by AFM, *Science 276*, 1109–1112.

251. Smith, D. A. and Radford, S. E. 2000. Protein folding: Pulling back the frontiers, *Curr Biol 10*, R662–R664.

252. Hinterdorfer, P., Baumgartner, W., Gruber, H. J., and Schilcher, K. 1996. Detection and localization of individual antibody–antigen recognition events by atomic force microscopy, *Proc Natl Acad Sci USA 93*, 3477–3481.

253. Lee, G. U., Chrisey, L. A., and Colton, R. J. 1994. Direct measurement of the forces between complementary strands of DNA, *Science 266*, 771–773.

254. Helenius, J., Heisenberg, C. P., Gaub, H. E., and Muller, D. J. 2008. Single-cell force spectroscopy, *J Cell Sci 121*, 1785–1791.

255. Linke, W. A. and Grutzner, A. 2008. Pulling single molecules of titin by AFM—Recent advances and physiological implications, *Pflugers Arch 456*, 101–115.

256. Kienberger, F., Ebner, A., Gruber, H. J., and Hinterdorfer, P. 2006. Molecular recognition imaging and force spectroscopy of single biomolecules, *Acc Chem Res 39*, 29–36.

257. Greulich, K. O. 2005. Single-molecule studies on DNA and RNA, *ChemPhysChem 6*, 2458–2471.

258. Alegre-Cebollada, J., Perez-Jimenez, R., Kosuri, P., and Fernandez, J. M. 2010. Single-molecule force spectroscopy approach to enzymatic catalysis, *J Biol Chem. 285*(25), 18961–18966.

259. Carrion-Vazquez, M., Oberhauser, A. F., Fisher, T. E., Marszalek, P. E., Li, H., and Fernandez, J. M. 2000. Mechanical design of proteins studied by single-molecule force spectroscopy and protein engineering, *Prog Biophys Mol Biol 74*, 63–91.

260. Fisher, T. E., Carrion-Vazquez, M., Oberhauser, A. F., Li, H., Marszalek, P. E., and Fernandez, J. M. 2000. Single molecular force spectroscopy of modular proteins in the nervous system, *Neuron 27*, 435–446.

261. Fisher, T. E., Marszalek, P. E., and Fernandez, J. M. 2000. Stretching single molecules into novel conformations using the atomic force microscope, *Nat Struct Biol 7*, 719–724.

262. Bell, G. I. 1978. Models for the specific adhesion of cells to cells, *Science 200*, 618–627.

263. Strunz, T., Oroszlan, K., Schumakovitch, I., Guntherodt, H. J., and Hegner, M. 2000. Model energy landscapes and the force-induced dissociation of ligand–receptor bonds, *Biophys J 79*(3), 1206–1212.

264. Merkel, R., Nassoy, P., Leung, A., Ritchie, K., and Evans, E. 1999. Energy landscapes of receptor-ligand bonds explored with dynamic force spectroscopy, *Nature 397*, 50–53.

265. Janovjak, H., Struckmeier, J., and Muller, D. J. 2005. Hydrodynamic effects in fast AFM single-molecule force measurements, *Eur Biophys J. 34*(1), 91–96.

266. Wagner, P. 1998. Immobilization strategies for biological scanning probe microscopy, *FEBS Lett 430*, 112–115.

267. Wadu-Mesthrige, K., Amro, N. A., and Liu, G. Y. 2000. Immobilization of proteins on self-assembled monolayers, *Scanning 22*, 380–388.

268. Schmitt, L., Ludwig, M., Gaub, H. E., and Tampe, R. 2000. A metal-chelating microscopy tip as a new toolbox for single-molecule experiments by atomic force microscopy, *Biophys J 78*, 3275–3285.

269. Ill, C. R., Keivens, V. M., Hale, J. E., Nakamura, K. K., Jue, R. A., Cheng, S., Melcher, E. D., Drake, B., and Smith, M. C. 1993. A COOH-terminal peptide confers regiospecific orientation and facilitates atomic force microscopy of an IGG1, *Biophys J 64*, 919–924.

270. Thomson, N. H., Smith, B. L., Almqvist, N., Schmitt, L., Kashlev, M., Kool, E. T., and Hansma, P. K. 1999. Oriented, active *Escherichia coli* RNA polymerase: An atomic force microscope study, *Biophys J 76*, 1024–1033.

271. Li, Q., Rukavishnikov, A. V., Petukhov, P. A., Zaikova, T. O., Jin, C., and Keana, J. F. 2003. Nanoscale tripodal 1,3,5,7-tetrasubstituted adamantanes for AFM applications, *J Org Chem 68*, 4862–4869.

272. Drew, M. E., Chworos, A., Oroudjev, E., Hansma, H., and Yamakoshi, Y. 2010. A tripod molecular tip for single molecule ligand–receptor force spectroscopy by AFM, *Langmuir 26*, 7117–7125.

273. Mukherjee, P. S., Das, N., and Stang, P. J. 2004. Self-assembly of nanoscopic coordination cages using a flexible tripodal amide containing linker, *J Org Chem 69*, 3526–3529.

274. Ganchev, D. N., Rijkers, D. T. S., Snel, M. M. E., Killian, J. A., and de Kruijff, B. 2004. Strength of integration of transmembrane alpha-helical peptides in lipid bilayers as determined by atomic force spectroscopy, *Biochemistry 43*, 14987–14993.

275. Stroh, C. M., Ebner, A., Geretschlager, M., Freudenthaler, G., Kienberger, F., Kamruzzahan, A. S., Smith-Gill, S. J., Gruber, H. J., and Hinterdorfer, P. 2004. Simultaneous topography and recognition imaging using force microscopy, *Biophys J 87*, 1981–1990.

276. Nevo, R., Stroh, C., Kienberger, F., Kaftan, D., Brumfeld, V., Elbaum, M., Reich, Z., and Hinterdorfer, P. 2003. A molecular switch between alternative conformational states in the complex of Ran and importin beta1, *Nat Struct Biol 10*, 553–557.

277. Kada, G., Blayney, L., Jeyakumar, L. H., Kienberger, F., Pastushenko, V. P., Fleischer, S., Schindler, H., Lai, F. A., and Hinterdorfer, P. 2001. Recognition force microscopy/spectroscopy of ion channels: Applications to the skeletal muscle Ca2+ release channel (ryr1), *Ultramicroscopy 86*, 129–137.

278. Schmidt, T., Hinterdorfer, P., and Schindler, H. 1999. Microscopy for recognition of individual bio-molecules, *Microsc Res Tech 44*, 339–346.

279. Raab, A., Han, W., Badt, D., Smith-Gill, S. J., Lindsay, S. M., Schindler, H., and Hinterdorfer, P. 1999. Antibody recognition imaging by force microscopy, *Nat Biotechnol 17*, 901–905.

280. Baumgartner, W., Hinterdorfer, P., Ness, W., Raab, A., Vestweber, D., Schindler, H., and Drenckhahn, D. 2000. Cadherin interaction probed by atomic force microscopy, *Proc Natl Acad Sci USA 97*, 4005–4010.

281. Baumgartner, W., Hinterdorfer, P., and Schindler, H. 2000. Data analysis of interaction forces measured with the atomic force microscope, *Ultramicroscopy 82*, 85–95.

282. Alsteens, D., Dague, E., Verbelen, C., Andre, G., Dupres, V., and Dufrene, Y. F. 2009. Nanoscale imaging of microbial pathogens using atomic force microscopy, *Wiley Interdiscip Rev Nanomed Nanobiotechnol 1*, 168–180.

283. Pelling, A. E., Li, Y. N., Shi, W. Y., and Gimzewski, J. K. 2005. Nanoscale visualization and charac-terization of *Myxococcus Xanthus* cells with atomic force microscopy, *Proc Natl Acad Sci, USA 102*, 6484–6489.

284. Puchner, E. M., Alexandrovich, A., Kho, A. L., Hensen, U., Schafer, L. V., Brandmeier, B., Grater, F., Grubmuller, H., Gaub, H. E., and Gautel, M. 2008. Mechanoenzymatics of titin kinase, *Proc Natl Acad Sci, USA 105*, 13385–13390.

285. Gaboriaud, F., Gee, M. L., Strugnell, R., and Duval, J. F. L. 2008. Coupled electrostatic, hydrodynamic, and mechanical properties of bacterial interfaces in aqueous media, *Langmuir 24*, 10988–10995.

286. Sheng, X. X., Ting, Y. P., and Pehkonen, S. O. 2007. Force measurements of bacterial adhesion on metals using a cell probe atomic force microscope, *J Colloid Interface Sci 310*, 661–669.

287. Lau, P. C. Y., Dutcher, J. R., Beveridge, T. J., and Lam, J. S. 2009. Absolute quantitation of bacterial biofilm adhesion and viscoelasticity by microbead force spectroscopy, *Biophys J 96*, 2935–2948.

288. Nussio, M. R., Oncins, G., Ridelis, I., Szili, E., Shapter, J. G., Sanz, F., and Voelcker, N. H. 2009. Nanomechanical characterization of phospholipid bilayer islands on flat and porous substrates: A force spectroscopy study, *J Phys Chem B 113*, 10339–10347.

289. Gaboriaud, F., Parcha, B. S., Gee, M. L., Holden, J. A., and Strugnell, R. A. 2008. Spatially resolved force spectroscopy of bacterial surfaces using force–volume imaging, *Colloids Surfaces B-Biointerfaces 62*, 206–213.

290. Kang, S. and Elimelech, M. 2009. Bioinspired single bacterial cell force spectroscopy, *Langmuir 25*, 9656–9659.

291. Cerf, A., Cau, J. C., Vieu, C., and Dague, E. 2009. Nanomechanical properties of dead or alive single-patterned bacteria, *Langmuir 25*, 5731–5736.

292. Gad, M., Itoh, A., and Ikai, A. 1997. Mapping cell wall polysaccharides of living microbial cells using atomic force microscopy, *Cell Biol Int 21*, 697–706.

293. Radmacher, M. 1997. Measuring the elastic properties of biological samples with the AFM, *IEEE Eng Med Biol Mag 16*, 47–57.

294. Shellenberger, K. and Logan, B. E. 2002. Effect of molecular scale roughness of glass beads on colloidal and bacterial deposition, *Environ Sci Technol 36*, 184–189.

295. van der Werf, K. O., Putman, C. A., de Grooth, B. G., and Greve, J. 1994. Adhesion force imaging in air and liquid by adhesion mode atomic force microscopy, *Appl Phys Lett 65*, 1195–1197.

296. Mizes, H. A., Loh, K.-G., Miller, R. J. D., Ahujy, S. K., and Grabowski, G. A. 1991. Submicron probe of polymer adhesion wtih atomic force microscopy. Dependence on topography and material inhomogenities, *Appl Phys Lett 59*, 2901–2903.

297. Nagao, E. and Dvorak, J. A. 1998. An integrated approach to the study of living cells by atomic force microscopy, *J Microsc 191 (Pt 1)*, 8–19.

298. Dupres, V., Menozzi, F. D., Locht, C., Clare, B. H., Abbott, N. L., Cuenot, S., Bompard, C., Raze, D., and Dufrene, Y. F. 2005. Nanoscale mapping and functional analysis of individual adhesins on living bacteria, *Nat Methods 2*, 515–520.

299. Francius, G., Alsteens, D., Dupres, V., Lebeer, S., De Keersmaecker, S., Vanderleyden, J., Gruber, H. J., and Dufrene, Y. F. 2009. Stretching polysaccharides on live cells using single molecule force spectroscopy, *Nat Protoc 4*, 939–946.

300. Francius, G., Lebeer, S., Alsteens, D., Wildling, L., Gruber, H. J., Hols, P., De Keersmaecker, S., Vanderleyden, J., and Dufrene, Y. F. 2008. Detection, localization, and conformational analysis of single polysaccharide molecules on live bacteria, *Acs Nano 2*, 1921–1929.

301. Dufrene, Y. F. and Hinterdorfer, P. 2008. Recent progress in AFM molecular recognition studies, *Pflugers Arch 456*, 237–245.

302. Hu, M., Wang, J., Cai, J., Wu, Y., and Wang, X. 2008. Nanostructure and force spectroscopy analysis of human peripheral blood CD4+ t cells using atomic force microscopy, *Biochem Biophys Res Commun 374*, 90–94.

303. Rosa-Zeiser, A., Weilandt, E., Hild, S., and Marti, O. 1997. The simultaneous measurement of elastic, electrostatic and adhesive properties by scanning force microscopy: Pulsed force mode operation, *Meas Sci Technol 8*, 1333–1338.

304. Okabe, Y., Furugori, M., Tani, Y., Akiba, U., and Fujihira, M. 2000. Chemical force microscopy of microcontact-printed self-assembled monolayers by pulsed-force-mode atomic force microscopy, *Ultramicroscopy 82*, 203–212.

305. Fujihira, M., Furugori, M., Akiba, U., and Tani, Y. 2001. Study of microcontact printed patterns by chemical force microscopy, *Ultramicroscopy 86*, 75–83.

306. Zhang, H., Grim, P. C. M., Vosch, T., Wiesler, U.-M., Berresheim, A. J., Mullen, K., and De Schryver, F. C. 2000. Discrimination of dendrimer aggregates on mica based on adhesion force: A pulsed mode atomic force microscopy study, *Langmuir 16*, 9294–9298.

307. Schneider, M., Zhu, M., Papastavrou, G., Akari, S., and Mohwald, H. 2002. Chemical pulsed-force microscopy of single polyethyleneimine molecules in aqueous solution, *Langmuir 18*, 602–606.

308. Kresz, N., Kokavecz, J., Smausz, T., Hopp, B., Csete, A., Hild, S., and Marti, O. 2004. Investigation of pulsed laser deposited crystalline PTFE thin layer with pulsed force mode AFM, *Thin Solid Films 453–454*, 239–244.

309. Stenert, M., Döring, A., and Bandermann, F. 2004. Poly(methyl methacrylate)-block-polystyrene and polystyrene-block-poly(*n*-butyl acrylate) as compatibilizers in PMMA/PNBA blends, *e-Polymers 15*, 1–16.

310. Evans, E. and Ritchie, K. 1999. Strength of a weak bond connecting flexible polymer chains, *Biophys J 76*, 2439–2447.

311. Dudko, O. K., Hummer, G., and Szabo, A. 2006. Intrinsic rates and activation free energies from single-molecule pulling experiments, *Phys Rev Lett 96*, 108101.

312. Ray, C., Guo, S., Brown, J., Li, N., and Akhremitchev, B. B. 2010. Kinetic parameters from detection probability in single molecule force spectroscopy, *Langmuir 26*(14), 11951–11957.

313. Li, N., Guo, S., and Akhremitchev, B. B. 2010. Apparent dependence of rupture force on loading rate in single-molecule force spectroscopy, *ChemPhysChem 11*(10), 2096–2098.

314. Grandbois, M., Beyer, M., Rief, M., Clausen-Schaumann, H., and Gaub, H. E. 1999. How strong is a covalent bond? *Science 283*, 1727–1730.

315. Haselgrubler, T., Amerstorfer, A., Schindler, H., and Gruber, H. J. 1995. Synthesis and applications of a new poly(ethylene glycol. derivative for the crosslinking of amines with thiols, *Bioconjug Chem 6*, 242–248.

316. Willemsen, O. H., Snel, M. M., van der Werf, K. O., de Grooth, B. G., Greve, J., Hinterdorfer, P., Gruber, H. J., Schindler, H., van Kooyk, Y., and Figdor, C. G. 1998. Simultaneous height and adhesion imaging of antibody–antigen interactions by atomic force microscopy, *Biophys J 75*, 2220–2228.

317. Wielert-Badt, S., Hinterdorfer, P., Gruber, H. J., Lin, J. T., Badt, D., Wimmer, B., Schindler, H., and Kinne, R. K. 2002. Single molecule recognition of protein binding epitopes in brush border membranes by force microscopy, *Biophys J 82*, 2767–2774.

318. Rivera, M., Lee, W., Ke, C., Marszalek, P. E., Cole, D. G., and Clark, R. L. 2008. Minimizing pulling geometry errors in atomic force microscope single molecule force spectroscopy, *Biophys J 95*, 3991–3998.

319. Ros, R., Schwesinger, F., Anselmetti, D., Kubon, M., Schafer, R., Pluckthun, A., and Tiefenauer, L. 1998. Antigen binding forces of individually addressed single-chain fv antibody molecules, *Proc Natl Acad Sci USA 95*, 7402–7405.

320. Allen, S., Davies, J., Davies, M. C., Dawkes, A. C., Roberts, C. J., Tendler, S. J., and Williams, P. M. 1999. The influence of epitope availability on atomic-force microscope studies of antigen-antibody interactions, *Biochem J 341 (Pt 1)*, 173–178.

321. Schwesinger, F., Ros, R., Strunz, T., Anselmetti, D., Guntherodt, H. J., Honegger, A., Jermutus, L., Tiefenauer, L., and Pluckthun, A. 2000. Unbinding forces of single antibody-antigen complexes correlate with their thermal dissociation rates, *Proc Natl Acad Sci USA 97*, 9972–9977.

322. Gergely, C., Voegel, J., Schaaf, P., Senger, B., Maaloum, M., Horber, J. K., and Hemmerle, J. 2000. Unbinding process of adsorbed proteins under external stress studied by atomic force microscopy spectroscopy, *Proc Natl Acad Sci USA 97*, 10802–10807.

323. Guzman, D. L., Randall, A., Baldi, P., and Guan, Z. 2010. Computational and single-molecule force studies of a macro domain protein reveal a key molecular determinant for mechanical stability, *Proc Natl Acad Sci USA 107*, 1989–1994.

324. Sharma, D., Perisic, O., Peng, Q., Cao, Y., Lam, C., Lu, H., and Li, H. 2007. Single-molecule force spectroscopy reveals a mechanically stable protein fold and the rational tuning of its mechanical stability, *Proc Natl Acad Sci USA 104*, 9278–9283.

325. Kim, T., Rhee, A., and Yip, C. M. 2006. Force-induced insulin dimer dissociation: A molecular dynamics study, *J Am Chem Soc 128*, 5330–5331.

326. Gao, M., Wilmanns, M., and Schulten, K. 2002. Steered molecular dynamics studies of titin i1 domain unfolding, *Biophys J 83*, 3435–3445.

327. Gao, M., Craig, D., Vogel, V., and Schulten, K. 2002. Identifying unfolding intermediates of FN-III[10] by steered molecular dynamics, *J Mol Biol 323*, 939–950.

328. Isralewitz, B., Gao, M., and Schulten, K. 2001. Steered molecular dynamics and mechanical functions of proteins, *Curr Opin Struct Biol 11*, 224–230.

329. Clementi, C., Carloni, P., and Maritan, A. 1999. Protein design is a key factor for subunit–subunit association, *Proc Natl Acad Sci USA 96*, 9616–9621.

330. Eom, K., Makarov, D. E., and Rodin, G. J. 2005. Theoretical studies of the kinetics of mechanical unfolding of cross-linked polymer chains and their implications for single-molecule pulling experiments, *Phys Rev E Stat Nonlin Soft Matter Phys 71*, 021904.

331. Qian, H. and Shapiro, B. E. 1999. Graphical method for force analysis: Macromolecular mechanics with atomic force microscopy, *Proteins 37*, 576–581.

332. Fisher, T. E., Marszalek, P. E., Oberhauser, A. F., Carrion-Vazquez, M., and Fernandez, J. M. 1999. The micro-mechanics of single molecules studied with atomic force microscopy, *J Physiol 520 Pt 1*, 5–14.

333. Vesenka, J., Manne, S., Giberson, R., Marsh, T., and Henderson, E. 1993. Collidal gold particles as an incompressible atomic force microscope imaging standard for assessing the compressibility of biomolecules, *Biochem J 65*, 992–997.

334. Engel, A., Gaub, H. E., and Muller, D. J. 1999. Atomic force microscopy: A forceful way with single molecules, *Curr Biol 9*, R133–136.

335. Fotiadis, D., Scheuring, S., Muller, S. A., Engel, A., and Muller, D. J. 2002. Imaging and manipulation of biological structures with the AFM, *Micron 33*, 385–397.

336. Muller, D. J., Fotiadis, D., and Engel, A. 1998. Mapping flexible protein domains at subnanometer resolution with the atomic force microscope, *FEBS Lett 430*, 105–111.

337. Schwaiger, I., Kardinal, A., Schleicher, M., Noegel, A. A., and Rief, M. 2004. A mechanical unfolding intermediate in an actin-crosslinking protein, *Nat Struct Mol Biol 11*, 81–85.

338. Williams, P. M., Fowler, S. B., Best, R. B., Toca-Herrera, J. L., Scott, K. A., Steward, A., and Clarke, J. 2003. Hidden complexity in the mechanical properties of titin, *Nature 422*, 446–449.

339. Kellermayer, M. S., Bustamante, C., and Granzier, H. L. 2003. Mechanics and structure of titin oligomers explored with atomic force microscopy, *Biochim Biophys Acta 1604*, 105–114.

340. Hertadi, R., Gruswitz, F., Silver, L., Koide, A., Koide, S., Arakawa, H., and Ikai, A. 2003. Unfolding mechanics of multiple ospa substructures investigated with single molecule force spectroscopy, *J Mol Biol 333*, 993–1002.

341. Carrion-Vazquez, M., Li, H., Lu, H., Marszalek, P. E., Oberhauser, A. F., and Fernandez, J. M. 2003. The mechanical stability of ubiquitin is linkage dependent, *Nat Struct Biol 10*(9), 738–743.

342. Rief, M. and Grubmuller, H. 2002. Force spectroscopy of single biomolecules, *ChemPhysChem 3*, 255–261.

343. Oberhauser, A. F., Badilla-Fernandez, C., Carrion-Vazquez, M., and Fernandez, J. M. 2002. The mechanical hierarchies of fibronectin observed with single-molecule afm, *J Mol Biol 319*, 433–447.

344. Muller, D. J., Kessler, M., Oesterhelt, F., Moller, C., Oesterhelt, D., and Gaub, H. 2002. Stability of bacteriorhodopsin alpha-helices and loops analyzed by single-molecule force spectroscopy, *Biophys J 83*, 3578–3588.

345. Best, R. B. and Clarke, J. 2002. What can atomic force microscopy tell us about protein folding?, *Chem Commun (Camb) Feb 7*,(3), 183–192.

346. Rief, M., Gautel, M., and Gaub, H. E. 2000. Unfolding forces of titin and fibronectin domains directly measured by AFM, *Adv Exp Med Biol 481*, 129–136; discussion 137–141.

347. Zhang, Y., Cui, F. Z., Wang, X. M., Feng, Q. L., and Zhu, X. D. 2002. Mechanical properties of skeletal bone in gene-mutated stopsel(dtl28d) and wild-type zebrafish (*Danio rerio*) measured by atomic force microscopy-based nanoindentation, *Bone 30*, 541–546.

348. Oberhauser, A. F., Hansma, P. K., Carrion-Vazquez, M., and Fernandez, J. M. 2001. Stepwise unfolding of titin under force-clamp atomic force microscopy, *Proc Natl Acad Sci USA 98*, 468–472.

349. Carrion-Vazquez, M., Marszalek, P. E., Oberhauser, A. F., and Fernandez, J. M. 1999. Atomic force microscopy captures length phenotypes in single proteins, *Proc Natl Acad Sci USA 96*, 11288–11292.

350. Marszalek, P. E., Lu, H., Li, H., Carrion-Vazquez, M., Oberhauser, A. F., Schulten, K., and Fernandez, J. M. 1999. Mechanical unfolding intermediates in titin modules, *Nature 402*, 100–103.

351. Becker, N., Oroudjev, E., Mutz, S., Cleveland, J. P., Hansma, P. K., Hayashi, C. Y., Makarov, D. E., and Hansma, H. G. 2003. Molecular nanosprings in spider capture-silk threads, *Nat Mater 2*, 278–283.

352. Yu, J., Malkova, S., and Lyubchenko, Y. L. 2008. Alpha-synuclein misfolding: Single molecule AFM force spectroscopy study, *J Mol Biol 384*, 992–1001.

353. Guo, S. and Akhremitchev, B. B. 2006. Packing density and structural heterogeneity of insulin amyloid fibrils measured by AFM nanoindentation, *Biomacromolecules 7*, 1630–1636.

354. Osada, T., Itoh, A., and Ikai, A. 2003. Mapping of the receptor-associated protein (RAP) binding proteins on living fibroblast cells using an atomic force microscope, *Ultramicroscopy 97*, 353–357.

355. Smith, J. F., Knowles, T. P., Dobson, C. M., Macphee, C. E., and Welland, M. E. 2006. Characterization of the nanoscale properties of individual amyloid fibrils, *Proc Natl Acad Sci USA 103*, 15806–15811.

356. Yan, C., Yersin, A., Afrin, R., Sekiguchi, H., and Ikai, A. 2009. Single molecular dynamic interactions between glycophorin A and lectin as probed by atomic force microscopy, *Biophys Chem 144*, 72–77.

357. Lesoil, C., Nonaka, T., Sekiguchi, H., Osada, T., Miyata, M., Afrin, R., and Ikai, A. 2010. Molecular shape and binding force of mycoplasma mobile's leg protein gli349 revealed by an afm study, *Biochem Biophys Res Commun 391*, 1312–1317.

358. Rief, M., Pascual, J., Saraste, M., and Gaub, H. E. 1999. Single molecule force spectroscopy of spectrin repeats: Low unfolding forces in helix bundles, *J Mol Biol 286*, 553–561.

359. Lenne, P. F., Raae, A. J., Altmann, S. M., Saraste, M., and Horber, J. K. 2000. States and transitions during forced unfolding of a single spectrin repeat, *FEBS Lett 476*, 124–128.

360. Yang, G., Cecconi, C., Baase, W. A., Vetter, I. R., Breyer, W. A., Haack, J. A., Matthews, B. W., Dahlquist, F. W., and Bustamante, C. 2000. Solid-state synthesis and mechanical unfolding of polymers of t4 lysozyme, *Proc Natl Acad Sci USA 97*, 139–144.

361. Clausen-Schaumann, H., Rief, M., Tolksdorf, C., and Gaub, H. E. 2000. Mechanical stability of single DNA molecules, *Biophys J 78*, 1997–2007.

362. Struckmeier, J., Wahl, R., Leuschner, M., Nunes, J., Janovjak, H., Geisler, U., Hofmann, G., Jahnke, T., and Muller, D. J. 2008. Fully automated single-molecule force spectroscopy for screening applications, *Nanotechnology 19*(38), 384020.

363. Zhang, B., and Evans, J. S. 2001. Modeling AFM-induced PEVK extension and the reversible unfolding of Ig/Fn III domains in single and multiple titin molecules, *Biophys J 80*, 597–605.

364. Paci, E. and Karplus, M. 2000. Unfolding proteins by external forces and temperature: The importance of topology and energetics, *Proc Natl Acad Sci USA 97*, 6521–6526.

365. Weisenhorn, A. L., Khorsandi, M., Kasas, S., Gotzos, V., and Butt, H.-J. 1993. Deformation and height anomaly of soft surfaces studied with an AFM, *Nanotechnology 4*, 106–113.

366. Vinckier, A., Dumortier, C., Engelborghs, Y., and Hellemans, L. 1996. Dynamical and mechanical study of immobilized microtubules with atomic force microscopy, *J Vac Sci Technol 14*, 1427–1431.

367. Laney, D. E., Garcia, R. A., Parsons, S. M., and Hansma, H. G. 1997. Changes in the elastic properties of cholinergic synaptic vesicles as measured by atomic force microscopy, *Biophys J 72*, 806–813.

368. Lekka, M., Laidler, P., Gil, D., Lekki, J., Stachura, Z., and Hrynkiewicz, A. Z. 1999. Elasticity of normal and cancerous human bladder cells studied by scanning force microscopy, *Eur Biophys J 28*, 312–316.

369. Parbhu, A. N., Bryson, W. G., and Lal, R. 1999. Disulfide bonds in the outer layer of keratin fibers confer higher mechanical rigidity: Correlative nano-indentation and elasticity measurement with an AFM, *Biochemistry 38*, 11755–11761.

370. Suda, H., Sasaki, Y. C., Oishi, N., Hiraoka, N., and Sutoh, K. 1999. Elasticity of mutant myosin subfragment-1 arranged on a functional silver surface, *Biochem Biophys Res Commun 261*, 276–282.

371. Cuenot, S., Demoustier-Champagne, S., and Nysten, B. 2000. Elastic modulus of polypyrrole nanotubes, *Phys Rev Lett 85*, 1690–1693.

372. Alhadlaq, A., Elisseeff, J. H., Hong, L., Williams, C. G., Caplan, A. I., Sharma, B., Kopher, R. A. et al. 2004. Adult stem cell driven genesis of human-shaped articular condyle, *Ann Biomed Eng 32*, 911–923.

373. Mathur, A. B., Truskey, G. A., and Reichert, W. M. 2000. Atomic force and total internal reflection fluorescence microscopy for the study of force transmission in endothelial cells, *Biophys J 78*, 1725–1735.

374. Velegol, S. B. and Logan, B. E. 2002. Contributions of bacterial surface polymers, electrostatics, and cell elasticity to the shape of AFM force curves, *Langmuir 18*, 5256–5262.

375. Touhami, A., Nysten, B., and Dufrene, Y. F. 2003. Nanoscale mapping of the elasticity of microbial cells by atomic force microscopy, *Langmuir 19*, 1745–1751.

376. Shroff, S. G., Saner, D. R., and Lal, R. 1995. Dynamic micromechanical properties of cultured rat atrial myocytes measured by atomic force microscopy, *Am J Physiol 269*, C286–292.

377. Ebenstein, D. M. and Pruitt, L. A. 2004. Nanoindentation of soft hydrated materials for application to vascular tissues, *J Biomed Mater Res 69A*, 222–232.

378. Thurner, P. J. 2009. Atomic force microscopy and indentation force measurement of bone, *Wiley Interdiscip Rev Nanomed Nanobiotechnol 1*, 624–649.

379. Grant, C. A., Brockwell, D. J., Radford, S. E., and Thomson, N. H. 2009. Tuning the elastic modulus of hydrated collagen fibrils, *Biophys J 97*, 2985–2992.

380. Lee, B., Han, L., Frank, E. H., Chubinskaya, S., Ortiz, C., and Grodzinsky, A. J. 2010. Dynamic mechanical properties of the tissue-engineered matrix associated with individual chondrocytes, *J Biomech 43*, 469–476.

381. Liao, X. and Wiedmann, T. S. 2004. Characterization of pharmaceutical solids by scanning probe microscopy, *J Pharm Sci 93*, 2250–2258.

382. Balooch, G., Marshall, G. W., Marshall, S. J., Warren, O. L., Asif, S. A., and Balooch, M. 2004. Evaluation of a new modulus mapping technique to investigate microstructural features of human teeth, *J Biomech 37*, 1223–1232.

383. Landman, U., Luedtke, W. D., Burnham, N. A., and Colton, R. J. 1990. Atomistic mechanisms and dynamics of adhesion, nanoindentation, and fracture, *Science 248*, 454–461.

384. Van Landringham, M. R., McKnight, S. H., Palmese, G. R., Bogetti, T. A., Eduljee, R. F., and Gillespie, J. W. J. 1997. Characterization of interphase regions using atomic force microscopy, *Mat Res Soc Symp Proc 458*, 313–318.

385. Van Landringham, M. R., McKnight, S. H., Palmese, G. R., Eduljee, R. F., Gillespie, J. W. J., and McCullough, R. L. 1997. Relating polymer indentation behavior to elastic modulus using atomic force microscopy, *Mat Res Soc Symp Proc 440*, 195–200.

386. Van Landringham, M. R., McKnight, S. H., Palmese, G. R., Huang, X., Bogetti, T. A., Eduljee, R. F., and Gillespie, J. W. J. 1997. Nanoscale indentation of polymer systems using the atomic force microscope, *J Adhesion 64*, 31–59.

387. Van Landringham, M. R., Dagastine, R. R., Eduljee, R. F., McCullough, R. L., and Gillespie, J. W. J. 1999. Characterization of nanoscale property variations in polymer composite systems: Part 1—experimental results, *Composites Part A 30*(1), 75–83.

388. Bogetti, T. A., Wang, T., Van Landringham, M. R., Eduljee, R. F., and Gillespie, J. W. J. 1999. Characterization of nanoscale property variations in polymer composite systems: Part 2—finite element modeling, *Composites Part A 30*, 85–94.

389. Bischel, M. S., Van Landringham, M. R., Eduljee, R. F., Gillespie, J. W. J., and Schultz, J. M. 2000. On the use of nanoscale indentation with the AFM in the identification of phases in blends on linear low density polyethylene and high density polyethylene, *J Mat Sci 35*, 221–228.

390. Cleveland, J. P., Manne, S., Bocek, D., and Hansma, P. K. 1993. A nondestructive method for determining the spring constant of cantilevers for scanning force microscopy, *Rev Sci Instrum 64*, 403–405.

391. Bogdanovic, G., Meurk, A., and Rutland, M. W. 2000. Tip friction—Torsional spring constant determination, *Colloids Surf B Biointerfaces 19*, 397–405.

392. Hutter, J. L. and Bechhoefer, J. 1993. Calibration of atomic-force microscope tips, *Rev Sci Instrum 64*, 1868–1873.

393. Sako, Y., Hibino, k., Miyauchi, T., Miyamoto, Y., Ueda, M., and Yanagida, T. 2000. Single-molecule imaging of signaling molecules in living cells, *Single Mol 2*, 159–163.

394. Sako, Y., Minoghchi, S., and Yanagida, T. 2000. Single-molecule imaging of egfr signalling on the surface of living cells, *Nat Cell Biol 2*, 168–172.

395. Ambrose, W. P., Goodwin, P. M., and Nolan, J. P. 1999. Single-molecule detection with total internal reflectance excitation: Comparing signal-to-background and total signals in different geometries, *Cytometry 36*, 224–231.

396. Osborne, M. A., Barnes, C. L., Balasubramanian, S., and Klenerman, D. 2001. Probing DNA surface attachment and local environment using single molecule spectroscopy, *J Phys Chem B 105*, 3120–3126.

397. Wakelin, S. and Bagshaw, C. R. 2003. A prism combination for near isotropic fluorescence excitation by total internal reflection, *J Microsc 209*, 143–148.

398. Michalet, X., Kapanidis, A. N., Laurence, T., Pinaud, F., Doose, S., Pflughoefft, M., and Weiss, S. 2003. The power and prospects of fluorescence microscopies and spectroscopies, *Annu Rev Biophys Biomol Struct 32*, 161–182.

399. Cannone, F., Chirico, G., and Diaspro, A. 2003. Two-photon interactions at single fluorescent molecule level, *J Biomed Opt 8*, 391–395.

400. Borisenko, V., Lougheed, T., Hesse, J., Fureder-Kitzmuller, E., Fertig, N., Behrends, J. C., Woolley, G. A., and Schutz, G. J. 2003. Simultaneous optical and electrical recording of single gramicidin channels, *Biophys J 84*, 612–622.

401. Sako, Y. and Uyemura, T. 2002. Total internal reflection fluorescence microscopy for single-molecule imaging in living cells, *Cell Struct Funct 27*, 357–365.

402. Ludes, M. D. and Wirth, M. J. 2002. Single-molecule resolution and fluorescence imaging of mixed-mode sorption of a dye at the interface of c18 and acetonitrile/water, *Anal Chem 74*, 386–393.

403. Harris, C. M. 2003. Shedding light on nsom, *Anal Chem 75*, 223A–228A.

404. Sekatskii, S. K., Shubeita, G. T., and Dietler, G. 2000. Time-gated scanning near-field optical microscopy, *Appl Phys Lett 77*, 2089–2091.

405. Muramatsu, H., Chiba, N., Umemoto, T., Homma, K., Nakajima, K., Ataka, T., Ohta, S., Kusumi, A., and Fujihira, M. 1995. Development of near-field optic/atomic force microscope for biological materials in aqueous solutions, *Ultramicroscopy 61*, 265–269.

406. Edidin, M. 2001. Near-field scanning optical microscopy, a siren call to biology, *Traffic 2*, 797–803.

407. de Lange, F., Cambi, A., Huijbens, R., de Bakker, B., Rensen, W., Garcia-Parajo, M., van Hulst, N., and Figdor, C. G. 2001. Cell biology beyond the diffraction limit: Near-field scanning optical microscopy, *J Cell Sci 114*, 4153–4160.

408. Betzig, E. and Chichester, R. J. 1993. Single molecules observed by near-field scanning optical microscopy, *Science 262*, 1422–1425.

409. Garcia-Parajo, M. F., Veerman, J. A., Segers-Nolten, G. M., de Grooth, B. G., Greve, J., and van Hulst, N. F. 1999. Visualising individual green fluorescent proteins with a near field optical microscope, *Cytometry 36*, 239–246.

410. van Hulst, N. F., Veerman, J. A., Garcia-Parajo, M. F., and Kuipers, J. 2000. Analysis of individual (macro)molecules and proteins using near-field optics, *J Chem Phys 112*, 7799–7810.

411. Moers, M. H., Ruiter, A. G., Jalocha, A., and van Hulst, N. F. 1995. Detection of fluorescence *in situ* hybridization on human metaphase chromosomes by near-field scanning optical microscopy, *Ultramicroscopy 61*, 279–283.

412. Micic, M., Radotic, K., Jeremic, M., Djikanovic, D., and Kammer, S. B. 2004. Study of the lignin model compound supramolecular structure by combination of near-field scanning optical microscopy and atomic force microscopy, *Colloids Surf B Biointerfaces 34*, 33–40.

413. Ianoul, A., Street, M., Grant, D., Pezacki, J., Taylor, R. S., and Johnston, L. J. 2004. Near-field scanning fluorescence microscopy study of ion channel clusters in cardiac myocyte membranes, *Biophys J 87*(5), 3525–3535.

414. Nagy, P., Jenei, A., Kirsch, A. K., Szollosi, J., Damjanovich, S., and Jovin, T. M. 1999. Activation-dependent clustering of the Erbb2 receptor tyrosine kinase detected by scanning near-field optical microscopy, *J Cell Sci 112 (Pt 11)*, 1733–1741.

415. Sommer, A. P. and Franke, R. P. 2002. Near-field optical analysis of living cells *in vitro, J Proteome Res 1*, 111–114.
416. Hosaka, N., and Saiki, T. 2001. Near-field fluorescence imaging of single molecules with a resolution in the range of 10 nm, *J Microsc 202*, 362–364.
417. Dunn, R. C., Holtom, G. R., Mets, L., and Xie, X. S. 1994. Near-field imaging and fluorescence lifetime measurement of light harvesting complexes in intact photosynthetic membranes, *J Phys Chem 98*, 3094–3098.
418. Ha, T., Enderle, T., Ogletree, D. F., Chemla, D. S., Selvin, P. R., and Weiss, S. 1996. Probing the interaction between two single molecules: Fluorescence resonance energy transfer between a single donor and a single acceptor, *Proc Natl Acad Sci USA 93*, 6264–6268.
419. Prikulis, J., Murty, K. V., Olin, H., and Kall, M. 2003. Large-area topography analysis and near-field Raman spectroscopy using bent fibre probes, *J Microsc 210*, 269–273.
420. Burgos, P., Lu, Z., Ianoul, A., Hnatovsky, C., Viriot, M. L., Johnston, L. J., and Taylor, R. S. 2003. Near-field scanning optical microscopy probes: A comparison of pulled and double-etched bent NSOM probes for fluorescence imaging of biological samples, *J Microsc 211*, 37–47.
421. Kitts, C. C., and Vanden Bout, D. A. 2009. Near-field scanning optical microscopy measurements of fluorescent molecular probes binding to insulin amyloid fibrils, *J Phys Chem B 113*, 12090–12095.
422. Tokumasu, F., Hwang, J., and Dvorak, J. A. 2004. Heterogeneous molecular distribution in supported multicomponent lipid bilayers, *Langmuir 20*, 614–618.
423. Vobornik, D., Rouleau, Y., Haley, J., Bani-Yaghoub, M., Taylor, R., Johnston, L. J., and Pezacki, J. P. 2009. Nanoscale organization of beta2-adrenergic receptor-venus fusion protein domains on the surface of mammalian cells, *Biochem Biophys Res Commun 382*, 85–90.
424. Ianoul, A. and Johnston, L. J. 2007. Near-field scanning optical microscopy to identify membrane microdomains, *Methods Mol Biol 400*, 469–480.
425. Nishida, S., Funabashi, Y., and Ikai, A. 2002. Combination of AFM with an objective-type total internal reflection fluorescence microscope (TIRFM) for nanomanipulation of single cells, *Ultramicroscopy 91*, 269–274.
426. Shaw, J. E., Slade, A., and Yip, C. M. 2003. Simultaneous *in situ* total internal reflectance fluorescence/atomic force microscopy studies of DPPC/DPOPC microdomains in supported planar lipid bilayers, *J Am Chem Soc 125*, 111838–111839.
427. Oreopoulos, J. and Yip, C. M. 2008. Combined scanning probe and total internal reflection fluorescence microscopy, *Methods 46*, 2–10.
428. Hugel, T., Holland, N. B., Cattani, A., Moroder, L., Seitz, M., and Gaub, H. E. 2002. Single-molecule optomechanical cycle, *Science 296*, 1103–1106.
429. Kellermayer, M. S. Z., Karsai, A., Kengyel, A., Nagy, A., Bianco, P., Huber, T., Kulcsar, A., Niedetzky, C., Proksch, R., and Grama, L. 2006. Spatially and temporally synchronized atomic force and total internal reflection fluorescence microscopy for imaging and manipulating cells and biomolecules, *Biophys J 91*, 2665–2677.
430. Kolodny, L. A., Willard, D. M., Carillo, L. L., Nelson, M. W., and Van Orden, A. 2001. Spatially correlated fluorescence/AFM of individual nanosized particles and biomolecules, *Anal Chem 73*, 1959–1966.
431. Shaw, J. E., Alattia, J. R., Verity, J. E., Prive, G. G., and Yip, C. M. 2006. Mechanisms of antimicrobial peptide action: Studies of indolicidin assembly at model membrane interfaces by *in situ* atomic force microscopy, *J Struct Biol 154*, 42–58.
432. Shaw, J. E., Epand, R. F., Epand, R. M., Li, Z., Bittman, R., and Yip, C. M. 2006. Correlated fluorescence-atomic force microscopy of membrane domains: Structure of fluorescence probes determines lipid localization, *Biophys J 90*, 2170–2178.
433. Deng, Z., Lulevich, V., Liu, F. T., and Liu, G. Y. 2010. Applications of atomic force microscopy in biophysical chemistry of cells, *J Phys Chem B 114*, 5971–5982.
434. Franz, C. M., and Muller, D. J. 2005. Analyzing focal adhesion structure by atomic force microscopy, *J Cell Sci 118*, 5315–5323.

435. Gradinaru, C. C., Martinsson, P., Aartsma, T. J., and Schmidt, T. 2004. Simultaneous atomic-force and two-photon fluorescence imaging of biological specimens *in vivo*, *Ultramicroscopy 99*, 235–245.

436. Yu, J. P., Wang, Q., Shi, X. L., Ma, X. Y., Yang, H. Y., Chen, Y. G., and Fang, X. H. 2007. Single-molecule force spectroscopy study of interaction between transforming growth factor beta 1 and its receptor in living cells, *J Phys Chem B 111*, 13619–13625.

437. Sun, Z., Juriani, A., Meininger, G. A., and Meissner, K. E. 2009. Probing cell surface interactions using atomic force microscope cantilevers functionalized for quantum dot-enabled Förster resonance energy transfer, *J Biomed Opt 14*(4), 040502.

438. Trache, A. and Meininger, G. A. 2005. Atomic force-multi-optical imaging integrated microscope for monitoring molecular dynamics in live cells, *J Biomed Opt 10*(6), 064023.

439. Trache, A. and Lim, S. M. 2009. Integrated microscopy for real-time imaging of mechanotransduction studies in live cells, *J Biomed Opt 14*, 034024.

440. Na, S., Trache, A., Trzeciakowski, J., Sun, Z., Meininger, G. A., and Humphrey, J. D. 2008. Time-dependent changes in smooth muscle cell stiffness and focal adhesion area in response to cyclic equibiaxial stretch, *Ann Biomed Eng 36*, 369–380.

441. Trache, A. and Meininger, G. A. 2005. Atomic force-multi-optical imaging integrated microscope for monitoring molecular dynamics in live cells, *J Biomed Opt 10*, 064023.

442. Hillenbrand, R., Taubner, T., and Keilmann, F. 2002. Phonon-enhanced light matter interaction at the nanometre scale, *Nature 418*, 159–162.

443. Anderson, M. S. and Gaimari, S. D. 2003. Raman-atomic force microscopy of the ommatidial surfaces of dipteran compound eyes, *J Struct Biol 142*, 364–368.

444. Knoll, A., Magerle, R., and Krausch, G. 2001. Tapping mode atomic force microscopy on polymers: Where is the true sample surface?, *Macromolecules 34*, 4159–4165.

445. Raschke, M. B., Molina, L., Elsaesser, T., Kim, D. H., Knoll, W., and Hinrichs, K. 2005. Apertureless near-field vibrational imaging of block-copolymer nanostructures with ultrahigh spatial resolution, *ChemPhysChem 6*, 2197–2203.

446. Knoll, B. and Keilmann, F. 1999. Mid-infrared scanning near-field optical microscope resolves 30 nm, *J Microsc 194*, 512–515.

447. Paulite, M., Fakhraai, Z., Akhremitchev, B. B., Mueller, K., and Walker, G. C. 2009. Assembly, tuning and use of an apertureless near field infrared microscope for protein imaging, *J Vis Exp Nov 25*, (33).

448. Mueller, K., Yang, X., Paulite, M., Fakhraai, Z., Gunari, N., and Walker, G. C. 2008. Chemical imaging of the surface of self-assembled polystyrene-b-poly(methyl methacrylate) diblock copolymer films using apertureless near-field IR microscopy, *Langmuir 24*, 6946–6951.

449. Dazzi, A., Prazeres, R., Glotin, F., Ortega, J. M., Al-Sawaftah, M., and de Frutos, M. 2008. Chemical mapping of the distribution of viruses into infected bacteria with a photothermal method, *Ultramicroscopy 108*, 635–641.

450. Dazzi, A., Prazeres, R., Glotin, F., and Ortega, J. M. 2007. Analysis of nano-chemical mapping performed by an AFM-based ("AFMIR") acousto-optic technique, *Ultramicroscopy 107*, 1194–1200.

451. Brucherseifer, M., Kranz, C., and Mizaikoff, B. 2007. Combined *in situ* atomic force microscopy-infrared-attenuated total reflection spectroscopy, *Anal Chem 79*, 8803–8806.

452. Wang, L., Kowalik, J., Mizaikoff, B., and Kranz, C. 2010. Combining scanning electrochemical microscopy with infrared attenuated total reflection spectroscopy for *in situ* studies of electrochemically induced processes, *Anal Chem 82*, 3139–3145.

453. Wang, L., Kranz, C., and Mizaikoff, B. 2010. Monitoring scanning electrochemical microscopy approach curves with mid-infrared spectroscopy: Toward a novel current-independent positioning mode, *Anal Chem 82*, 3132–3138.

454. Verity, J. E., Chhabra, N., Sinnathamby, K., and Yip, C. M. 2009. Tracking molecular interactions in membranes by simultaneous ATR-FTIR-AFM, *Biophys J 97*, 1225–1231.

17

Parenteral Infusion Devices

Gregory I. Voss
IVAC Corporation

Robert D.
Butterfield
IVAC Corporation

The circulatory system is the body's primary pathway for both the distribution of oxygen and other nutrients and the removal of carbon dioxide and other waste products. Since the entire blood supply in a healthy adult completely circulates within 60 s, substances introduced into the circulatory system are distributed rapidly. Thus intravenous (IV) and intraarterial access routes provide an effective pathway for the delivery of fluid, blood, and medicants to a patient's vital organs. Consequently, about 80% of hospitalized patients receive infusion therapy. Peripheral and central veins are used for the majority of infusions. Umbilical artery delivery (in neonates), enteral delivery of nutrients, and epidural delivery of anesthetics and analgesics comprise smaller patient populations. A variety of devices can be used to provide flow through an intravenous catheter. An intravenous delivery system typically consists of three major components: (1) fluid or drug reservoir, (2) catheter system for transferring the fluid or drug from the reservoir into the vasculature through a venipuncture, and (3) device for regulation and/or generating flow (see Figure 17.1).

This chapter is separated into five sections. Section 17.1 describes the clinical needs associated with intravenous drug delivery that determine device performance criteria. Section 17.2 reviews the principles of flow through a tube; Section 17.3 introduces the underlying electromechanical principles for flow regulation and/or generation and their ability to meet the clinical performance criteria. Section 17.4 reviews complications associated with intravenous therapy, and Section 17.5 concludes with a short list of articles providing more detailed information.

17.1 Performance Criteria for IV Infusion Devices

The IV pathway provides an excellent route for continuous drug therapy. The ideal delivery system regulates drug concentration in the body to achieve and maintain a desired result. When the drug's effect cannot be monitored directly, it is frequently assumed that a specific blood concentration or infusion

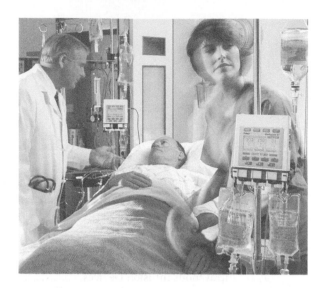

FIGURE 17.1 Typical IV infusion system.

rate will achieve the therapeutic objective. Although underinfusion may not provide sufficient therapy, overinfusion can produce even more serious toxic side effects.

The therapeutic range and risks associated with under- and overinfusion are highly drug and patient dependent. Intravenous delivery of fluids and electrolytes often does not require very accurate regulation. Low-risk patients can generally tolerate well infusion rate variability of ±30% for fluids. In some situations, however, specifically for fluid-restricted patients, prolonged under- or overinfusion of fluids can compromise the patient's cardiovascular and renal systems.

The infusion of many drugs, especially potent cardioactive agents, requires high accuracy. For example, postcoronary-artery-bypass-graft patients commonly receive sodium nitroprusside to lower arterial blood pressure. Hypertension, associated with underinfusion, subjects the graft sutures to higher stress with an increased risk for internal bleeding. Hypotension associated with overinfusion can compromise the cardiovascular state of the patient. Nitroprusside's potency, short onset delay, and short half-life (30–180 s) provide for very tight control, enabling the clinician to quickly respond to the many events that alter the patient's arterial pressure. The fast response of drugs such as nitroprusside creates a need for short-term flow uniformity as well as long-term accuracy.

The British Department of Health employs *Trumpet curves* in their Health Equipment Information reports to compare flow uniformity of infusion pumps. For a prescribed flow rate, the trumpet curve is the plot of the maximum and minimum measured percentage flow rate error as a function of the accumulation interval (Figure 17.2). Flow is measured gravimetrically in 30-s blocks for 1 h. These blocks are summed to produce 120-s, 300-s, and other longer total accumulation intervals. Though the 120-s window may not detect flow variations important in delivery of the fastest acting agents, the trumpet curve provides a helpful means for performance comparison among infusion devices. Additional statistical information such as standard deviations may be derived from the basic trumpet flow measurements.

The short half-life of certain pharmacologic agents and the clotting reaction time of blood during periods of stagnant flow require that fluid flow be maintained without significant interruption. Specifically, concern has been expressed in the literature that the infusion of sodium nitroprusside and other short half-life drugs occur without interruption exceeding 20 s. Thus, minimization of false alarms and rapid detection of occlusions are important aspects of maintaining a constant vascular concentration. Accidental occlusions of the IV line due to improper positioning of stopcocks or clamps, kinked tubing, and clotted catheters are common.

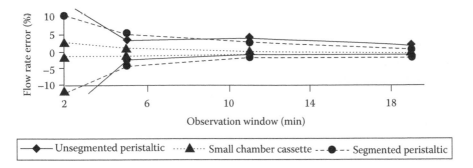

FIGURE 17.2 Trumpet curve for several representative large-volume infusion pumps operated at 5 mL/h. Note that peristaltic pumps were designed for low-risk patients.

Occlusions between pump and patient present a secondary complication in maintaining serum drug concentration. Until detected, the pump will infuse, storing fluid in the delivery set. When the occlusion is eliminated, the stored volume is delivered to the patient in a bolus. With concentrated pharmaceutic agents, this bolus can produce a large perturbation in the patient's status.

Occlusions of the pump intake also interrupt delivery. If detection is delayed, inadequate flow can result. During an intake occlusion, in some pump designs removal of the delivery set can produce abrupt aspiration of blood. This event may precipitate clotting and cause injury to the infusion site.

The common practice of delivering multiple drugs through a single venous access port produces an additional challenge to maintaining uniform drug concentration. Although some mixing will occur in the venous access catheter, fluid in the catheter more closely resembles a first-in/first-out digital queue: during delivery, drugs from the various infusion devices mix at the catheter input, an equivalent fluid volume discharges from the outlet. Rate changes and flow nonuniformity cause the mass flow of drugs at the outlet to differ from those at the input. Consider a venous access catheter with a volume of 2 mL and a total flow of 10 mL/h. Due to the digital queue phenomenon, an incremental change in the intake flow rate of an individual drug will not appear at the output for 12 min. In addition, changing flow rates for one drug will cause short-term marked swings in the delivery rate of drugs using the same access catheter. When the delay becomes significantly larger than the time constant for a drug that is titrated to a measurable patient response, titration becomes extremely difficult leading to large oscillations.

As discussed, the performance requirements for drug delivery vary with multiple factors: drug, fluid restriction, and patient risk. Thus the delivery of potent agents to fluid-restricted patients at risk requires the highest performance standards defined by flow rate accuracy, flow rate uniformity, and ability to minimize risk of IV-site complications. These performance requirements need to be appropriately balanced with the device cost and the impact on clinician productivity.

17.2 Flow through an IV Delivery System

The physical properties associated with the flow of fluids through cylindrical tubes provide the foundation for understanding flow through a catheter into the vasculature. Hagen–Poiseuille's equation for laminar flow of a Newtonian fluid through a rigid tube states

$$Q = \pi \cdot r^4 \cdot \frac{(P_1 - P_2)}{8 \cdot \eta \cdot L} \tag{17.1}$$

where Q is the flow; P_1 and P_2 are the pressures at the inlet and outlet of the tube, respectively; L and r are the length and internal radius of the tube, respectively; and η is fluid viscosity. Although many drug delivery systems do not strictly meet the flow conditions for precise application of the laminar flow

TABLE 17.1   Resistance Measurements for Catheter Components Used for Infusion

Component	Length, cm	Flow Resistance, Fluid ohm, mmHg/(L/h)
Standard administration set	91–213	4.3–5.3
Extension tube for CVP monitoring	15	15.5
19-gauge epidural catheter	91	290.4–497.1
18-gauge needle	6–9	14.1–17.9
23-gauge needle	2.5–9	165.2–344.0
25-gauge needle	1.5–4.0	525.1–1412.0
Vicra Quick-Cath 18-gauge catheter	5	12.9
Extension set with 0.22 μm air-eliminating filter		623.0
0.2 μm filter		555.0

Note: Mean values are presented over a range of infusions (100, 200, and 300 mL/h) and sample size ($n = 10$).

equation, it does provide insight into the relationship between flow and pressure in a catheter. The fluid analog of Ohms Law describes the resistance to flow under constant flow conditions:

$$R = \frac{P_1 - P_2}{Q} \tag{17.2}$$

Thus, resistance to flow through a tube correlates directly with catheter length and fluid viscosity and inversely with the fourth power of catheter diameter. For steady flow, the delivery system can be modeled as a series of resistors representing each component, including administration set, access catheter, and circulatory system. When dynamic aspects of the delivery system are considered, a more detailed model including catheter and venous compliance, fluid inertia, and turbulent flow is required. Flow resistance may be defined with units of mm Hg/(L/h), so that 1 fluid ohm $= 4.8 \times 10^{-11}$ Pa s/m^3. Studies determining flow resistance for several catheter components with distilled water for flow rates of 100, 200, and 300 mL/h appear in Table 17.1.

17.3 Intravenous Infusion Devices

From Hagen–Poiselluie's equation, two general approaches to intravenous infusion become apparent. First, a hydrostatic pressure gradient can be used with adjustment of delivery system resistance controlling flow rate. Complications such as partial obstructions result in reduced flow which may be detected by an automatic flow monitor. Second, a constant displacement flow source can be used. Now complications may be detected by monitoring elevated fluid pressure and/or flow resistance. At the risk of overgeneralization, the relative strengths of each approach will be presented.

17.3.1 Gravity Flow/Resistance Regulation

The simplest means for providing regulated flow employs gravity as the driving force with a roller clamp as controlled resistance. Placement of the fluid reservoir 60–100 cm above the patient's right atrium provides a hydrostatic pressure gradient P_h equal to 1.34 mm Hg/cm of elevation. The modest physiologic mean pressure in the veins, P_v, minimally reduces the net hydrostatic pressure gradient. The equation for flow becomes

$$Q = \frac{P_h - P_v}{R_{mfr} + R_n} \tag{17.3}$$

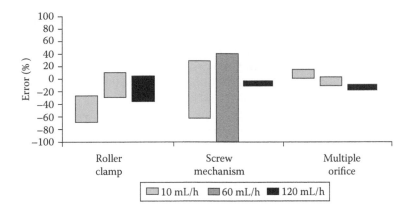

FIGURE 17.3 Drift in flow rate (mean ± standard deviation) over a 4-h period for three mechanical flow regulators at initial flow rates of 10, 60, and 120 mL/h with distilled water at constant hydrostatic pressure gradient.

where R_{mfr} and R_n are the resistance to flow through the mechanical flow regulator and the remainder of the delivery system, respectively. Replacing the variables with representative values for an infusion of 5% saline solution into a healthy adult at 100 mL/h yields

$$100 \text{ mL/h} = \frac{(68 - 8) \text{ mmHg}}{(550 + 50) \text{ mmHg/(L/h)}} \tag{17.4}$$

Gravity flow cannot be used for arterial infusions since the higher vascular pressure exceeds available hydrostatic pressure.

Flow stability in a gravity infusion system is subject to variations in hydrostatic and venous pressure as well as catheter resistance. However, the most important factor is the change in flow regulator resistance caused by viscoelastic creep of the tubing wall (see Figure 17.3). Caution must be used in assuming that a preset flow regulator setting will accurately provide a predetermined rate. The clinician typically estimates flow rate by counting the frequency of drops falling through an in-line drip-forming chamber, adjusting the clamp to obtain the desired drop rate. The cross-sectional area of the drip chamber orifice is the major determinant of drop volume. Various manufacturers provide minidrip sets designed for pediatric (e.g., 60 drops/mL) and regular sets designed for adult (10–20 drops/mL) patients. Tolerances on the drip chamber can cause a 3% error in minidrip sets and a 17% error in regular sets at 125 mL/h flow rate with 5% dextrose in water. Mean drop size for rapid rates increased by as much as 25% over the size of drops which form slowly. In addition, variation in the specific gravity and surface tension of fluids can provide an additional large source of drop size variability.

Some mechanical flow regulating devices incorporate the principle of a Starling resistor. In a Starling device, resistance is proportional to hydrostatic pressure gradient. Thus, the device provides a negative feedback mechanism to reduce flow variation as the available pressure gradient changes with time.

Mechanical flow regulators comprise the largest segment of intravenous infusion systems, providing the simplest means of operation. Patient transport is simple, since these devices require no electric power. Mechanical flow regulators are most useful where the patient is not fluid restricted and the acceptable therapeutic rate range of the drug is relatively wide with minimal risk of serious adverse sequelae. The most common use for these systems is the administration of fluids and electrolytes.

17.3.2 Volumetric Infusion Pumps

Active pumping infusion devices combine electronics with a mechanism to generate flow. These devices have higher performance standards than simple gravity flow regulators. The Association for the

Advancement of Medical Instrumentation (AAMI) recommends that long-term rate accuracy for infusion pumps remain within ±10% of the set rate for general infusion and, for the more demanding applications, that long-term flow remains within ±5%. Such requirements typically extend to those agents with narrow therapeutic indices and/or low flow rates, such as the neonatal population or other fluid-restricted patients. The British Department of Health has established three main categories for hospital-based infusion devices: neonatal infusions, high-risk infusions, and low-risk infusions. Infusion control for neonates requires the highest performance standards, because their size severely restricts fluid volume. A fourth category, ambulatory infusion, pertains to pumps worn by patients.

17.3.3 Controllers

These devices automate the process of adjusting the mechanical flow regulator. The most common controllers utilize sensors to count the number of drops passing through the drip chamber to provide flow feedback for automatic rate adjustment. Flow rate accuracy remains limited by the rate and viscosity dependence of drop size. Delivery set motion associated with ambulation and improper angulation of the drip chamber can also hinder accurate rate detection.

An alternative to the drop counter is a volumetric metering chamber. A McGaw Corporation controller delivery set uses a rigid chamber divided by a flexible membrane. Instrument-controlled valves allow fluid to fill one chamber from the fluid reservoir, displacing the membrane driving the fluid from the second chamber toward the patient. When inlet and outlet valves reverse state, the second chamber is filled while the first chamber delivers to the patient. The frequency of state change determines the average flow rate. Volumetric accuracy demands primarily on the dimensional tolerances of the chamber. Although volumetric controllers may provide greater accuracy than drop-counting controllers, their disposables are inherently more complex, and maximum flow is still limited by head height and system resistance.

Beyond improvements in flow rate accuracy, controllers should provide an added level of patient safety by quickly detecting IV-site complications. The IVAC Corporation has developed a series of controllers employing pulsed modulated flow providing for monitoring of flow resistance as well as improved accuracy.

The maximum flow rate achieved by gravimetric based infusion systems can become limited by R_n and by concurrent infusion from other sources through the same catheter. In drop-counting devices, flow rate uniformity suffers at low flow rates from the discrete nature of the drop detector.

In contrast with infusion controllers, pumps generate flow by mechanized displacement of the contents of a volumetric chamber. Typical designs provide high flow rate accuracy and uniformity for a wide rate range (0.1–1000.0 mL/h) of infusion rates. Rate error correlates directly with effective chamber volume, which, in turn, depends on both instrument and disposable repeatability, precision, and stability under varying load. Stepper or servo-controlled dc motors are typically used to provide the driving force for the fluid. At low flow rates, dc motors usually operate in a discrete stepping mode. On average, each step propels a small quanta of fluid toward the patient. Flow rate uniformity therefore is a function of both the average volume per quanta and the variation in volume. Mechanism factors influencing rate uniformity include: stepping resolution, gearing and activator geometries, volumetric chamber coupling geometry, and chamber elasticity. When the quanta volume is not inherently uniform over the mechanism's cycle, software control has been used to compensate for the variation.

17.3.4 Syringe Pumps

These pumps employ a syringe as both reservoir and volumetric pumping chamber. A precision lead-screw is used to produce constant linear advancement of the syringe plunger. Except for those ambulatory systems that utilize specific microsyringes, pumps generally accept syringes ranging in size from 5 to 100 mL. Flow rate accuracy and uniformity are determined by both mechanism displacement characteristics and tolerance on the internal syringe diameter. Since syringe mechanisms can generate a specified linear travel with less than 1% error, the manufacturing tolerance on the internal cross-sectional area of the syringe largely determines flow rate accuracy. Although syringes can be manufactured to tighter tolerances, standard plastic syringes provide long-term accuracy of ±5%. Flow rate uniformity, however, can benefit from the ability to select syringe size (see Figure 17.4). Since many syringes have similar stroke length, diameter variation provides control of volume. Also the linear advancement per step is typically fixed. Therefore selection of a lower-volume syringe provides smaller-volume quanta. This allows tradeoffs among drug concentration, flow rate, and duration of flow per syringe. Slack in the gear train and drive shaft coupling as well as plunger slip cause rate inaccuracies during the initial stages of delivery (see Figure 17.5a).

Since the syringe volumes are typically much smaller than reservoirs used with other infusion devices, syringe pumps generally deliver drugs in either fluid-restricted environments or for short duration. With high-quality syringes, flow rate uniformity in syringe pumps is generally superior to that accomplished by other infusion pumps. With the drug reservoir enclosed within the device, syringe pumps manage patient transport well, including the operating room environment.

Cassette pumps conceptually mimic the piston type action of the syringe pump but provide an automated means of repeatedly emptying and refilling the cassette. The process of refilling the cassette in single piston devices requires an interruption in flow (see Figure 17.5b). The length of interruption relative to the drug's half-life determines the impact of the refill period on hemodynamic stability. To eliminate the interruption caused by refill, dual piston devices alternate refill and delivery states, providing nearly continuous output. Others implement cassettes with very small volumes which can refill in less than a second (see Figure 17.2). Tight control of the internal cross-sectional area of the pumping chamber provides exceptional flow rate accuracy. Manufacturers have recently developed remarkably small cassette pumps that can still generate the full spectrum of infusion rate (0.1–999.0 mL/h). These systems combine pumping chamber, inlet and outlet valving, pressure sensing, and air detection into a single complex component.

Peristaltic pumps operate on a short segment of the IV tubing. Peristaltic pumps can be separated into two subtypes. Rotary peristaltic mechanisms operate by compressing the pumping segment against the rotor housing with rollers mounted on the housing. With rotation, the rollers push fluid from the container through the tubing toward the patient. At least one of the rollers completely occludes the tubing against the housing at all times precluding free flow from the reservoir to the patient. During a portion of the revolution, two rollers trap fluid in the intervening pumping segment. The captured volume between the rollers determines volumetric accuracy. Linear peristaltic pumps hold the pumping segment in a channel pressed against a rigid backing plate. An array of cam-driven actuators sequentially occlude the segment starting with the section nearest the reservoir forcing fluid toward the patient with a sinusoidal wave action. In a typical design using uniform motor step intervals, a characteristic flow wave resembling a positively biased sine wave is produced (see Figure 17.5c).

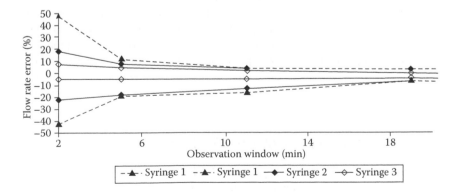

FIGURE 17.4   Effect of syringe type on trumpet curve of a syringe pump at 1 mL/h.

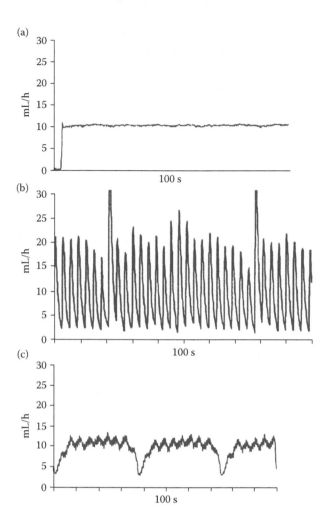

FIGURE 17.5 Continuous flow pattern for a representative, (a) syringe, (b) cassette, and (c) linear peristaltic pump at 10 mL/h.

Infusion pumps provide significant advantages over both manual flow regulators and controllers in several categories. Infusion pumps can provide accurate delivery over a wide range of infusion rates (0.1–999.0 mL/h). Neither elevated system resistance nor distal line pressure limit the maximum infusion rate. Infusion pumps can support a wider range of applications including arterial infusions, spinal and epidural infusions, and infusions into pulmonary artery or central venous catheters. Flow rate accuracy of infusion pumps is highly dependent on the segment employed as the pumping chamber (see Figure 17.2). Incorporating special syringes or pumping segments can significantly improve flow rate accuracy (see Figure 17.6). Both manufacturing tolerances and segment material composition significantly dictate flow rate accuracy. Time- and temperature-related properties of the pumping segment further impact long-term drift in flow rate.

17.4 Managing Occlusions of the Delivery System

One of the most common problems in managing an IV delivery system is the rapid detection of occlusion in the delivery system. With a complete occlusion, the resistance to flow approaches infinity. In this condition, gravimetric-based devices cease to generate flow. Mechanical flow regulators have no

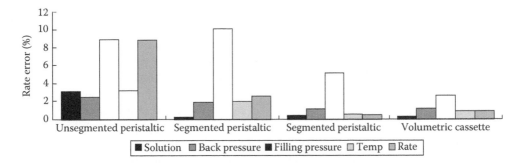

FIGURE 17.6 Impact of five variables on flow rate accuracy in four different infusion pumps. Variables tested included solution: Distilled water and 25% dextrose in water, back pressure: −100 and 300 mm Hg, pumping segment filling pressure: −30 inches of water and +30 inches of water, temperature: 10°C and 40°C, and infusion rate: 5 mL/h and 500 mL/h. Note: First and second peristaltic mechanism qualified for low-risk patients, while the third peristaltic device qualified for high-risk patients.

mechanism for adverse event detection and thus must rely on the clinician to identify an occlusion as part of routine patient care. Electronic controllers sense the absence of flow and alarm in response to their inability to sustain the desired flow rate.

The problem of rapidly detecting an occlusion in an infusion pump is more complex. Upstream occlusions that occur between the fluid reservoir and the pumping mechanism impact the system quite differently than downstream occlusions which occur between the pump and the patient. When an occlusion occurs downstream from an infusion pump, the pump continues to propel fluid into the section of tubing between the pump and the occlusion. The time rate of pressure rise in that section increases in direct proportion to flow rate and inversely with tubing compliance (compliance, C, is the volume increase in a closed tube per mm Hg pressure applied). The most common approach to detecting downstream occlusion requires a pressure transducer immediately below the pumping mechanism. These devices generate an alarm when either the mean pressure or rate of change in pressure exceeds a threshold. For pressure-limited designs, the time to downstream alarm (TTA) may be estimated as

$$\text{TTA} = \frac{P_\text{alarm} \cdot C_\text{delivery-set}}{\text{flow rate}} \tag{17.5}$$

Using a representative tubing compliance of 1 μL/mm Hg, flow rate of 1 mL/h, and a fixed alarm threshold set of 500 mm Hg, the time to alarm becomes

$$\text{TTA} = \frac{500_\text{mmHg} \cdot 1000 \text{ mL/mmHg}}{1 \text{ mL/h}} = 30 \text{ min} \tag{17.6}$$

where TTA is the time from occlusion to alarm detection. Pressure-based detection algorithms depend on accuracy and stability of the sensing system. Lowering the threshold on absolute or relative pressure for occlusion alarm reduces the TTA, but at the cost of increasing the likelihood of false alarms. Patient movement, patient-to-pump height variations, and other clinical circumstances can cause wide perturbations in line pressure. To optimize the balance between fast TTA and minimal false alarms, some infusion pumps allow the alarm threshold to be set by the clinician or be automatically shifted upward in response to alarms; other pumps attempt to optimize performance by varying pressure alarm thresholds with flow rate.

A second approach to detection of downstream occlusions uses motor torque as an indirect measure of the load seen by the pumping mechanism. Although this approach eliminates the need for a pressure sensor, it introduces additional sources for error including friction in the gear mechanism or pumping mechanism that requires additional safety margins to protect against false alarms. In syringe pumps, where the coefficient of static friction of the syringe bung (rubber end of the syringe plunger) against the syringe wall can be substantial, occlusion detection can exceed 1 h at low flow rates.

Direct, continuous measurement of downstream flow resistance may provide a monitoring modality which overcomes the disadvantages of pressure-based alarm systems, especially at low infusion rates. Such a monitoring system would have the added advantage of performance unaffected by flow rate, hydrostatic pressure variations, and motion artifacts.

Upstream occlusions can cause large negative pressures as the pumping mechanism generates a vacuum on the upstream tubing segment. The tube may collapse and the vacuum may pull air through the tubing walls or form cavitation bubbles. A pressure sensor situated above the mechanism or a pressure sensor below the mechanism synchronized with filling of the pumping chamber can detect the vacuum associated with an upstream occlusion. Optical or ultrasound transducers, situated below the mechanism, can detect air bubbles in the catheter, and air-eliminating filters can remove air, preventing large air emboli from being introduced into the patient.

Some of the most serious complications of IV therapy occur at the venipuncture site; these include extravasation, postinfusion phlebitis (and thrombophlebitis), IV-related infections, ecchymosis, and hematomas. Other problems that do not occur as frequently include speed shock and allergic reactions.

Extravasation (or infiltration) is the inadvertent perfusion of infusate into the interstitial tissue. Reported percentage of patients to whom extravasation has occurred ranges from 10% to over 25%. Tissue damage does not occur frequently, but the consequences can be severe, including skin necrosis requiring significant plastic and reconstructive surgery and amputation of limbs. The frequency of extravasation injury correlates with age, state of consciousness, and venous circulation of the patient as well as the type, location, and placement of the intravenous cannula. Drugs that have high osmolality, vessicant properties, or the ability to induce ischemia correlate with frequency of extravasation injury. Neonatal and pediatric patients who possess limited communication skills, constantly move, and have small veins that are difficult to cannulate require superior vigilance to protect against extravasation.

Since interstitial tissue provides a greater resistance to fluid flow than the venous pathway, infusion devices with accurate and precise pressure monitoring systems have been used to detect small pressure increases due to extravasation. To successfully implement this technique requires diligence by the clinician, since patient movement, flow rate, catheter resistance, and venous pressure variations can obscure the small pressure variations resulting from the extravasation. Others have investigated the ability of a pumping mechanism to withdraw blood as indicative of problems in a patent line. The catheter tip, however, may be partially in and out of the vein such that infiltration occurs yet blood can be withdrawn from the patient. A vein might also collapse under negative pressure in a patent line without successful blood withdrawal. Techniques currently being investigated which monitor infusion impedance (resistance and compliance) show promise for assisting in the detection of extravasation.

When a catheter tip wedges into the internal lining of the vein wall, it is considered positional. With the fluid path restricted by the vein wall, increases in line resistance may indicate a positional catheter. With patient movement, for example wrist flexation, the catheter may move in and out of the positional state. Since a positional catheter is thought to be more prone toward extravasation than other catheters, early detection of a positional catheter and appropriate adjustment of catheter position may be helpful in reducing the frequency of extravasation.

Postinfusion phlebitis is acute inflammation of a vein used for IV infusion. The chief characteristic is a reddened area or red streak that follows the course of the vein with tenderness, warmth, and edema at the venipuncture site. The vein, which normally is very compliant, also hardens. Phlebitis positively correlates with infusion rate and with the infusion of vesicants.

Fluid overload and speed shock result from the accidental administration of a large fluid volume over a short interval. Speed shock associates more frequently with the delivery of potent medications, rather than fluids. These problems most commonly occur with manually regulated IV systems, which do not provide the safety features of instrumented lines. Many IV sets designed for instrumented operation will free flow when the set is removed from the instrument without manual clamping. To protect against this possibility, some sets are automatically placed in the occluded state on disengagement. Although an apparent advantage, reliance on such automatic devices may create a false sense of security and lead to manual errors with sets not incorporating these features.

17.5 Summary

Intravenous infusion has become the mode of choice for delivery of a large class of fluids and drugs both in hospital and alternative care settings. Modern infusion devices provide the clinician with a wide array of choices for performing intravenous therapy. Selection of the appropriate device for a specified application requires understanding of drug pharmacology and pharmacokinetics, fluid mechanics, and device design and performance characteristics. Continuing improvements in performance, safety, and cost of these systems will allow even broader utilization of intravenous delivery in a variety of settings.

References

Association for the Advancement of Medical Instrumentation. 1992. *Standard for Infusion Devices.* Arlington.

Bohony J. 1993. Nine common intravenous complications and what to do about them. *Am. J. Nurs.* 10: 45.

British Department of Health. 1990. *Evaluation of Infusion Pumps and Controllers.* HEI Report #198.

Glass P.S.A., Jacobs J.R., Reves J.G. 1991. Technology for continuous infusions in anesthesia. Continuous infusions in anesthesia. *Int. Anesthesiol. Clin.* 29: 39.

MacCara M. 1983. Extravasation: A hazard of intravenous therapy. *Drug Intell. Clin. Pharm.* 17: 713.

Further Information

Peter Glass provides a strong rationale for intravenous therapy including pharmacokinetic and pharmaco-dynamic bases for continuous delivery. Clinical complications around intravenous therapy are well summarized by MacCara (1983) and Bohony (1993). The AAMI Standard for Infusion Devices provides a comprehensive means of evaluating infusion device technology, and the British Department of Health OHEI Report #198 provides a competitive analysis of pumps and controllers.

18

Clinical Laboratory: Separation and Spectral Methods

Richard L. Roa
Baylor University Medical Center

18.1 Introduction

The purpose of the clinical laboratory is to analyze body fluids and tissues for specific substances of interest and to report the results in a form which is of value to clinicians in the diagnosis and treatment of disease. A large range of tests has been developed to achieve this purpose. Four terms commonly used to describe tests are *accuracy, precision, sensitivity,* and *specificity*. An accurate test, on average, yields true values. Precision is the ability of a test to produce identical results upon repeated trials. Sensitivity is a measure of how small an amount of substance can be measured. Specificity is the degree to which a test measures the substance of interest without being affected by other substances which may be present in greater amounts.

The first step in many laboratory tests is to separate the material of interest from other substances. This may be accomplished through extraction, filtration, and centrifugation. Another step is derivatization, in which the substance of interest is chemically altered through addition of reagents to change it into a substance which is easily measured. For example, one method for measuring glucose is to add otoluidine which, under proper conditions, forms a green-colored solution with an absorption maximum at 630 nm. Separation and derivatization both improve the specificity required of good tests.

18.2 Separation Methods

Centrifuges are used to separate materials on the basis of their relative densities. The most common use in the laboratory is the separation of cells and platelets from the liquid part of the blood. This requires a relative centrifugal force (RCF) of roughly 1000*g* (1000 times the force of gravity) for a period of 10 min.

Relative centrifugal force is a function of the speed of rotation and the distance of the sample from the center of rotation as stated in Equation 18.1

$$RCF = (1.12 \times 10^{-5}) \, r(rpm)^2 \tag{18.1}$$

where RCF is the relative centrifugal force in g, and r is the radius in cm.

Some mixtures require higher g-loads in order to achieve separation in a reasonable period of time. Special rotors contain the sample tubes inside a smooth container, which minimizes air resistance to allow faster rotational speeds. Refrigerated units maintain the samples at a cool temperature throughout long high-speed runs which could lead to sample heating due to air friction on the rotor. Ultracentrifuges operate at speeds on the order of 100,000 rpm and provide relative centrifugal forces of up to 600,000g. These usually require vacuum pumps to remove the air which would otherwise retard the rotation and heat the rotor.

18.3 Chromatographic Separations

Chromatographic separations depend upon the different rates at which various substances moving in a stream (mobile phase) are retarded by a stationary material (stationary phase) as they pass over it. The mobile phase can be a volatilized sample transported by an inert carrier gas such as helium or a liquid transported by an organic solvent such as acetone. Stationary phases are quite diverse depending upon the separation being made, but most are contained within a long, thin tube (column). Liquid stationary phases may be used by coating them onto inert packing materials. When a sample is introduced into a chromatographic column, it is carried through it by the mobile phase. As it passes through the column, the substances which have greater affinity for the stationary phase fall behind those with less affinity. The separated substances may be detected as individual peaks by a suitable detector placed at the end of the chromatographic column.

18.4 Gas Chromatography

The most common instrumental chromatographic method used in the clinical laboratory is the gas–liquid chromatograph. In this system the mobile phase is a gas, and the stationary phase is a liquid coated onto either an inert support material, in the case of a packed column, or the inner walls of a very thin tube, in the case of a capillary column. Capillary columns have the greatest resolving power but cannot handle large sample quantities. The sample is injected into a small heated chamber at the beginning of the column, where it is volatilized if it is not already a gaseous sample. The sample is then carried through the column by an inert carrier gas, typically helium or nitrogen. The column is completely housed within an oven. Many gas chromatographs allow for the oven temperature to be programmed to slowly increase for a set time after the sample injection is made. This produces peaks which are spread more uniformly over time.

Four detection methods commonly used with gas chromatography are thermal conductivity, flame ionization, nitrogen/phosphorous, and mass spectrometry. The thermal conductivity detector takes advantage of variations in thermal conductivity between the carrier gas and the gas being measured. A heated filament immersed in the gas leaving the chromatographic column is part of a Wheatstone bridge circuit. Small variations in the conductivity of the gas cause changes in the resistance of the filament, which are recorded. The flame ionization detector measures the current between two plates with a voltage applied between them. When an organic material appears in the flame, ions which contribute to the current are formed. The NP detector, or nitrogen/phosphorous detector, is a modified flame ionization detector (see Figure 18.1) which is particularly sensitive to nitrogen- and phosphorous-containing compounds.

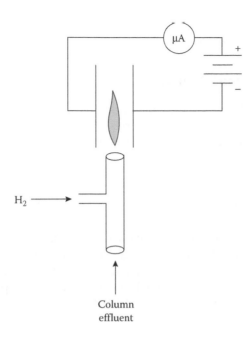

FIGURE 18.1   Flame ionization detector. Organic compounds in the column effluent are ionized in the flame, producing a current proportional to the amount of the compound present.

Mass spectrometry (MS) provides excellent sensitivity and selectivity. The concept behind these devices is that the volatilized sample molecules are broken into ionized fragments which are then passed through a mass analyzer that separates the fragments according to their mass/charge (m/z) ratios. A mass spectrum, which is a plot of the relative abundance of the various fragments versus m/z, is produced. The mass spectrum is characteristic of the molecule sampled. The mass analyzer most commonly used with gas chromatographs is the quadrupole detector, which consists of four rods that have dc and RF voltages applied to them. The m/z spectrum can be scanned by appropriate changes in the applied voltages. The detector operates in a manner similar to that of a photomultiplier tube except that the collision of the charged particles with the cathode begins the electron cascade, resulting in a measurable electric pulse for each charged particle captured. The MS must operate in a high vacuum, which requires good pumps and a porous barrier between the GC and MS that limits the amount of carrier gas entering the MS.

18.5 High-Performance Liquid Chromatography

In liquid chromatography, the mobile phase is liquid. High-performance liquid chromatography (HPLC) refers to systems which obtain excellent resolution in a reasonable time by forcing the mobile phase at high pressure through a long thin column. The most common pumps used are pistons driven by asymmetrical cams. By using two such pumps in parallel and operating out of phase, pressure fluctuations can be minimized. Typical pressures are 350–1500 psi, though the pressure may be as high as 10,000 psi. Flow rates are in the 1–10 mL/min range.

A common method for placing a sample onto the column is with a loop injector, consisting of a loop of tubing which is filled with the sample. By a rotation of the loop, it is brought in seriés with the column, and the sample is carried onto the column. A UV/visible spectrophotometer is often used as a detector for this method. A mercury arc lamp with the 254-nm emission isolated is useful for detection of aromatic compounds, while diode array detectors allow a complete spectrum from 190 to 600 nm in 10 ms.

This provides for detection and identification of compounds as they come off the column. Fluorescent, electrochemical, and mass analyzer detectors are also used.

18.6 Basis for Spectral Methods

Spectral methods rely on the absorption or emission of electromagnetic radiation by the sample of interest. Electromagnetic radiation is often described in terms of frequency or wavelength. Wavelengths are those obtained in a vacuum and may be calculated with the formula

$$\lambda = c/v \tag{18.2}$$

where λ is the wavelength in meters, c the speed of light in vacuum (3×10^8 m/s), and v the frequency in Hz.

The frequency range of interest for most clinical laboratory work consists of the visible (390–780 nm) and the ultraviolet or UV (180–390 nm) ranges. Many substances absorb different wavelengths preferentially. When this occurs in the visible region, they are colored. In general, the color of a substance is the complement of the color it absorbs, for example, absorption in the blue produces a yellow color. For a given wavelength or bandwidth, transmittance is defined as

$$T = \frac{I_t}{I_i} \tag{18.3}$$

where T is the transmittance ratio (often expressed as %), I_i the incident light intensity, and I_t the transmitted light intensity. Absorbance is defined as

$$A = -\log_{10} 1/T \tag{18.4}$$

Under suitable conditions, the absorbance of a solution with an absorbing compound dissolved in it is proportional to the concentration of that compound as well as the path length of light through it. This relationship is expressed by Beer's law:

$$A = abc \tag{18.5}$$

where A is the absorbance, a a constant, b the path length, and c the concentration.

A number of situations may cause deviations from Beer's law, such as high concentration or mixtures of compounds which absorb at the wavelength of interest. From an instrumental standpoint, the primary causes are stray light and excessive spectral bandwidth. Stray light refers to any light reaching the detector other than light from the desired pass-band which has passed through sample. Sources of stray light may include room light leaking into the detection chamber, scatter from the cuvette, and undesired *fluorescence*.

A typical spectrophotometer consists of a light source, some form of wavelength selection, and a detector for measuring the light transmitted through the samples. There is no single light source that covers the entire visible and UV spectrum. The source most commonly used for the visible part of the spectrum is the tungsten–halogen lamp, which provides continuous radiation over the range of 360–950 nm. The deuterium lamp has become the standard for much UV work. It covers the range from 220 to 360 nm. Instruments which cover the entire UV/visible range use both lamps with a means for switching from one lamp to the other at a wavelength of approximately 360 nm (Figure 18.2).

Wavelength selection is accomplished with filters, prisms, and diffraction gratings. Specially designed interference filters can provide bandwidths as small as 5 nm. These are useful for instruments which do

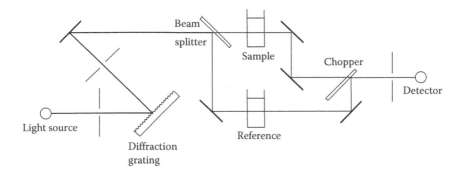

FIGURE 18.2 Dual-beam spectrophotometer. The diffraction grating is rotated to select the desired wavelength. The beam splitter consists of a half-silvered mirror which passes half the light while reflecting the other half. A rotating mirror with cut-out sections (chopper) alternately directs one beam and then the other to the detector.

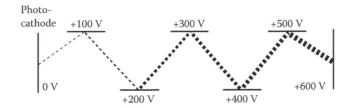

FIGURE 18.3 Photomultiplier tube. Incident photons cause the photocathode to emit electrons which collide with the first dynode which emits additional electrons. Multiple dynodes provide sufficient gain to produce an easily measurable electric pulse from a single photon.

not need to scan a range of wavelengths. Prisms produce a nonlinear dispersion of wavelengths with the longer wavelengths closer together than the shorter ones. Since the light must pass through the prism material, they must be made of quartz for UV work. Diffraction gratings are surfaces with 1000–3000 grooves/mm cut into them. They may be transmissive or reflective; the reflective ones are more popular since there is no attenuation of light by the material. They produce a linear dispersion. By proper selection of slit widths, pass bands of 0.1 nm are commonly achieved.

The most common detector is the photomultiplier tube, which consists of a photosensitive cathode that emits electrons in proportion to the intensity of light striking it (Figure 18.3). A series of 10–15 dynodes, each at 50–100 V greater potential than the preceding one, produce an electron amplification of 4–6 per stage. Overall gains are typically a million or more. Photomultiplier tubes respond quickly and cover the entire spectral range. They require a high voltage supply and can be damaged if exposed to room light while the high voltage is applied.

18.7 Fluorometry

Certain molecules absorb a photon's energy and then emit a photon with less energy (longer wavelength). When the reemission occurs in less than 10^{-8} s, the process is known as fluorescence. This physical process provides the means for assays which are 10–100 times as sensitive as those based on absorption measurements. This increase in sensitivity is largely because the light measured is all from the sample of interest. A dim light is easily measured against a black background, while it may be lost if added to an already bright background.

Fluorometers and spectrofluorometers are very similar to photometers and spectrophotometers but with two major differences. Fluorometers and spectrofluorometers use two monochrometers, one for

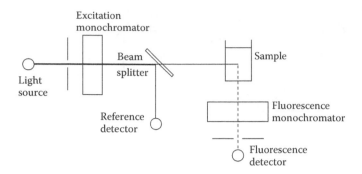

FIGURE 18.4   Spectrofluorometer. Fluorescence methods can be extremely sensitive to the low background interference. Since the detector is off-axis from the incident light and a second monochromator blocks light of wavelengths illuminating the sample, virtually no signal reaches the detector other than the desired fluorescence.

excitation light and one for emitted light. By proper selection of the bandpass regions, all the light used to excite the sample can be blocked from the detector, assuring that the detector sees only fluorescence. The other difference is that the detector is aligned off-axis, commonly at 90°, from the excitation source. At this angle, scatter is minimal, which helps ensure a dark background for the measured fluorescence. Some spectrofluorometers use polarization filters both on the input and output light beams, which allows for fluorescence polarization studies (Figure 18.4). An intense light source in the visible-to-UV range is desirable. A common source is the xenon or mercury arc lamps, which provide a continuum of radiation over this range.

18.8 Flame Photometry

Flame photometry is used to measure sodium, potassium, and lithium in body fluids. When these elements are heated in a flame they emit characteristic wavelengths of light. The major emission lines are 589 nm (yellow) for sodium, 767 nm (violet) for potassium, and 671 nm (red) for lithium. An atomizer introduces a fine mist of the sample into a flame. For routine laboratory use, a propane and compressed air flame is adequate. High-quality interference filters with narrow pass bands are often used to isolate the major emission lines. The narrow band pass is necessary to maximize the signal-to-noise ratio. Since it is impossible to maintain stable aspiration, atomization, and flame characteristics, it is necessary to use an internal standard of known concentration while making measurements of unknowns. In this way the ratio of the unknown sample's emission to the internal standard's emission remains stable even as the total signal fluctuates. An internal standard is usually an element which is found in very low concentration in the sample fluid. By adding a high concentration of this element to the sample, its concentration can be known to a high degree of accuracy. Lithium, potassium, and cesium all may be used as internal standards depending upon the particular assay being conducted.

18.9 Atomic Absorption Spectroscopy

Atomic absorption spectroscopy is based on the fact that just as metal elements have unique emission lines, they have identical absorption lines when in a gaseous or dissociated state. The atomic absorption spectrometer takes advantage of these physical characteristics in a clever manner, producing an instrument with approximately 100 times the sensitivity of a flame photometer for similar elements. The sample is aspirated into a flame, where the majority of the atoms of the element being measured remain in the ground state, where they are capable of absorbing light at their characteristic wavelengths. An intense source of exactly these wavelengths is produced by a hollow cathode lamp. These lamps are constructed so that the cathode is made from the element to be measured, and the lamps are filled with a low pressure of argon or neon gas. When a current is passed through the lamp, metal atoms are sputtered off the cathode and collide with the argon or neon in the tube, producing emission of the characteristic wavelengths. A monochromator and photodetector complete the system.

Light reaching the detector is a combination of that which is emitted by the sample (undesirable) and light from the hollow cathode lamp which was not absorbed by the sample in the flame (desirable). By pulsing the light from the lamp either by directly pulsing the lamp or with a chopper, and using a detector which is sensitive to ac signals and insensitive to dc signals, the undesirable emission signal is eliminated. Each element to be measured requires a lamp with that element present in the cathode. Multielement lamps have been developed to minimize the number of lamps required. Atomic absorption spectrophotometers may be either single beam or double beam; the double-beam instruments have greater stability.

There are various flameless methods for atomic absorption spectroscopy in which the burner is replaced with a method for vaporizing the element of interest without a flame. The graphite furnace which heats the sample to 2700° consists of a hollow graphite tube which is heated by passing a large current through it. The sample is placed within the tube, and the light beam is passed through it while the sample is heated.

18.10 Turbidimetry and Nephelometry

Light scattering by particles in solution is directly proportional to both concentration and molecular weight of the particles. For small molecules the scattering is insignificant, but for proteins, immunoglobulins, immune complexes, and other large particles, light scattering can be an effective method for the detection and measurement of particle concentration. For a given wavelength λ of light and particle size d, scattering is described as Raleigh ($d < \lambda/10$), Raleigh–Debye ($d \approx \lambda$), or Mie ($d > 10\,\lambda$). For particles that are small compared to the wavelength, the scattering is equal in all directions. However, as the particle size becomes larger than the wavelength of light, it becomes preferentially scattered in the forward direction. Light-scattering techniques are widely used to detect the formation of antigen–antibody complexes in immunoassays.

When light scattering is measured by the attenuation of a beam of light through a solution, it is called *turbidimetry*. This is essentially the same as absorption measurements with a photometer except that a large passband is acceptable. When maximum sensitivity is required a different method is used—direct measurement of the scattered light with a detector placed at an angle to the central beam. This method is called *nephelometry*. A typical nephelometer will have a light source, filter, sample cuvette, and detector set at an angle to the incident beam (Figure 18.5).

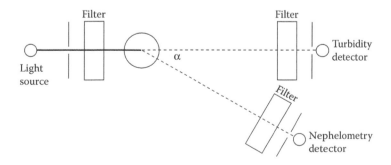

FIGURE 18.5 Nephelometer. Light scattered by large molecules is measured at an angle α away from the axis of incident light. The filters select the wavelength range desired and block undesired fluorescence. When $\alpha = 0$, the technique is known as turbidimetry.

Defining Terms

Accuracy: The degree to which the average value of repeated measurements approximate the true value being measured.

Fluorescence: Emission of light by an atom or molecule following absorption of a photon by greater energy. Emission normally occurs within 10^{-8} of absorption.

Nephelometry: Measurement of the amount of light scattered by particles suspended in a fluid.

Precision: A measure of test reproducibility.

Sensitivity: A measure of how small an amount or concentration of an analyte can be detected.

Specificity: A measure of how well a test detects the intended analyte without being "fooled" by other substances in the sample.

Turbidimetry: Measurement of the attenuation of a light beam due to light lost to scattering by particles suspended in a fluid.

References

1. Burtis C.A. and Ashwood E.R. (Eds.) 1994. *Tietz Textbook of Clinical Chemistry*, 2nd ed., Philadelphia, W.B. Saunders.
2. Hicks M.R., Haven M.C., and Schenken J.R. et al. (Eds.) 1987. *Laboratory Instrumentation*, 3rd ed., Philadelphia, Lippincott.
3. Kaplan L.A. and Pesce A.J. (Eds.) 1989. *Clinical Chemistry: Theory, Analysis, and Correlation*, 2nd ed., St. Louis, Mosby.
4. Tietz N.W. (Ed.) 1987. *Fundamentals of Clinical Chemistry*, 3rd ed., Philadelphia, W.B. Saunders.
5. Ward J.M., Lehmann C.A., and Leiken A.M. 1994. *Clinical Laboratory Instrumentation and Automation: Principles, Applications, and Selection*, Philadelphia, W.B. Saunders.

19

Clinical Laboratory: Nonspectral Methods and Automation

Richard L. Roa
Baylor University Medical Center

19.1 Particle Counting and Identification

The Coulter principle was the first major advance in automating blood cell counts. The cells to be counted are drawn through a small aperture between two fluid compartments, and the electric imped-ance between the two compartments is monitored (see Figure 19.1). As cells pass through the aperture, the impedance increases in proportion to the volume of the cell, allowing large numbers of cells to be counted and sized rapidly. Red cells are counted by pulling diluted blood through the aperture. Since red cells greatly outnumber white cells, the contribution of white cells to the red cell count is usu-ally neglected. White cells are counted by first destroying the red cells and using a more concentrated sample.

Modern cell counters using the Coulter principle often use *hydrodynamic focusing* to improve the performance of the instrument. A sheath fluid is introduced which flows along the outside of a channel with the sample stream inside it. By maintaining laminar flow conditions and narrowing the channel, the sample stream is focused into a very thin column with the cells in single file. This eliminates prob-lems with cells flowing along the side of the aperture or sticking to it and minimizes problems with having more than one cell in the aperture at a time.

Flow cytometry is a method for characterizing, counting, and separating cells which are suspended in a fluid. The basic flow cytometer uses hydrodynamic focusing to produce a very thin stream of fluid containing cells moving in single file through a quartz flow chamber (Figure 19.2). The cells are char-acterized on the basis of their scattering and fluorescent properties. This simultaneous measurement of scattering and fluorescence is accomplished with a sophisticated optical system that detects light from the sample both at the wavelength of the excitation source (scattering) as well as at longer wavelengths (fluorescence) at more than one angle. Analysis of these measurements produces parameters related

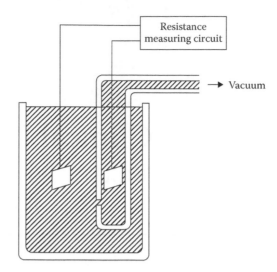

FIGURE 19.1 Coulter method. Blood cells are surrounded by an insulating membrane, which makes them non-conductive. The resistance of electrolyte-filled channel will increase slightly as cells flow through it. This resistance variation yields both the total number of cells which flow through the channel and the volume of each cell.

to the cells' size, granularity, and natural or tagged fluorescence. High-pressure mercury or xenon arc lamps can be used as light sources, but the argon laser (488 nm) is the preferred source for high-performance instruments.

One of the more interesting features of this technology is that particular cells may be selected at rates that allow collection of quantities of particular cell types adequate for further chemical testing. This is accomplished by breaking the outgoing stream into a series of tiny droplets using piezoelectric vibration. By charging the stream of droplets and then using deflection plates controlled by the cell analyzer, the cells of interest can be diverted into collection vessels.

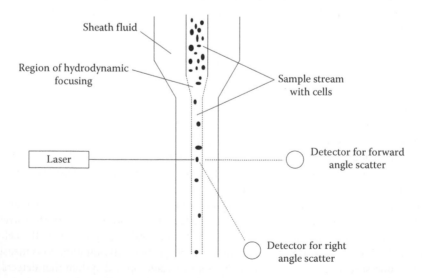

FIGURE 19.2 Flow cytometer. By combining hydrodynamic focusing, state-of-the-art optics, fluorescent labels, and high-speed computing, large numbers of cells can be characterized and sorted automatically.

The development of monoclonal antibodies coupled with flow cytometry allows for quantitation of T and B cells to assess the status of the immune system as well as characterization of leukemias, lymphomas, and other disorders.

19.2 Electrochemical Methods

Electrochemical methods are increasingly popular in the clinical laboratory, for measurement not only of electrolytes, blood gases, and pH but also of simple compounds such as glucose. *Potentiometry* is a method in which a voltage is developed across electrochemical cells as shown in Figure 19.3. This voltage is measured with little or no current flow.

Ideally, one would like to measure all potentials between the reference solution in the indicator electrode and the test solution. Unfortunately there is no way to do that. Interface potentials develop across any metal–liquid boundary, across liquid junctions, and across the ion-selective membrane. The key to making potentiometric measurements is to ensure that all the potentials are constant and do not vary with the composition of the test solution except for the potential of interest across the ion-selective membrane. By maintaining the solutions within the electrodes constant, the potential between these solutions and the metal electrodes immersed in them is constant. The liquid junction is a structure which severely limits bulk flow of the solution but allows free passage of all ions between the solutions. The reference electrode commonly is filled with saturated KCl, which produces a small, constant liquid-junction potential. Thus, any change in the measured voltage (V) is due to a change in the ion concentration in the test solution for which the membrane is selective.

The potential which develops across an ion-selective membrane is given by the Nernst equation:

$$V = \left(\frac{RT}{zF}\right)\ln\frac{a_2}{a_1} \tag{19.1}$$

where R is the gas constant = 8.314 J/K mol, T = the temperature in K, z = the ionization number, F = the Faraday constant = 9.649×10^4 C/mol, a_n = the activity of ion in solution n. When one of the solutions is a reference solution, this equation can be rewritten in a convenient form as

$$V = V_0 + \frac{N}{z}\log_{10} a \tag{19.2}$$

where V_0 is the constant voltage due to reference solution and N the Nernst slope $\approx$ 59 mV/decade at room temperature. The actual Nernst slope is usually slightly less than the theoretical value. Thus, the typical

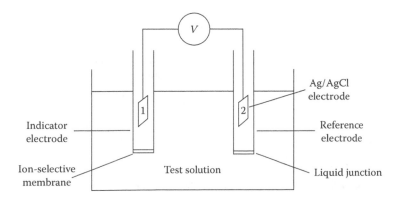

FIGURE 19.3 Electrochemical cell.

pH meter has two calibration controls. One adjusts the offset to account for the value of V_0, and the other adjusts the range to account for both temperature effects and deviations from the theoretical Nernst slope.

19.3 Ion-Specific Electrodes

Ion-selective electrodes use membranes which are permeable only to the ion being measured. To the extent that this can be done, the specificity of the electrode can be very high. One way of overcoming a lack of specificity for certain electrodes is to make multiple simultaneous measurement of several ions which include the most important interfering ones. A simple algorithm can then make corrections for the interfering effects. This technique is used in some commercial electrolyte analyzers. A partial list of the ions that can be measured with ion-selective electrodes includes H^+ (pH), Na^+, K^+, Li^+, Ca^{2+}, Cl^-, F^-, NH_4^+, and CO_2.

NH_4^+, and CO_2 are both measured with a modified ion-selective electrode. They use a pH electrode modified with a thin layer of a solution (sodium bicarbonate for CO_2 and ammonium chloride for NH_4^+) whose pH varies depending on the concentration of ammonium ions or CO_2 it is equilibrated with. A thin membrane holds the solution against the pH glass electrode and provides for equilibration with the sample solution. Note that the CO_2 electrode in Figure 19.4 is a combination electrode. This means that both the reference and indicating electrodes have been combined into one unit. Most pH electrodes are made as combination electrodes.

The Clark electrode measures pO_2 by measuring the current developed by an electrode with an applied voltage rather than a voltage measurement. This is an example of *amperometry*. In this electrode a voltage of approximately -0.65 V is applied to a platinum electrode relative to an Ag/AgCl electrode in an electrolyte solution. The reaction

$$O_2 + 2H^+ + 2e^- \rightarrow H_2O_2$$

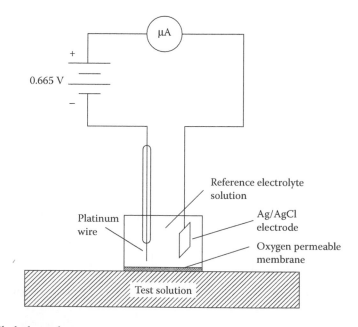

FIGURE 19.4 Clark electrode.

proceeds at a rate proportional to the partial pressure of oxygen in the solution. The electrons involved in this reaction form a current which is proportional to the rate of the reaction and thus to the pO_2 in the solution.

19.4 Radioactive Methods

Isotopes are atoms which have identical atomic number (number of protons) but different atomic mass numbers (protons + neutrons). Since they have the same number of electrons in the neutral atom, they have identical chemical properties. This provides an ideal method for labeling molecules in a way that allows for detection at extremely low concentrations. Labeling with radioactive isotopes is extensively used in radioimmunoassays where the amount of antigen bound to specific antibodies is measured. The details of radioactive decay are complex, but for our purposes there are three types of emission from decaying nuclei: *alpha, beta,* and *gamma radiation*. Alpha particles are made up of two neutrons and two protons (helium nucleus). Alpha emitters are rarely used in the clinical laboratory. Beta emission consists of electrons or positrons emitted from the nucleus. They have a continuous range of energies up to a maximum value characteristic of the isotope. *Beta radiation* is highly interactive with matter and cannot penetrate very far in most materials. Gamma radiation is a high-energy form of electromagnetic radiation. This type of radiation may be continuous, discrete, or mixed depending on the details of the decay process. It has greater penetrating ability than beta radiation (see Figure 19.5).

The kinetic energy spectrum of emitted radiation is characteristic of the isotope. The energy is commonly measured in electron volts (eV). One electron volt is the energy acquired by an electron falling through a potential of 1 V. The isotopes commonly used in the clinical laboratory have energy spectra which range from 18 keV to 3.6 MeV.

The activity of a quantity of radioactive isotope is defined as the number of disintegrations per second which occur. The usual units are the curie (Ci), which is defined as 3.7×10^{10} dps, and the becquerel (Bq), defined as 1 dps. Specific activity for a given isotope is defined as activity per unit mass of the isotope.

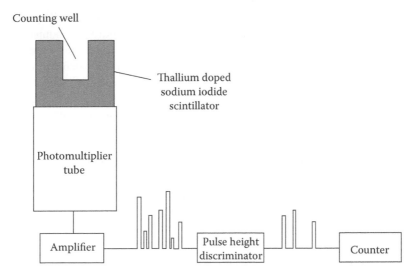

FIGURE 19.5 Gamma counted. The intensity of the light flash produced when a gamma photon interacts with a scintillator is proportional to the energy of the photon. The photomultiplier tube converts these light flashes into electric pulses which can be selected according to size (gamma energy) and counted.

The rate of decay for a given isotope is characterized by the decay constant λ, which is the proportion of the isotope which decays in unit time. Thus, the rate of loss of radioactive isotope is governed by the equation

$$\frac{dN}{dt} = -\lambda N \tag{19.3}$$

where N is the amount of radioactive isotope present at time t. The solution to this differential equation is

$$N = N_0\,e^{-\lambda t} \tag{19.4}$$

It can easily be shown that the amount of radioactive isotope present will be reduced by half after time

$$t_{1/2} = \frac{0.693}{\lambda} \tag{19.5}$$

This is known as the half-life for the isotope and can vary widely; for example, carbon-14 has a half-life of 5760 years, and iodine-131 has a half-life of 8.1 days.

The most common method for detection of radiation in the clinical laboratory is by *scintillation*. This is the conversion of radiation energy into photons in the visible or near-UV range. These are detected with photomultiplier tubes.

For gamma radiation, the scintillating crystal is made of sodium iodide doped with about 1% thallium, producing 20–30 photons for each electron-volt of energy absorbed. The photomultiplier tube and amplifier circuit produce voltage pulses proportional to the energy of the absorbed radiation. These voltage pulses are usually passed through a pulse-height analyzer which eliminates pulses outside a preset energy range (window). Multichannel analyzers can discriminate between two or more isotopes if they have well-separated energy maxima. There generally will be some spill down of counts from the higher-energy isotope into the lower-energy isotope's window, but this effect can be corrected with a simple algorithm. Multiple well detectors with up to 64 detectors in an array are available which increase the throughput for counting systems greatly. Counters using the sodium iodide crystal scintillator are referred to as gamma counters or well counters.

The lower energy and short penetration ability of beta particles requires a scintillator in direct contact with the decaying isotope. This is accomplished by dissolving or suspending the sample in a liquid fluor. Counters which use this technique are called beta counters or liquid scintillation counters.

Liquid scintillation counters use two photomultiplier tubes with a coincidence circuit that prevents counting of events seen by only one of the tubes. In this way, false counts due to chemiluminescence and noise in the phototube are greatly reduced. Quenching is a problem in all liquid scintillation counters. Quenching is any process which reduces the efficiency of the scintillation counting process, where efficiency is defined as

$$\text{Efficiency} = \text{counts per minute/decays per minute} \tag{19.6}$$

A number of techniques have been developed that automatically correct for quenching effects to produce estimates of true decays per minute from the raw counts. Currently there is a trend away from beta-emitting isotopic labels, but these assays are still used in many laboratories.

19.5 Coagulation Timers

Screening for and diagnosis of coagulation disorders is accomplished by assays that determine how long it takes for blood to clot following initiation of the clotting cascade by various reagents. A variety of instruments have been designed to automate this procedure. In addition to increasing the speed and throughput of such testing, these instruments improve the reproducibility of such tests. All the instruments provide precise introduction of reagents, accurate timing circuits, and temperature control. They differ in the method for detecting clot formation. One of the older methods still in use is to dip a small metal hook into the blood sample repeatedly and lift it a few millimeters above the surface. The electric resistance between the hook and the sample is measured, and when fibrin filaments form, they produce a conductive pathway which is detected as clot formation. Other systems detect the increase in viscosity due to fibrin formation or the scattering due to the large polymerized molecules formed. Absorption and fluorescence spectroscopy can also be used for clot detection.

19.6 Osmometers

The *colligative properties* of a solution are a function of the number of solute particles present regardless of size or identity. Increased solute concentration causes an increase in osmotic pressure and boiling point and a decrease in vapor pressure and freezing point. Measuring these changes provides information on the total solute concentration regardless of type. The most accurate and popular method used in clinical laboratories is the measurement of freezing point depression. With this method, the sample is supercooled to a few degrees below 0°C while being stirred gently. Freezing is then initiated by vigorous stirring. The heat of fusion quickly brings the solution to a slushy state where an equilibrium exists between ice and liquid, ensuring that the temperature is at the freezing point. This temperature is measured. A solute concentration of 1 osmol/kg water produces a freezing point depression of 1.858°C. The measured temperature depression is easily calibrated in units of milliosmols/kg water.

The vapor pressure depression method has the advantage of smaller sample size. However, it is not as precise as the freezing point method and cannot measure the contribution of volatile solutes such as ethanol. This method is not used as widely as the freezing point depression method in clinical laboratories.

Osmolality of blood is primarily due to electrolytes such as Na^+ and Cl^-. Proteins with molecular weights of 30,000 or more atomic mass units (amu) contribute very little to total osmolality due to their smaller numbers (a single Na^+ ion contributes just as much to osmotic pressure as a large protein molecule). However, the contribution to osmolality made by proteins is of great interest when monitoring conditions leading to pulmonary edema. This value is known as colloid osmotic pressure, or oncotic pressure, and is measured with a membrane permeable to water and all molecules smaller than about 30,000 amu. By placing a reference saline solution on one side and the unknown sample on the other, an osmotic pressure is developed across the membrane. This pressure is measured with a pressure transducer and can be related to the true colloid osmotic pressure through a calibration procedure using known standards.

19.7 Automation

Improvements in technology coupled with increased demand for laboratory tests as well as pressures to reduce costs have led to the rapid development of highly automated laboratory instruments. Typical automated instruments contain mechanisms for measuring, mixing, and transport of samples and reagents, measurement systems, and one or more microprocessors to control the entire system. In addition to system control, the computer systems store calibration curves, match test results to specimen IDs, and generate reports. Automated instruments are dedicated to complete blood counts, coagulation studies, microbiology assays, and immunochemistry, as well as high-volume instruments used in clinical chemistry laboratories. The chemistry analyzers tend to fall into one of four classes: continuous flow, centrifugal, pack-based, and dry-slide-based systems. The continuous flow systems pass successive samples and reagents through a single set of tubing, where they are directed to appropriate mixing, dialyzing, and measuring stations. Carry-over from one sample to the next is minimized by the introduction of air bubbles and wash solution between samples.

Centrifugal analyzers use plastic rotors which serve as reservoirs for samples and reagents and also as cuvettes for optical measurements. Spinning the plastic rotor mixes, incubates, and transports the test solution into the cuvette portion of the rotor, where the optical measurements are made while the rotor is spinning.

Pack-based systems are those in which each test uses a special pack with the proper reagents and sample preservation devices built-in. The sample is automatically introduced into as many packs as tests required. The packs are then processed sequentially.

Dry chemistry analyzers use no liquid reagents. The reagents and other sample preparation methods are layered onto a slide. The liquid sample is placed on the slide, and after a period of time the color developed is read by reflectance photometry. Ion-selective electrodes have been incorporated into the same slide format.

There are a number of technological innovations found in many of the automated instruments. One innovation is the use of fiberoptic bundles to channel excitation energy toward the sample as well as transmitted, reflected, or emitted light away from the sample to the detectors. This provides a great deal of flexibility in instrument layout. Multiwavelength analysis using a spinning filter wheel or diode array detectors is commonly found. The computers associated with these instruments allow for innovative improvements in the assays. For instance, when many analytes are being analyzed from one sample, the interference effects of one analyte on the measurement of another can be predicted and corrected before the final report is printed.

19.8 Trends in Laboratory Instrumentation

Predicting the future direction of laboratory instrumentation is difficult, but there seem to be some clear trends. Decentralization of the laboratory functions will continue with more instruments being located in or around ICUs, operating rooms, emergency rooms, and physician offices. More electrochemistry-based tests will be developed. The flame photometer is already being replaced with ion-selective electrode methods. Instruments which analyze whole blood rather than *plasma* or *serum* will reduce the amount of time required for sample preparation and will further encourage testing away from the central laboratory. Dry reagent methods increasingly will replace wet chemistry methods. Radioimmunoassays will continue to decline with the increasing use of methods for performing immunoassays that do not rely upon radioisotopes such as enzyme-linked fluorescent assays. Books by Burtis and Ashwood (1994), Hicks et al. (1987), Kaplan and Pesce (1989), and Tietz (1987) give an overview of the concepts in this chapter.

Defining Terms

Alpha radiation: Particulate radiation consisting of a helium nucleus emitted from a decaying a nucleus.
Amperometry: Measurements based on current flow produced in an electrochemical cell by an applied voltage.
Beta radiation: Particulate radiation consisting of an electron or positron emitted from a decaying nucleus.
Colligative properties: Physical properties that depend on the number of molecules present rather than on their individual properties.
Gamma radiation: Electromagnetic radiation emitted from an atom undergoing nuclear decay.
Hydrodynamic focusing: A process in which a fluid stream is first surrounded by a second fluid and then narrowed to a thin stream by a narrowing of the channel.
Isotopes: Atoms with the same number of protons but differing numbers of neutrons.
Plasma: The liquid portion of blood.
Potentiometry: Measurement of the potential produced by electrochemical cells under equilibrium conditions with no current flow.

Scintillation: The conversion of the kinetic energy of a charged particle or photon to a flash of light.
Serum: The liquid portion of blood remaining after clotting has occurred.

References

Burtis C.A. and Ashwood E.R. (Eds.) 1994. *Tietz Textbook of Clinical Chemistry,* 2nd ed., Philadelphia, Saunders Company.

Hicks M.R., Haven M.C., Schenken J.R. et al. (Eds.) 1987. *Laboratory Instrumentation*, 3rd ed., Philadelphia, Lippincott Company, 1987.

Kaplan L.A. and Pesce A.J. (Eds.) 1989. *Clinical Chemistry: Theory, Analysis, and Correlation*, 2nd ed., St. Louis, Mosby.

Tietz N.W. (Ed.). 1987. *Fundamentals of Clinical Chemistry,* 3rd ed., Philadelphia, W.B. Saunders.

Ward J.M., Lehmann C.A., and Leiken A.M. 1994. *Clinical Laboratory Instrumentation and Automation: Principles, Applications, and Selection*, Philadelphia, W.B. Saunders.

20

Noninvasive Optical Monitoring

Ross Flewelling
Nellcor Inc.

20.1 Introduction

Optical measures of physiologic status are attractive because they can provide a simple, noninvasive, yet real-time assessment of medical condition. Noninvasive optical monitoring is taken here to mean the use of visible or near-infrared light to directly assess the internal physiologic status of a person without the need of extracting a blood of tissue sample or using a catheter. Liquid water strongly absorbs ultraviolet and infrared radiation, and thus these spectral regions are useful only for analyzing thin surface layers or respiratory gases, neither of which will be the subject of this review. Instead, it is the visible and near-infrared portions of the electromagnetic spectrum that provide a unique "optical window" into the human body, opening new vistas for noninvasive monitoring technologies.

Various molecules in the human body possess distinctive spectral absorption characteristics in the visible or near-infrared spectral regions and therefore make optical monitoring possible. The most strongly absorbing molecules at physiologic concentrations are the hemoglobins, myoglobins, *cytochromes*, melanins, carotenes, and bilirubin (see Figure 20.1 for some examples). Perhaps less appreciated are the less distinctive and weakly absorbing yet ubiquitous materials possessing spectral characteristics in the near-infrared: water, fat, proteins, and sugars. Simple optical methods are now available to quantitatively and noninvasively measure some of these compounds directly in intact tissue. The most successful methods to date have used hemoglobins to assess the oxygen content of blood, cytochromes to assess the respiratory status of cells, and possibly near-infrared to assess endogenous concentrations of metabolites, including glucose.

20.2 Oximetry and Pulse Oximetry

Failure to provide adequate oxygen to tissues—*hypoxia*—can in a matter of minutes result in reduced work capacity of muscles, depressed mental activity, and ultimately cell death. It is therefore of considerable interest to reliably and accurately determine the amount of oxygen in blood or tissues. *Oximetry* is

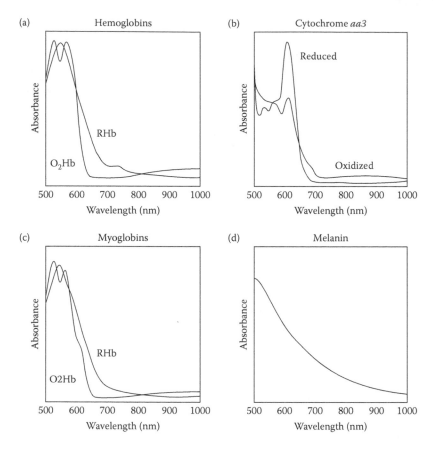

FIGURE 20.1   Absorption spectra of some endogenous biologic materials: (a) hemoglobins, (b) cytochrome *aa3*, (c) myoglobins, and (d) melanin.

the determination of the oxygen content of blood of tissues, normally by optical means. In the clinical laboratory the oxygen content of whole blood can be determined by a bench-top cooximeter or blood gas analyzer. But the need for timely clinical information and the desire to minimize the inconvenience and cost of extracting a blood sample and later analyze it in the lab has led to the search for alternative non-invasive optical methods. Since the 1930s, attempts have been made to use multiple wavelengths of light to arrive at a complete spectral characterization of a tissue. These approaches, although somewhat successful, have remained of limited utility owing to the awkward instrumentation and unreliable results.

It was not until the invention of *pulse oximetry* in the 1970s and its commercial development and application in the 1980s that noninvasive oximetry became practical. Pulse oximetry is an extremely easy-to-use, noninvasive, and accurate measurement of real-time arterial oxygen saturation. Pulse oximetry is now used routinely in clinical practice, has become a standard of care in all U.S. operating rooms, and is increasingly used wherever critical patients are found. The explosive growth of this new technology and its considerable utility led John Severinghaus and Poul Astrup (1986, p. 287) in an excellent historical review to conclude that pulse oximetry was "arguably the most significant technological advance ever made in monitoring the well-being and safety of patients during anesthesia, recovery and critical care."

20.2.1 Background

The partial pressure of oxygen (pO_2) in tissues need only be about 3 mmHg to support basic metabolic demands. This tissue level, however, requires capillary pO_2 to be near 40 mmHg, with a corresponding arterial pO_2 of about 95 mmHg. Most of the oxygen carried by blood is stored in red blood cells reversibly bound to hemoglobin molecules. Oxygen saturation (SaO_2) is defined as the percentage of hemoglobin-bound oxygen compared to the total amount of hemoglobin available for reversible oxygen binding. The relationship between the oxygen partial pressure in blood and the oxygen saturation of blood is given by the hemoglobin oxygen dissociation curve as shown in Figure 20.2. The higher the pO_2 in blood, the higher the SaO_2. But due to the highly cooperative binding of four oxygen molecules to each hemoglobin molecule, the oxygen binding curve is sigmoidal, and consequently the SaO_2 value is particularly sensitive to dangerously low pO_2 levels. With a normal arterial blood pO_2 above 90 mmHg, the oxygen saturation should be at least 95%, and a pulse oximeter can readily verify a safe oxygen level. If oxygen content falls, say to a pO_2 below 40 mmHg, metabolic needs may not be met, and the corresponding oxygen saturation will drop below 80%. Pulse oximetry therefore provides a direct measure of oxygen sufficiency and will alert the clinician to any danger of imminent hypoxia in a patient.

Although endogenous molecular oxygen is not optically observable, hemoglobin serves as an oxygen-sensitive "dye" such that when oxygen reversibly binds to the iron atom in the large heme prosthetic group, the electron distribution of the heme is shifted, producing a significant color change. The optical absorption of hemoglobin in its oxygenated and deoxygenated states is shown in Figure 20.1. Fully oxygenated blood absorbs strongly in the blue and appears bright red; deoxygenated blood absorbs through the visible region and is very dark (appearing blue when observed through tissue due to light scattering effects). Thus the optical absorption spectra of oxyhemoglobin (O_2Hb) and "reduced" deoxyhemoglobin (RHb) differ substantially, and this difference provides the basis for spectroscopic determinations of the proportion of the two hemoglobin states. In addition to these two normal functional hemoglobins, there are also *dysfunctional hemoglobins*—carboxyhemoglobin, methemoglobin, and sulfhemoglobin—which are spectroscopically distinct but do not bind oxygen reversibly. Oxygen saturation is therefore defined in Equation 20.1 only in terms of the *functional saturation* with respect to O_2Hb and RHb:

$$SaO_2 = \frac{O_2Hb}{RHb + O_2Hb} \times 100\% \tag{20.1}$$

Cooximeters are bench-top analyzers that accept whole blood samples and utilize four or more wavelengths of monochromatic light, typically between 500 and 650 nm, to spectroscopically determine the various individual hemoglobins in the sample. If a blood sample can be provided, this spectroscopic method is accurate and reliable. Attempts to make an equivalent quantitative analysis noninvasively

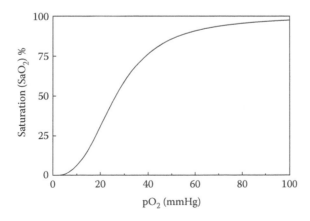

FIGURE 20.2 Hemoglobin oxygen dissociation curve showing the sigmoidal relationship between the partial pressure of oxygen and the oxygen saturation of blood. The curve is given approximately by $\%SaO_2 = 100\%/[1 + P_{50}/pO_2^n]$, with $n = 2.8$ and $P_{50} = 26$ mmHg.

through intact tissue have been fraught with difficulty. The problem has been to contend with the wide variation in scattering and nonspecific absorption properties of very complex heterogeneous tissue. One of the more successful approaches, marketed by Hewlett–Packard, used eight optical wavelengths transmitted through the pinna of the ear. In this approach a "bloodless" measurement is first obtained by squeezing as much blood as possible from an area of tissue; the arterial blood is then allowed to flow back, and the oxygen saturation is determined by analyzing the change in the spectral absorbance characteristics of the tissue. While this method works fairly well, it is cumbersome, operator dependent, and does not always work well on poorly perfused or highly pigmented subjects.

In the early 1970s, Takuo Aoyagi recognized that most of the interfering nonspecific tissue effects could be eliminated by utilizing only the change in the signal during an arterial pulse. Although an early prototype was built in Japan, it was not until the refinements in implementation and application by Biox (now Ohmeda) and Nellcor Incorporated in the 1980s that the technology became widely adopted as a safety monitor for critical care use.

20.2.2 Theory

Pulse oximetry is based on the fractional change in light transmission during an arterial pulse at two different wavelengths. In this method the fractional change in the signal is due only to the arterial blood itself, and therefore the complicated nonpulsatile and highly variable optical characteristics of tissue are eliminated. In a typical configuration, light at two different wavelengths illuminating one side of a finger will be detected on the other side, after having traversed the intervening vascular tissues (Figure 20.3). The transmission of light at each wavelength is a function of the thickness, color, and structure of the skin, tissue, bone, blood, and other material through which the light passes. The absorbance of light by a sample is defined as the negative logarithm of the ratio of the light intensity in the presence of the sample (I) to that without (I_0): $A = -\log(I/I_0)$. According to the *Beer–Lambert law*, the absorbance of a sample at a given wavelength with a molar absorptivity (ε) is directly proportional to both the concentration (c) and pathlength (l) of the absorbing material: $A = \varepsilon cl$. (In actuality, biologic tissue is highly scattering, and the Beer–Lambert law is only approximately correct; see the references for further elaboration). Visible or near-infrared light passing through about one centimeter of tissue (e.g., a finger) will be attenuated by about one or two orders of magnitude for a typical emitter–detector geometry, corresponding to an effective optical density (OD) of 1–2 OD (the detected light intensity is decreased by one order of magnitude for each OD unit). Although hemoglobin in the blood is the single strongest absorbing molecule, most of the total attenuation is due to the scattering of light away from the detector by the highly heterogeneous tissue. Since human tissue contains about 7% blood, and since

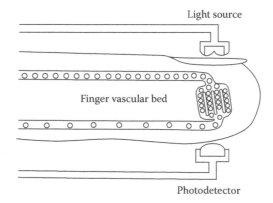

FIGURE 20.3 Typical pulse oximeter sensing configuration on a finger. Light at two different wavelengths is emitted by the source, diffusely scattered through the finger, and detected on the opposite side by a photodetector.

blood contains typically about 14 g/dL hemoglobin, the effective hemoglobin concentration in tissue is about 1 g/dL (~150 µM). At the wavelengths used for pulse oximetry (650–950 nm), the oxy- and deoxyhemoglobin molar absorptivities fall in the range of 100–1000 $M^{-1}cm^{-1}$, and consequently hemoglobin accounts for less than 0.2 OD of the total observed optical density. Of this amount, perhaps only 10% is pulsatile, and consequently pulse signals of only a few percent are ultimately measured, at times even one-tenth of this.

A mathematical model for pulse oximetry begins by considering light at two wavelengths, λ_1 and λ_2, passing through tissue and being detected at a distant location as in Figure 20.3. At each wavelength the total light attenuation is described by four different component absorbances: oxyhemoglobin in the blood (concentration c_o, molar absorptivity ε_o, and effective pathlength l_o), "reduced" deoxyhemoglobin in the blood (concentration c_r, molar absorptivity ε_r, and effective pathlength l_r), specific variable absorbances that are not from the arterial blood (concentration c_x, molar absorptivity ε_x, and effective pathlength l_x), and all other nonspecific sources of optical attenuation, combined as A_y, which can include light scattering, geometric factors, and characteristics of the emitter and detector elements. The total absorbance at the two wavelengths can then be written:

$$\begin{cases} A_{\lambda_1} = \varepsilon_{o_1} c_o l_o + \varepsilon_{r_1} c_r l_r + \varepsilon_{x_1} c_x l_x + A_{y_1} \\ A_{\lambda_2} = \varepsilon_{o_2} c_o l_o + \varepsilon_{r_2} c_r l_r + \varepsilon_{x_2} c_x l_x + A_{y_2} \end{cases} \tag{20.2}$$

The blood volume change due to the arterial pulse results in a modulation of the measured absorbances. By taking the time rate of change of the absorbances, the two last terms in each equation are effectively zero, since the concentration and effective pathlength of absorbing material outside the arterial blood do not change during a pulse [$d(c_x l_x)/dt = 0$], and all the nonspecific effects on light attenuation are also effectively invariant on the time scale of a cardiac cycle ($dA_y/dt = 0$). Since the extinction coefficients are constant, and the blood concentrations are constant on the time scale of a pulse, the time-dependent changes in the absorbances at the two wavelengths can be assigned entirely to the change in the blood pathlength (dl_o/dt and dl_r/dt). With the additional assumption that these two blood pathlength changes are equivalent (or more generally, their ratio is a constant), the ratio R of the time rate of change of the absorbance at wavelength 1 to that at wavelength 2 reduces to the following:

$$R = \frac{dA_{\lambda_1}/dt}{dA_{\lambda_2}/dt} = \frac{-d\log(I_1/I_o)/dt}{-d\log(I_2/I_o)/dt} = \frac{(\Delta I_1/I_1)}{(\Delta I_2/I_2)} = \frac{\varepsilon_{o_1} c_o + \varepsilon_{r_1} c_r}{\varepsilon_{o_2} c_o + \varepsilon_{r_2} c_r} \tag{20.3}$$

Observing that functional oxygen saturation is given by $S = c_o/(c_o + c_r)$, and that $(1 - S) = c_r/(c_o + c_r)$, the oxygen saturation can then be written in terms of the ratio R as follows

$$S = \frac{\varepsilon_{r1} - \varepsilon_{r2} R}{(\varepsilon_{r1} - \varepsilon_{o1}) - (\varepsilon_{r2} - \varepsilon_{o2})R} \tag{20.4}$$

Equation 20.4 provides the desired relationship between the experimentally determined ratio R and the clinically desired oxygen saturation S. In actual use, commonly available LEDs are used as the light sources, typically a red LED near 660 nm and a near-infrared LED selected in the range 890–950 nm. Such LEDs are not monochromatic light sources, typically with bandwidths between 20 and 50 nm, and therefore standard molar absorptivities for hemoglobin cannot be used directly in Equation 20.4. Further, the simple model presented above is only approximately true; for example, the two wavelengths do not necessarily have the exact same pathlength changes, and second-order scattering effects have

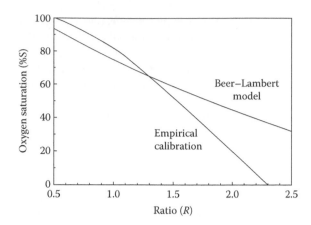

FIGURE 20.4   Relationship between the measured ratio of fractional changes in light intensity at two wavelengths, R, and the oxygen saturation S. Beer–Lambert model is from Equation 20.4 with $\varepsilon_{o1} = 100$, $\varepsilon_{o2} = 300$, $\varepsilon_{r1} = 800$, and $\varepsilon_{r2} = 200$. Empirical calibration is based on $\%S = 100\% \times (a - bR)/(c - dR)$ with $a = 1000$, $b = 550$, $c = 900$, and $d = 350$, with a linear extrapolation below 70%.

been ignored. Consequently the relationship between S and R is instead determined empirically by fitting the clinical data to a generalized function of the form $S = (a - bR)/(c - dR)$. The final empirical calibration will ultimately depend on the details of an individual sensor design, but these variations can be determined for each sensor and included in unique calibration parameters. A typical empirical calibration for R vs. S is shown in Figure 20.4, together with the curve that standard molar absorptivities would predict.

In this way the measurement of the ratio of the fractional change in signal intensity of the two LEDs is used along with the empirically determined calibration equation to obtain a beat-by-beat measurement of the arterial oxygen saturation in a perfused tissue—continuously, noninvasively, and to an accuracy of a few percent.

20.2.3 Application and Future Directions

Pulse oximetry is now routinely used in nearly all operating rooms and critical care areas in the United States and increasingly throughout the world. It has become so pervasive and useful that it is now being called the "fifth" vital sign (for an excellent review of practical aspects and clinical applications of the technology see Kelleher (1989)).

The principal advantages of pulse oximetry are that it provides continuous, accurate, and reliable monitoring of arterial oxygen saturation on nearly all patients, utilizing a variety of convenient sensors, reusable as well as disposable. Single-patient-use adhesive sensors can easily be applied to fingers for adults and children and to arms for legs or neonates. Surface reflectance sensors have also been developed based on the same principles and offer a wider choice for sensor location, though they tend to be less accurate and prone to more types of interference.

Limitations of pulse oximetry include sensitivity to high levels of optical or electric interference, errors due to high concentrations of dysfunctional hemoglobins (methemoglobin or carboxyhemoglobin) or interference from physiologic dyes (such as methylene blue). Other important factors, such as total hemoglobin content, fetal hemoglobin, or sickle cell trait, have little or no effect on the measurement except under extreme conditions. Performance can also be compromised by poor signal quality, as may occur for poorly perfused tissues with weak pulse amplitudes or by motion artifact.

Hardware and software advances continue to provide more sensitive signal detection and filtering capabilities, allowing pulse oximeters to work better on more ambulatory patients. Already some pulse oximeters incorporate ECG synchronization for improved signal processing. A pulse oximeter for use in labor and delivery is currently under active development by several research groups and companies. A likely implementation may include use of a reflectance surface sensor for the fetal head to monitor the adequacy of fetal oxygenation. This application is still in active development, and clinical utility remains to be demonstrated.

20.3 Nonpulsatile Spectroscopy

20.3.1 Background

Nonpulsatile optical spectroscopy has been used for more than half a century for noninvasive medical assessment, such as in the use of multiwavelength tissue analysis for oximetry and skin reflectance measurement for bilirubin assessment in jaundiced neonates. These early applications have found some limited use, but with modest impact. Recent investigations into new nonpulsatile spectroscopy methods for assessment of deep-tissue oxygenation (e.g., cerebral oxygen monitoring), for evaluation of respiratory status at the cellular level, and for the detection of other critical analytes, such as glucose, may yet prove more fruitful. The former applications have led to spectroscopic studies of cytochromes in tissues, and the latter has led to considerable work into new approaches in near-infrared analysis of intact tissues.

20.3.2 Cytochrome Spectroscopy

Cytochromes are electron-transporting, heme-containing proteins found in the inner membranes of mitochondria and are required in the process of oxidative phosphorylation to convert metabolites and oxygen into CO_2 and high-energy phosphates. In this metabolic process the cytochromes are reversibly oxidized and reduced, and consequently the oxidation–reduction states of cytochromes c and aa_3 in particular are direct measures of the respiratory condition of the cell. Changes in the absorption spectra of these molecules, particularly near 600 and 830 nm for cytochrome aa_3, accompany this shift. By monitoring these spectral changes, the cytochrome oxidation state in the tissues can be determined (see, e.g., Jöbsis 1977 and Jöbsis et al. 1977). As with all nonpulsatile approaches, the difficulty is to remove the dependence of the measurements on the various nonspecific absorbing materials and highly variable scattering effects of the tissue. To date, instruments designed to measure cytochrome spectral changes can successfully track relative changes in brain oxygenation, but absolute quantitation has not yet been demonstrated.

20.3.3 Near-Infrared Spectroscopy and Glucose Monitoring

Near-infrared (NIR), the spectral region between 780 and 3000 nm, is characterized by broad and overlapping spectral peaks produced by the overtones and combinations of infrared vibrational modes. Figure 20.5 shows typical NIR absorption spectra of fat, water, and starch. Exploitation of this spectral region for *in vivo* analysis has been hindered by the same complexities of nonpulsatile tissue spectroscopy described above and is further confounded by the very broad and indistinct spectral features characteristic of the NIR. Despite these difficulties, NIR spectroscopy has garnered considerable attention, since it may enable the analysis of common analytes.

Karl Norris and coworkers pioneered the practical application of NIR spectroscopy, using it to evaluate water, fat, and sugar content of agricultural products (see Burns and Cuirczak 1992; Osborne et al. 1993). The further development of sophisticated *multivariate analysis* techniques, together with new scattering models (e.g., Kubelka–Munk theory) and high-performance instrumentation, further extended the application of NIR methods. Over the past decade, many research groups and companies have touted the use of NIR techniques for medical monitoring, such as for determining the relative fat, protein, and water content of tissue, and more recently for noninvasive glucose measurement. The body

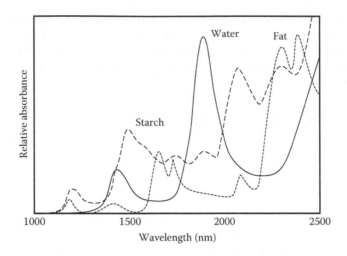

FIGURE 20.5   Typical near-infrared absorption spectra of several biologic materials.

composition analyses are useful but crude and are mainly limited to applications in nutrition and sports medicine. Noninvasive glucose monitoring, however, is of considerable interest.

More than 2 million diabetics in the United States lance their fingers three to six times a day to obtain a drop of blood for chemical glucose determination. The ability of these individuals to control their glucose levels, and the quality of their life generally, would dramatically improve if a simple, noninvasive method for determining blood glucose levels could be developed. Among the noninvasive optical methods proposed for this purpose are optical rotation, NIR analysis, and Raman spectroscopy. The first two have received the most attention. Optical rotation methods aim to exploit the small optical rotation of polarized light by glucose. To measure physiologic glucose levels in a 1-cm thick sample to an accuracy of 25 mg/dL would require instrumentation that can reliably detect an optical rotation of at least 1 millidegree. Finding an appropriate *in vivo* optical path for such measurements has proved most difficult, with most approaches looking to use either the aqueous humor or the anterior chamber of the eye (Coté et al., 1992; Rabinovitch et al., 1982). Although several groups have developed laboratory analyzers that can measure such a small effect, so far *in vivo* measurement has not been demonstrated, due both to unwanted scattering and optical activity of biomaterials in the optical path and to the inherent difficulty in developing a practical instrument with the required sensitivity.

NIR methods for noninvasive glucose determination are particularly attractive, although the task is formidable. Glucose has spectral characteristics near 1500 nm and in the 2000–2500 nm band where many other compounds also absorb, and the magnitude of the glucose absorbance in biologic samples is typically two orders of magnitude lower than those of water, fat, or protein. The normal detection limit for NIR spectroscopy is on the order of one part in 10^3, whereas a change of 25 mg/dL in glucose concentration corresponds to an absorbance change of 10^{-4}–10^{-5}. In fact, the temperature dependence of the NIR absorption of water alone is at least an order of magnitude greater than the signal from glucose in solution. Indeed, some have suggested that the apparent glucose signature in complex NIR spectra may actually be the secondary effect of glucose on the water.

Sophisticated chemometric (particularly multivariate analysis) methods have been employed to try to extract the glucose signal out of the noise (for methods reviews see Martens and Næs (1989) and Haaland (1992)). Several groups have reported using multivariate techniques to quantitate glucose in whole blood samples, with encouraging results (Haaland et al., 1992). And despite all theoretical disputations to the contrary, some groups claim the successful application of these multivariate analysis methods to noninvasive *in vivo* glucose determination in patients (Robinson et al., 1992). Yet even with the many groups working in this area, much of the work remains unpublished, and few if any of the reports have been independently validated.

20.3.4 Time-Resolved Spectroscopy

The fundamental problem in making quantitative optical measurements through intact tissue is dealing with the complex scattering phenomena. This scattering makes it difficult to determine the effective pathlength for the light, and therefore attempts to use the Beer–Lambert law, or even to determine a consistent empirical calibration, continue to be thwarted. Application of new techniques in time-resolved spectroscopy may be able to tackle this problem. Thinking of light as a packet of photons, if a single packet from a light source is sent through tissue, then a distant receiver will detect a photon distribution over time—the photons least scattered arriving first and the photons most scattered arriving later. In principle, the first photons arriving at the detector passed directly through the tissue. For these first photons the distance between the emitter and the detector is fixed and known, and the Beer–Lambert law should apply, permitting determination of an *absolute* concentration for an absorbing component. The difficulty in this is, first, that the measurement time scale must be on the order of the photon transit time (subnanosec), and second, that the number of photons getting through without scattering will be extremely small, and therefore the detector must be exquisitely sensitive. Although these considerable technical problems have been overcome in the laboratory, their implementation in a practical instrument applied to a real subject remains to be demonstrated. This same approach is also being investigated for noninvasive optical imaging, since the unscattered photons should produce sharp images (see Chance et al. 1988, Chance 1991, and Yoo and Alfano 1989).

20.4 Conclusions

The remarkable success of pulse oximetry has established noninvasive optical monitoring of vital physiologic functions as a modality of considerable value. Hardware and algorithm advances in pulse oximetry are beginning to broaden its use outside the traditional operating room and critical care areas. Other promising applications of noninvasive optical monitoring are emerging, such as for measuring deep tissue oxygen levels, determining cellular metabolic status, or for quantitative determination of other important physiologic parameters such as blood glucose. Although these latter applications are not yet practical, they may ultimately impact noninvasive clinical monitoring just as dramatically as pulse oximetry.

Defining Terms

Beer–Lambert law: Principle stating that the optical absorbance of a substance is proportional to both the concentration of the substance and the pathlength of the sample.

Cytochromes: Heme-containing proteins found in the membranes of mitochondria and required for oxidative phosphorylation, with characteristic optical absorbance spectra.

Dysfunctional hemoglobins: Those hemoglobin species that cannot reversibly bind oxygen (carboxyhemoglobin, methemoglobin, and sulfhemoglobin).

Functional saturation: The ratio of oxygenated hemoglobin to total nondysfunctional hemoglobins (oxyhemoglobin plus deoxyhemoglobin).

Hypoxia: Inadequate oxygen supply to tissues necessary to maintain metabolic activity.

Multivariate analysis: Empirical models developed to relate multiple spectral intensities from many calibration samples to known analyte concentrations, resulting in an optimal set of calibration parameters.

Oximetry: The determination of blood or tissue oxygen content, generally by optical means.

Pulse oximetry: The determination of functional oxygen saturation of pulsatile arterial blood by ratiometric measurement of tissue optical absorbance changes.

References

Burns, D.A. and Ciurczak, E.W. (Eds.). 1992. *Handbook of Near-Infrared Analysis*. New York, Marcel Dekker.

Chance, B. 1991. Optical method. *Annu. Rev. Biophys. Biophys. Chem.* 20: 1.

Chance, B., Leigh, J.S., Miyake, H. et al. 1988. Comparison of time-resolved and -unresolved measurements of deoxyhemoglobin in brain. *Proc. Natl Acad. Sci. USA* 85: 4971.

Coté G.L., Fox M.D., and Northrop, R.B. 1992. Noninvasive optical polarimetric glucose sensing using a true phase measurement technique. *IEEE Trans. Biomed. Eng.* 39: 752.

Haaland, D.M. 1992. Multivariate calibration methods applied to the quantitative analysis of infrared spectra. In P.C. Jurs (Ed.), *Computer-Enhanced Analytical Spectroscopy*, Vol. 3, pp. 1–30. New York, Plenum Press.

Haaland, D.M., Robinson, M.R., Koepp, G.W. et al. 1992. Reagentless near-infrared determination of glucose in whole blood using multivariate calibration. *Appl. Spectros.* 46: 1575.

Jöbsis, F.F. 1977. Noninvasive, infrared monitoring of cerebral and myocardial oxygen sufficiency and circulatory parameters. *Science* 198: 1264.

Jöbsis, F.F., Keizer, L.H., LaManna, J.C. et al. 1977. Reflectance spectrophotometry of cytochrome aa_3 in vivo. *J. Appl. Physiol.* 43: 858.

Kelleher, J.F. 1989. Pulse oximetry. *J. Clin. Monit.* 5: 37.

Martens, H. and Næs, T. 1989. *Multivariate Calibration*. New York, John Wiley & Sons.

Osborne, B.G., Fearn, T., and Hindle, P.H. 1993. *Practical NIR Spectroscopy with Applications in Food and Beverage Analysis*. Essex, England, Longman Scientific & Technical.

Payne, J.P. and Severinghaus, J.W. (Eds.). 1986. *Pulse Oximetry*. New York, Springer-Verlag.

Rabinovitch, B., March, W.F., and Adams, R.L. 1982. Noninvasive glucose monitoring of the aqueous humor of the eye: Part I. Measurement of very small optical rotations. *Diabetes Care* 5: 254.

Robinson, M.R., Eaton, R.P., Haaland, D.M. et al. 1992. Noninvasive glucose monitoring in diabetic patients: A preliminary evaluation. *Clin. Chem.* 38: 1618.

Severinghaus, J.W. and Astrup, P.B. 1986. History of blood gas analysis. VI. Oximetry. *J. Clin. Monit.* 2: 135.

Severinghaus, J.W. and Honda, Y. 1987a. History of blood gas analysis. VII. Pulse oximetry. *J. Clin. Monit.* 3: 135.

Severinghaus, J.W. and Honda, Y. 1987b. Pulse oximetry. *Int. Anesthesiol. Clin.* 25: 205.

Severinghaus, J.W. and Kelleher, J.F. 1992. Recent developments in pulse oximetry. *Anesthesiology* 76: 1018.

Tremper, K.K. and Barker, S.J. 1989. Pulse oximetry. *Anesthesiology* 70: 98.

Wukitsch, M.W., Petterson, M.T., Tobler, D.R. et al. 1988. Pulse oximetry: Analysis of theory, technology, and practice. *J. Clin. Monit.* 4: 290.

Yoo, K.M. and Alfano, R.R. 1989. Photon localization in a disordered multilayered system. *Phys. Rev. B* 39: 5806.

Further Information

Two collections of papers on pulse oximetry include a book edited by J.P. Payne and J.W. Severinghaus, *Pulse Oximetry* (New York, Springer-Verlag, 1986), and a journal collection—*International Anesthesiology Clinics* (25, 1987). For technical reviews of pulse oximetry, see J.A. Pologe's, 1987 "Pulse Oximetry" (*Int. Anesthesiol. Clin.* 25: 137), Kevin K. Tremper and Steven J. Barker's, 1989 "Pulse Oximetry" (*Anesthesiology* 70: 98), and Michael W. Wukitsch, Michael T. Patterson, David R. Tobler, and coworkers' 1988 "Pulse Oximetry: Analysis of Theory, Technology, and Practice" (*J. Clin. Monit.* 4: 290).

For a review of practical and clinical applications of pulse oximetry, see the excellent review by Joseph K. Kelleher 1989 and John Severinghaus and Joseph F. Kelleher 1992. John Severinghaus and Yoshiyuki Honda have written several excellent histories of pulse oximetry (1987a, 1987b).

For an overview of applied near-infrared spectroscopy, see Donald A. Burns and Emil W. Ciurczak 1992 and B.G. Osborne, T. Fearn, and P.H. Hindle 1993. For a good overview of multivariate methods, see Harald Martens and Tormod Næs 1989.

Index

F